THE
PIERCING
BIBLE

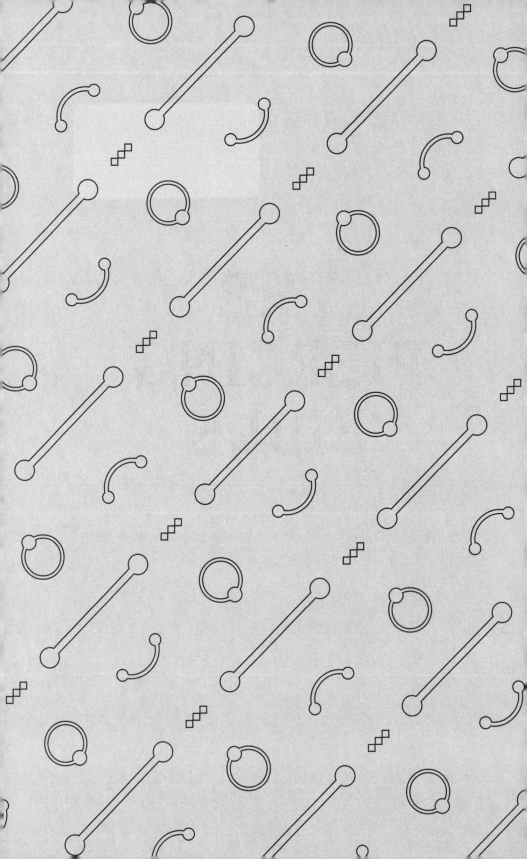

REVISED AND EXPANDED

THE PIERCING BIBLE

THE DEFINITIVE GUIDE TO SAFE PIERCING

ELAYNE ANGEL

WITH
JEF SAUNDERS

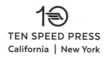

TEN SPEED PRESS
California | New York

Copyright © 2009, 2021 by Elayne Angel
Illustrations copyright © 2009, 2021 by Jennifer Klepacki

All rights reserved.
Published in the United States by Ten Speed Press, an imprint of Random House, a division of Penguin Random House LLC, New York. www.tenspeed.com

Ten Speed Press and the Ten Speed Press colophon are registered trademarks of Penguin Random House LLC.

Originally published in slightly different form as *The Piercing Bible: The Definitive Guide to Safe Body Piercing* by Crossing Press, an imprint of Random House, a division of Penguin Random House LLC, in 2009.

Photos of jewelry on pages 89, 90, 294, and 296 reprinted by permission of J.D. Lorenz of Industrial Strength Body Jewelry, www.isbodyjewelry.com.

Photos of jewelry and tools on pages 69, 71, 72, 80, 82, 122, 124, 273, and 274 reprinted by permission of Paul King of Cold Steel America, www.coldsteelpiercing.com.

Photo of jewelry on page 122 reprinted by permission of Gale Shub of Body Circle Designs, www.bodycircle.com.

Photos of threadless jewelry on page 90 reprinted by permission of John Kittel of NeoMetal, www.neometal.com.

Photos of jewelry on pages 80, 82, 85, 86, 91, 118, and 163 reprinted by permission of Rich Hartwick of Iconic Tattoo & Piercing, www.richhartwick.com.

Photo of jewelry on page 81 reprinted by permission of James Weber of Infinite Body Piercings, www.infinitebody.com.

Photo of jewelry on page 122 reprinted by permission of Kaylee Heaps and Jef Saunders of Gamma Piercing, www.gammapiercing.com.

Diagrams on pages 77, 83, 84, and 88 reprinted by permission of Danielle Greenwood and Jef Saunders.

Photos on page 364 reprinted by permission of Todd Friedman.

Library of Congress Cataloging-in-Publication Data

Names: Angel, Elayne, author.

Title: The piercing bible : the definitive guide to safe piercing / Elayne Angel with Jef Saunders.
Description: First revised edition. | California : Ten Speed Press, 2021.
    | Originally published in slightly different form in 2009 as The Piercing Bible:
    The Definitive Guide to Safe Body Piercing. | Includes
    bibliographical references and index.
Identifiers: LCCN 2020055865 (print) | LCCN 2020055866 (ebook) | ISBN
    9781984859327 (trade paperback) | ISBN 9781984859334 (ebook)
Subjects: LCSH: Body piercing—Safety measures. | Body piercing—Health aspects.
Classification: LCC RD119.5.B82 A54 2021 (print) | LCC RD119.5.B82
    (ebook) | DDC 391.6/5—dc23

LC record available at https://lccn.loc.gov/2020055865

LC ebook record available at https://lccn.loc.gov/2020055866

Trade Paperback ISBN 978-1-9848-5932-7
eBook ISBN 978-1-9848-5933-4

Printed in the United States of America

Acquiring Editor: Lisa Westmoreland | Project Editor: Shaida Boroumand
Cover Designer: Annie Marino | Book Designers: Jeff Brandenburg and Annie Marino |
    Production designers: Mari Gill and Faith Hague
Production Manager: Dan Myers
Copyeditor: Jennifer Traig | Proofreader: Carolyn Keating | Indexer: Ken DellaPenta
Publicist: Leilani Zee | Marketer: Monica Stanton

3rd Printing

Revised Edition

To my past and future clients:
I am honored by your trust, and grateful for your
role in making it possible to live my passion.

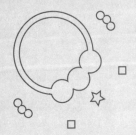

CONTENTS

Acknowledgments viii

Preface ix

Introduction: Piercing 101 x

PART 1 THE NEW PIERCING

1   Motivations 2

2   Piercing Past to Present 8

PART 2 GROUNDWORK AND PRELIMINARY CONSIDERATIONS

3   Risks, Myths, and Warnings 20

4   Is Piercing Right for You? 30

5   Is Piercing Right for Your Child? 36

6   You and Your Piercer 40

PART 3 PIERCING PREPARATION

7   Picking and Preparing 54

8   At the Studio 59

9   Piercing Procedures 68

10 Jewelry 101: Sizes, Shapes, and Materials 78

PART 4 THE HOLES

11 Holes in Your Head: Ear, Nose, and Facial Piercings 102

12 Kiss of the Needle: Tongue and Oral Piercings 132

13 Torso Piercings: Nipple and Navel Piercings 151

14 Below the Belt: Genital Piercings 166

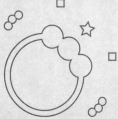

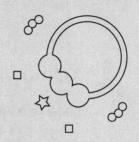

PART 5 HEALING, AFTERCARE, AND TROUBLESHOOTING

15   Essential Guide to Healing and Aftercare 222

16   Trouble and Troubleshooting 246

PART 6 LIVING WITH YOUR PIERCINGS

17   Upkeep and Stretching 268

18   Advanced Jewelry and Practices 285

19   Special Situations 302

20   Sex! 311

PART 7 PIERCING IN MODERN CULTURE

21   Piercees and the Establishment 320

22   A Career in Professional Piercing 324

23   The Future of Piercing 329

Appendix A: Gauge Conversion Chart 332

Appendix B: Minimum Healing Times Chart 333

Appendix C: The Piercer Survey 334

Notes 338

Glossary 349

Select Bibliography 363

About the Author and Contributor 364

Index 365

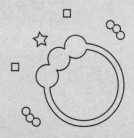

Acknowledgments

Immense thanks to Carolyn Ward for a lifetime of friendship, encouragement, and indispensable editing advice.

I am so grateful to my esteemed colleagues for all their valuable input. An extra loud shout-out to Jef Saunders, whose guidance and contributions were instrumental to this revised edition. You rock! I'm profoundly thankful for my cherished piercer and sweetheart, Rich Hartwick (the best boyfriend ever), for all the support and unconditional love.

Much obliged to the cadre of talented and dedicated piercers who answered my many questions: Cale DiFrancesco, Bridgett Celeste Dearing, Becky Dill, Luis Garcia, Miro Hernandez, John Johnson, Paul King, Jane-Marie Martinez, Ryan Ouellette, Pablo Perelmuter, Bethrah Szumski, James Weber, and David Vidra. Much appreciation to Erica Skadsen for information on natural jewelry, and Jason Pfohl for facts about glass. Kudos to the many piercers who contributed to this project but are not mentioned by name, including everyone who shared in the Piercing Bible Updates Group.

Cheers, applause, and high praise to Dr. Stephanie Hutter Thomas, Becky Dill, and the Board of the Association of Professional Piercers for their collaboration on the groundbreaking Piercer Survey. We did it!

Hats off to my respected supporters from the health care professions: Dr. Stanley Steinberg (my dad), Dr. Robert Winn; Betsy Reynolds, RDH; Scott DeBoer, RN; and Dr. Myrna Armstrong.

Mi más profundo agradecimiento y amor a mis ángeles yucatecos, Lulú y su hijo Ángel, por cuidarme siempre y por darme la oportunidad de concentrarme completamente en mi trabajo. (My deepest appreciation and love to my Yucatecan angels, Lulu and her son Angel, for always taking care of me, giving me the freedom to focus on my work.)

Much gratitude to Ten Speed Press and their marvelous team for all their expertise and hard work, especially my editor, Shaida Boroumand, for making this a better book. Big props to my agent, Jim Donovan, for his know-how and unflappability. A thousand thanks to Jennifer Klepacki for her stunning job on the illustrations, unwavering dedication, and patience. A thousand more to Jef Saunders and Danielle Greenwood for the wonderful diagrams. Credit to J.D. Lorenz of Industrial Strength Body Jewelry, Paul King of Cold Steel America, Gale Shub of Body Circle Designs, Rich Hartwick of Iconic Tattoo & Piercing, James Weber of Infinite Body Piercing, Kaylee Heaps and Jef Saunders of Gamma Piercing, and John Kittell of NeoMetal for their photos of jewelry and tools.

And, finally, thanks to Lee Bass for providing the initial foundation and impetus for this book.

Preface

It has been truly remarkable to observe—and cultivate—the evolution of piercing from a rare practice to a thriving facet of our contemporary culture. When I became a professional piercer in the 1980s, there was just *one* specialty studio, and I was its manager. Back then, piercing was so uncommon that people found it shocking and thought it was just a bizarre fad. How wrong they were! Piercing has never been more prevalent and accepted than it is today.

Following a five-year-long journey writing *The Piercing Bible*, it was published in 2009. I felt confident that easy access to comprehensive, reliable information would raise the overall level of safety and competency in the field. Unfortunately, as an online consultant, I bear witness (and offer professional advice) to a plethora of piercees suffering unnecessary pain, complications, and frustration from botched piercings at the hands of incompetent practitioners. To get a high-quality job, consumers still need to be discerning, diligent, and well educated. (I can help with that if you keep turning the pages.)

Changes in the piercing world have been fast and frequent, so just a decade later, parts of my original book are like a historical document. This fully renovated version contains the most up-to-date, relevant material available on the subject, including new content on piercing placements, techniques, aftercare, and much more.

For years I've specialized exclusively in nipple and genital work as a touring "guest piercer." So, I enlisted my esteemed colleague, Jef Saunders, to provide input, especially on the aspects that are no longer in my purview. I also queried hundreds of other piercers through social media groups for feedback and contributions. To gather data about the industry, I conducted the first large-scale piercer survey in conjunction with the Association of Professional Piercers. This is far more of a group compendium and combined effort than the original, and is surely better for it.

This edition's journey was a wild ride. As a perfectionist, I wrestle vigorously with the process of writing. I can easily recognize an ideal piercing, but flawlessness is far more subjective in a sentence or paragraph. To compound an already formidable challenge, the COVID-19 pandemic began its rampage several months before my deadline to deliver the completed manuscript. As a science nerd and research fanatic, I was riveted to the endless outpouring of news, studies, and analysis, while also attempting to focus on the task at hand. Though distracted and worried about family, friends, and civilization as we know it, I managed to complete the project.

I am thrilled to share it with you and feel certain you'll find practical, valuable information within these pages. It is my hope that all piercings are safe, successful, and bring great joy to those who wear them.

—*Elayne Angel, Mérida, Mexico*

Introduction: Piercing 101

Whether it fascinates or repels, something *is* captivating about hard metal worn through tender flesh. Piercing is thrilling. Literally. The word *thrill* originates from the Middle English word *thrillen*, "To perforate by a pointed instrument. Hence, to cause a shivering, throbbing, tingling, or exquisite sensation; to pierce; to penetrate."[1] By that account, piercing sounds quite exciting. And so it is! Piercing is among the most ancient *and* current practices for ornamenting and customizing the human form.

THE ART OF MODERN PIERCING

Except for traditional earrings and a rare nostril stud or hoop, piercing was virtually unheard of just a few decades ago. As body piercing initially came into the light from the far-flung fringes of society, people perceived it as radical, deviant, and even disgusting. Over time it has fully blossomed as a mode of personal expression nearly anyone may use to enhance their appearance, self-image, and quality of life. Professional piercing has come into its own, and it has been accepted as a part of our modern culture.

In some areas, it seems more people have visible piercings than don't! In conjunction with talented and creative body jewelry designers and manufacturers, piercing has been elevated to a legitimate art form. We're now in the second generation, with Millennial and Gen X parents bringing their children to studios for safe ear piercings, instead of the mall to be pierced by a gun.

The practice of piercing is one of the activities grouped under the term *body modification*. These pursuits include tattooing, scarification, branding, and other body art. The number of possible placements on the body; the array of jewelry styles, sizes, and materials; and the necessary aftercare all distinguish piercing from other types of body modification. Because piercing breaks the protective barrier of the skin and leaves a foreign object in the tissue, there are risks of infection and other potential dangers. If all aspects are not handled appropriately, complications are more likely.

The spectacular rise in the popularity of piercing has resulted in a proliferation of piercers and jewelry. Some of the products and services are excellent, but unfortunately, many are of inferior quality. Piercing establishments range from inexpensive jewelry kiosks at shopping malls to high-end specialty studios staffed with expert practitioners, the latest equipment, and top-quality jewelry. There is a big difference between them! You significantly increase your chance of uneventful healing by choosing the right piercer and jewelry. The relative newness of professional piercing—it has been widely practiced only since the 1990s—has many ramifications for consumers. There are still no standardized regulations, piercer training, or competency requirements in the United States. A few states now require practical exams for piercers, but many laws merely mandate hygiene requirements or restrict the piercing of minors. In some areas, however, basic regulations do not exist; in others, local laws are not enforced.

Even the most egregious cases of piercer negligence and malpractice seldom result in litigation, fines, or other consequences.

The art of piercing is continuing to evolve, and its practitioners are still experimenting with its limits and possibilities. The information in this book is intended to distill the most sensible piercing advice available. By educating yourself, you can get a flawless first—or twentieth—piercing or find the information you need to deal with a bungled job.

HOW TO USE THIS BOOK

The Piercing Bible is directed primarily toward piercees. However, it also contains a wealth of information for the parents of children who want to get pierced or are already pierced, teachers who work with pierced students, and health care professionals dealing with pierced patients (whether treating problem piercings or performing unrelated medical procedures). Apprentices and piercers will also find an authoritative reference work containing plenty of hints and tips, and an educational tool for clients.

Part 1 touches on the ancient and modern history of this art form and contains general information about who is getting pierced and what commonly motivates them. The novice piercee should carefully read parts 2 and 3, which provide a rundown on everything that should be taken into consideration when deciding to get pierced. Part 4 delves into each of the most common piercings in detail. Piercees can use it as a reference, and apprentices and piercers will also find pointers here. This portion includes information about jewelry sizes, styles, and piercing placements, as well as the techniques that are commonly used to perform each piercing. Next, part 5 offers in-depth aftercare advice and provides practical information on troubleshooting healing complications. Part 6 explains the maintenance of healed piercings, discusses special situations encountered when living with piercings, and explores advanced practices for healed piercings, including stretching. Finally, part 7 takes a look at the future of piercing and includes a section on becoming a piercer.

The appendices include a table with jewelry size conversions (gauge, inch, and millimeter), and a chart of minimum healing time ranges for popular piercings. You'll find a summary of data gathered in the first major survey of US body piercers in Appendix C, page 334, and a sprinkling of stats from it throughout the chapters. There's also a handy glossary of piercing-related terms.

WHY THIS BOOK?

Piercing can be dangerous, and it is far more complicated than most people realize. The hazards range from tearing, scarring, migration, and rejection to localized bacterial invasions and, though rare, severe infections. Consumers need facts about the risks, choices, and best practices involved. People who interact with piercees also need to be informed about various aspects of piercing. Many myths have persisted, including in academic and medical literature; they are finally dispelled here too.

Piercing and tattooing are often linked, as they are frequently performed in the same establishments. However, tattoos are comparatively straightforward; healing is rapid, and there are seldom complications. The same is not true of piercings. They require aftercare throughout the healing period, plus regular maintenance once healed. The array of options can be confusing: where to pierce, what jewelry to wear, and how to care for the wound. Many people get the bulk of their "facts" about piercing online. Unfortunately, the web can be unreliable, offering contradictory ideas from questionable sources. Countless piercees have experienced needless pain, avoidable healing problems, and undesirable outcomes from a lack of sound information.

Will your pierced body part turn green and fall off if you don't follow every rule and guideline in the book? Probably not, but by educating yourself and being conscientious, you will have a much higher chance of having a healthy piercing that heals well, gives you a minimum of trouble, and provides maximum enjoyment. Admittedly, not every piercee who fails to adhere to sound practices has a terrible catastrophe—but some do. This book takes a cautionary tone because the risks are real.

DISCLAIMERS AND SOUND ADVICE

The Piercing Bible is deliberately limited in scope to provide detailed, useful information about the most common piercings. Related subjects such as "play" (temporary) piercings, implants, and suspensions, which are all part of the broader piercing scene, are touched on only in passing. Tattoos and other forms of body modification, such as scarification, branding, tongue splitting, and so on, are not addressed.

This book is *not* an instructional manual on how to perform piercings on yourself or others. Visit a competent professional piercer for all permanent piercings. If you want to become a piercer, I urge you to seek appropriate training under the guidance of an experienced mentor before attempting to do any piercings. Learn more in "A Career in Professional Piercing," page 324.

Some piercers exercise poor judgment and lack ethics. So, you must maintain your own: never request that a piercer work on an animal, someone who is intoxicated, or any other unsuitable candidate.

The Piercing Bible does not cover every possible situation, but it deals with all of the areas I'm most frequently asked about. Popular terminology and names for piercings vary by region and change over time, so don't get too preoccupied with the labels. The modern piercing industry is still a relatively new and growing field: changes are fast, frequent, and sometimes drastic. The industry is dynamic, but books are static; so I can present only information that is current at the time of publication.

Substantive research studies, statistical analyses, and other definitive resource materials related to modern piercing are in short supply. Therefore, the information, practices, and procedures described in this book are primarily based on my own extensive clinical experience, and input from respected colleagues. I've integrated industry standards where they exist, but there is still precious little that is truly standard, so my opinions are a primary component of many chapters.

There are few absolutes when it comes to piercing, since each individual is unique. For the sake of accuracy, I use words such as "frequently," "commonly," "generally," and so on throughout.

I respect and support all individual gender expressions and identities. For clarity, the terms "male" and "female" are occasionally used in this book to refer to the predominant biological configurations and their common physical characteristics. It is my intention to be a supportive ally to transgender and gender nonbinary individuals.

The novel coronavirus (SARS-CoV-2) emerged, and the COVID-19 pandemic began, just months before the completion of this book. I will not be addressing the subject since it is too soon to know what effects the virus might have on the industry.

Finally, and importantly, I am a professional in the field of piercing, not medicine; this book is not intended to provide medical advice, diagnosis, or treatment. There is no substitute for a hands-on consultation with an experienced piercer or, when needed, the counsel of a health care provider. This book is intended to support—not replace—the relationships that exist between piercee and piercer or doctor.

PART 1

THE NEW PIERCING

MOTIVATIONS 2

PIERCING PAST TO PRESENT 8

1

MOTIVATIONS

*To me style is just the outside of content and content the
inside of style, like the outside and the inside of the human
body—both go together, they can't be separated.*
—JEAN-LUC GODARD

The urge to decorate the body and control one's appearance is a universal human trait. Each of us uses clothing, hairstyle, and so on to express our individuality. In this way, we make the most of the gifts or curses—perceived or real—bestowed by nature. Nowadays, we have more choices than ever to manipulate our looks. The options range from minor adjustments such as hair dye and teeth whitener to more extreme but still socially acceptable practices such as liposuction and breast implants. Although body modification was at the fringes of culture not long ago, it has become prevalent in today's world.

Piercing and other types of body modification are methods of changing the actual physical form, which is empowering in a way that may not be fully understood by those who have never participated. Women, in particular, are bombarded by the media's unrealistic notions of beauty, which profoundly affect self-esteem and body image. We may turn to piercing or other forms of body art to help us embrace a positive attitude about ourselves. While there is no unanimous consensus about whether body jewelry enhances appearance, aesthetics is a widespread motivating factor for piercing.

WHO GETS PIERCED AND WHY?

I have pierced people from all professions and socioeconomic backgrounds—rocket scientists, clergy, and empty-nest retirees among them. Getting pierced can even be a multi-generational event, as families sometimes join in the bonding of mother and daughter, and sometimes grandmother, too. There's no single type of person who gets pierced; we represent a tremendously diverse and growing population.

Years ago, before piercing became so widespread, people would frequently approach me, point to one or more of my visible piercings, and ask two primary questions. One was "Didn't that hurt?" and the other was "Why would you do that to yourself?" Now piercing has become so mainstream, the question of motivation is raised less frequently. Yet there are a multitude of reasons for getting pierced, from the superficial to the profound. It might be all about expressing independence, attracting attention, the sensation of metal through flesh, or the opportunity to wear some gorgeous jewelry. For others, piercing is a response to deep internal triggers. These are all valid inspirations.

There is sometimes a marked difference in age between the visibly adorned and those more discreetly pierced in intimate locations below the neck. Younger people are frequently motivated by a desire to fit in with peers or the need to establish autonomy from their parents. Visible piercings offer a perfect means for fulfilling these desires. Young piercees tend to be more heavily influenced by popular music, social media, and fashion, and they are frequently limited in their piercing options by regulations for those under the age of majority.

Older people are obviously not subject to these prohibitions, nor are we typically motivated by the same impulses. Some adults endure trauma or other life experiences that lead us to turn to body modification for self-realization and healing purposes. The increased popularity of piercings has brought greater acceptance, and some employees are permitted to wear visible body jewelry while on the job. But for working adults whose employers favor a more conservative look, torso and genital piercings are easily concealed under everyday clothing.

> "After birthing two girls (who weighed over eight pounds each) and passing forty, I needed something to make me feel like 'me' again, not just a mom, and a wife, and a nurse, etc. I chose a navel piercing 'cause I've always thought they were sexy. I knew there was a sexy part of me somewhere inside, and my piercings helped bring that out again."—J.
> "My [VCH] piercing has been life-changing. After being molested as a child, having this piercing has been a way to reclaim my body. It helped me get my confidence back."—G.

GROUP IDENTIFICATION
Piercing and body modification have long been used to indicate and solidify one's cultural identity. For a time in the late 1980s and into the '90s, some Western piercees described themselves as "Modern Primitives" and were proud to wear jewelry made of natural materials such as horn, wood, and stone that echoed indigenous designs and ancient adornments. As the West becomes more sensitive to cultural appropriation, this movement has faded, but beautiful natural jewelry remains available. Conversely, some traditional peoples make use of modern human-made materials. The herdsmen of northern Kenya, for example, have used the metals found in telephone wires to make lip and ear ornaments.[1]

People have visibly aligned themselves with rave, punk, goth, hip-hop, skater, swinger, gender nonbinary, and other identities and subcultures through piercings.

It may seem contradictory, but piercing can be a statement of rebellion and conformity at the same time.

MAGICAL AND SYMBOLIC HEALING

People often use piercing as a path to restore physical and spiritual health after a trauma or to exercise some control while struggling with illness or feelings of vulnerability. They may get pierced with the intention of exchanging bad for good, turning to this type of symbolic healing to reclaim their bodies by getting a piercing after childbearing, sexual assault, or an abusive relationship. Through the deliberate act of breaking skin and shedding blood, these people feel whole, connected with their bodies, and in control of their lives again. Getting pierced following a breakup, divorce, or the death of a spouse is also common, and very therapeutic for many recently single souls. Piercing to exert command of the body and cope with the changes of menopause has been cited more recently as a motivation. Piercing a part of the body that is not your favorite can help you to embrace and accept it. This can be especially effective for transgender people and those with body-image challenges. Some people seek piercing to distract themselves from stress and difficult times or circumvent the desire to self-harm.

> "I had a very bad breakup . . . and needed to get myself together and learn to love myself. I went into therapy and made great strides. I started to deal with sexual trauma from early in life. As part of marking my new beginning and taking ownership of my body and sexuality I got a vertical clitoral hood piercing. Thankfully I had a very open-minded therapist who respected my self-determination and recognized my piercing as a positive step. Funny thing, my last boyfriend had pressured me to get nipple piercings and got abusive when I refused. Long after our (very bad) breakup I became enamored with the idea and got both nipples pierced. Now I love them because they are entirely mine! . . . [E]very time I look at them, they remind me of who I am now."—N.

> "Personally, I made the choice to take control of the needles. Because of my blood disorder, I am a human pincushion . . . So, my piercings are a way for me to dictate when, where, and why I am being poked with a sharp needle! For me it is a reclaiming of me; my body is not just a pincushion for medical uses . . . It is a piece of artwork!"—S.

RITES OF PASSAGE

Ceremonial practices have provided structure and meaning to human existence throughout the ages. Unfortunately, modern society retains few of these traditions, so people often struggle to create their own rites to mark the changes in their lives. Piercing accomplishes this when it is used to commemorate a milestone. Many visit a piercing or tattoo studio soon after or even on the very date of their eighteenth birthday to celebrate finally having legal possession of their own skin. Whether or not the piercing experience is consciously approached in a ritual manner, getting a piercing does effect a physical—and possibly an emotional or spiritual—transformation.

I have performed piercings to mark births, deaths, graduations, divorces, clean-and-sober time, relationship commitments, anniversaries of all kinds, and other special occasions in people's lives. One young woman memorialized the death of her peers with a piercing:

> "I wanted to get a piercing done to remember my senior year because a lot happened that I don't want to forget—most importantly, the passing of three members of my senior class . . . I also wanted to get either a piercing or tattoo to show that—hey, I'm eighteen, I can do it now!"—M.

EROTIC INSPIRATIONS

Many adults are motivated to get pierced for sexual gratification. The presence of piercings and jewelry in specific locations results in increased physical stimulation for piercees or their partners. Couples sometimes use piercings to revitalize their sensual focus and reignite the flames in relationships that have lost some of their spark. Intimate piercings can bolster confidence in the bedroom and oneself as a sexual being.

People may not find their private parts attractive or appealing. A large percentage of the population from Western nations have had their penises altered through nonconsensual circumcision during infancy. When an individual chooses to modify the appearance of their genitals by piercing and adorning them with jewelry, it can be highly liberating. For many it inspires harmony with their bodies that could not be achieved through any other means.

> "One of the main reasons [I got a genital piercing] was that I've always had confidence issues, and I felt that if I could drop my pants in front of a stranger and get a needle shoved through it, I could do damn near anything and everything else."—J.

> "I saw a picture of a guy with a genital piercing on the internet . . . and it intrigued me. I wondered, like most guys would, *why* would a sensible guy go and have a piece of metal stuck through a sensitive part of his body? Well, at the time I was still coming to terms with my sexuality, and I wondered how anyone could like me if even I wasn't sure about myself . . . I now feel more self-confident about who I am and am more comfortable with myself and the identity I present to the public."—C.

A SPECIAL CONNECTION

A piercing client and close friend of mine named Cliff willed his body jewelry to his friends when he knew the end of his life was imminent. After he passed away, I carefully sterilized his jewelry and inserted it into the piercings of the people who loved him. Cliff's friends maintain a special connection with him by wearing his jewelry. A part of him carries on, literally inside of them. (This took place in 1992, before we'd seen studies showing that biological residue can remain after autoclave sterilization.)

CONTEMPORARY CONSIDERATIONS

By getting pierced, people make bold statements about personal freedom and combat the impersonality and pressures of modern life. Piercing can be an effective way to exert control over one's existence. Even if their modifications are not visible to the public, people working in conservative environments sometimes use piercings to remind themselves that they are individuals despite the conventionality of their outward appearance. One man living in the Midwest explained, "I was about fifty when I got my first. I live in a place where ignorance and poverty are a 'career choice.' Almost everyone is religious, conservative, and tends to believe that everyone else shares that viewpoint. Bigotry is rampant. I needed to make a statement that said, in effect, 'I might be one of you, but I'm not one with you.' Piercing was, and is, that statement."

WHICH EAR IS THE GAY EAR?

This question reflects uncertainty about piercings and what they may suggest about the sexual orientation of the wearer. Some people fear that being pierced may cause others to mistakenly believe they are gay or participate in an alternative lifestyle such as BDSM (consensual bondage and discipline and sadomasochism). Piercing, however, has evolved a great deal since a pierced right ear was used as a coded message by gay men in the 1970s, and it's now a practice embraced by all types of people. In other words, it doesn't matter whether you pierce your ear or some other body part, or which side you choose; it doesn't mean you're gay.

While many people who engage in unconventional forms of sexual expression *do* have piercings, being pierced does not signify anything in particular—except for any meaning *you* wish to ascribe to it. Nor, of course, does getting pierced turn you gay, as was the misguided concern of one client from Atlanta. He stormed back into the piercing studio the day after he received an ear piercing and angrily reported, "You pierced the wrong ear, and now I've caught the gay!"

WELL, WHY NOT?

Many people don't spend a lot of time considering why they choose this form of self-expression. Doing it simply because you like it and it makes you feel good about yourself are some of the best reasons for getting pierced. Upon reflection, sometimes a deeper reason becomes apparent, but this isn't required for piercing to be gratifying.

> "I am a trans man, and I got a pair of Duke piercings. It was a life-changing experience for me. That part of my body has been the one thing I've still struggled with since transitioning, and the Dukes have given me so much confidence and presence in my body. I didn't think it was possible for me to feel this way. My friend who was with me has noticed such a difference that we call it my 'Big Duke Energy.' The piercings have given me a gift of being more comfortable in my body."—A.

2

PIERCING PAST TO
PRESENT

From the prehistoric era to the present, piercing has been an essential part of the tradition of permanent body decoration. Museums are full of piercing ornaments and depictions of the practice from every part of the world. Piercing jewelry is made from the most mundane to truly precious materials. We can better appreciate the uniqueness and diversity of modern piercing by acknowledging the ways humans have pierced themselves in the past.

HISTORICAL INACCURACY

Unfortunately, records on the history of piercing are scant, often sensationalized, and filled with inaccuracies. Without intact human remains, the intended purpose of many surviving relics remains ambiguous. For example, is an object a talismanic artifact, or a piece of septum piercing jewelry? References to piercing in written records are scarce, and scholarly interpretations are often contradictory. One source, for example, says that traditional nostril piercings worn by Indian women are a sign of beauty and status. But another claims they are meant to induce submissiveness in women.[1] These inconsistencies may demonstrate that motivations for piercing are multifaceted even within a group, and that they change over time. Further, no researcher or historian is free from personal bias affecting their work.

Social anthropologists and historians have only recently begun to treat body decoration with any seriousness. Clarifying the history of piercing has been made even more difficult because many of the colorful stories about its origins were entirely fabricated by an influential early modern enthusiast, Doug Malloy (see page 15). His myths were widely circulated and repeated until they were considered facts. Almost every account of piercing history—even the most scholarly—reiterates some of his fictitious tales.

Since the focus of *The Piercing Bible* is on helping the consumer with day-to-day piercing questions and concerns, it is beyond the scope of this book to provide a detailed historical study of piercing. The emphasis of this chapter is on the development of the modern piercing industry in the late twentieth century. Therefore, I will present only a brief overview of what is reliably known about piercing in the ancient world and indigenous societies.

THE ANCIENT WORLD

Here are some of the oldest documented references to piercing:

o A crafted piece of bone from 44,000 BCE found in Australia appears designed to be worn in the nasal septum, making it what is believed to be the oldest bone body jewelry belonging to *Homo sapiens* to be identified anywhere in the world.[2]

o A skull from a man who lived over 12,000 years ago in Tanzania, Africa, shows erosion patterns on the teeth consistent with wearing plugs over one inch in diameter in labret and bilateral cheek piercings.[3]

o India's ancient religious texts, the Vedas, dating from about 1500 BCE, describe the goddess Lakshmi wearing earlobe and nose piercings.[4]

o The gold funerary mask of ancient Egyptian pharaoh Tutankhamun ("King Tut," d. 1323 BCE) has enlarged ear piercings.[5]

o Ötzi the Iceman, the 5,300-year-old mummy found in the Austrian Alps, had stretched earlobe piercings as well as numerous tattoos.

o In northern Iraq, Assyrian stone sculptures from the ninth century BCE depict bearded figures wearing large pendant earrings.[6]

o The tomb of the Ukok Princess was unearthed on the border of China and Russia in the 1990s. Artifacts included sophisticated gold jewelry for pierced ears dating from the fifth century BCE.[7]

o Jewelry for pierced ears has been found in ancient Greece, Cyprus, China, Italy, and many other countries, as well as early sculptures depicting individuals with pierced ears.

o *Infibulation* (mechanical restriction of sexual activity) was extensively practiced on men in antiquity, usually by passing a *fibula* (fastening device) through two sides of the foreskin. This was often performed in ancient Rome on enslaved people to assure their chastity, and on gladiators to prevent loss of strength due to "sexual excesses."[8] Actors and singers would also undergo infibulation, since intercourse was believed to be harmful to the voice.[9]

9

o In his medical encyclopedia, the writer Celsus (25–50 CE) describes the infibulation procedure which commences with something like a modern piercing: "The foreskin covering the glans is stretched forward and the point for perforation marked on each side with ink."[10] An echo of this practice was carried out in modern Europe to prevent the "harmful effects of masturbation" in young men.[11]

o From Peru to Mexico, ancient Mesoamerica and South America had rich traditions of personal adornment, including elaborate plugs for enlarged earlobe piercings, and septum jewelry. Ritual piercings, primarily of the tongue and penis, were practiced in the Olmec, Maya, and Aztec cultures.

o The oldest known written reference to piercing the glans of the penis is in the *Kama Sutra*, an ancient Sanskrit text on the art of love dating back to around the first century CE. It describes in detail a variety of penis inserts and pins as a means of enhancing sexual enjoyment for the wearer and their partner.[12]

TRIBAL CULTURES

Among the body parts commonly pierced today, a few have substantial tribal antecedents from around the globe:

o **Labret:** The word *labret* refers to an ornament worn through a perforation in the lip. It is not French (and the *t* is *not* silent); rather, it is English and derived from Latin. The term has been in our dictionaries since explorers interacted with the Tlingit people of Alaska in the nineteenth century. Labret piercing has been practiced in diverse areas, including Papua New Guinea, Ethiopia, Amazonia, and the northwest coast of the United States.

o **Nostril:** This traditional piercing placement in India has also been favored by indigenous tribes in both North and South America, the Middle East, and Africa.

o **Nasal septum:** A prevalent piercing in Mesoamerica, South America, Papua New Guinea, Borneo, and elsewhere. Septum jewelry can be particularly frightening and impressive, making this a common ornament in many warrior cultures.

o **Ear cartilage:** Popular among African tribal peoples such as the Fulani and Maasai, upper-ear piercings were also widespread among the Iban Dayaks of Borneo. They wore their ornaments for a fearsome appearance and to denote their status.[13] The claws and teeth of leopards and bears were placed through the upper ears of successful hunters.[14]

○ **Tongue:** Shamans of aboriginal tribes in central Australia, including the Aranda, wore tongue piercings. A spirit's lance ostensibly left a hole the size of a small finger as proof of the encounter and attainment of shamanic status. A shaman was not to practice for a year after receiving the piercing. If it closed, they would know their power was gone, and would not practice at all.[15]

○ **Penis:** Various penis piercings and modifications have been practiced worldwide. In Southeast Asia, beads, gold bells, or other foreign objects are implanted in the tissue of the penis. The Japanese have a tradition of inserting pearls under the skin. Australian aboriginal people sometimes insert small stones into incisions in the penis.[16]

WESTERN CIVILIZATION

Unlike indigenous cultures, Western societies have not been fertile ground for piercing practices. Religion has had a powerful puritanical effect on our relationship to our bodies, even though there are mentions of ear and nose piercing in the Bible. Passages have been interpreted to mean that marking the skin is prohibited because the body belongs to God.

Westerners' attitudes toward body art changed during the early fifteenth through seventeenth centuries as travelers and explorers returned with tales from faraway lands where the "savages" painted, poked, and decorated their bodies. Sailors came home sporting earrings and tattoos. Among sailors' favorite ornaments were gold earrings, which were reputed to pay for proper burial if the seaman washed ashore.[17] These masculine decorations eventually spread to soldiers, miners, and stevedores. There is also evidence that a number of upper-class men and women, particularly in the Victorian era, were inspired to flirt with piercings. A "breast-piercing craze" hit London in the 1890s, and the practice reportedly became popular among "seemingly sane, civilized Englishwomen."[18] This risqué trend also reached Paris and New York, which is all the more shocking considering that single earlobe piercings were not acceptable on adult women in Western culture until Queen Elizabeth popularized the style in the 1950s.[19]

SAILORS, FREAKS, AND FETISHISTS

Seafaring men had been decorating themselves for centuries, but before World War II, body art was still mostly limited to sailors and sideshow entertainers. During this time, however, there were a few body-art pioneers who carried it further, mostly in secret. Ethel Granger (1905–1982), whose famous thirteen-inch corseted waist echoed the practice of decades past, was one notable fan of piercing. Ethel's husband, Will Granger, assisted her by piercing her nostrils, septum, nipples, and ear cartilage. She was the first Western woman recorded in modern history to be so extensively pierced.[20] Piercing was also practiced in the 1930s by the Great Omi, a famous sideshow performer, born Horace Ridler. He wanted something more extreme than the tattoos that covered his entire body and face, so he had his septum pierced by a veterinarian and inserted a variety of ivory tusks. He also had his earlobes pierced and stretched until the holes could accommodate jewelry the size of a silver dollar.[21]

PUNKS AND PRIMITIVES

During the 1980s, two divergent philosophies emerged about piercing and other forms of body art. One harkens back to traditional cultures by paying tribute to the spiritual and ritual meanings of body modification. The other philosophy, more visceral and modern, emphasizes the use of piercing for pleasure, pain, and rebellion. These approaches are not always conscious, nor are they mutually exclusive, and they both still have relevance today.

One of the most influential figures in the rise of contemporary piercing was Fakir Musafar (1930–2018), the father of the "Modern Primitive" movement. Born Roland Loomis, he grew up close to Native American communities in South Dakota, which inspired his imagination at an early age. Fakir was one of a few modern pioneers whose fascination with body adornment and modification and a compulsion to experiment on his own body contributed to the existence of piercing as we know it today. He coined the term *modern primitives* to represent what he felt to be the connection between body modification and the spiritual use of piercing and other rituals, which were often taken directly from indigenous traditions. He viewed modern primitivism as an antidote to the superficiality of contemporary life. Fakir, along with a handful of other individuals, was deeply affected by the images of body art that appeared in old *National Geographic* magazines. A number of these early devotees were inspired to emulate some of the modifications they viewed in those pages.

In 1989, Re/Search Publications released a book containing a series of interviews with body modification enthusiasts, who were considered radical at the time. The book, *Modern Primitives: An Investigation of Contemporary Adornment & Ritual*, was highly influential. In it are interviews with Fakir Musafar and my mentor Jim Ward, and there's even a photograph showing the outline of my angel wings after my first major tattooing session. The interviewees frankly discuss their body modifications as expressions of their alternative sexuality. *Modern Primitives* was the first mass-market publication to address these subjects in a thoughtful and nonjudgmental manner, and it had a significant impact on the early growth of piercing.

Fakir's followers and other piercees enjoy exploring the mystical side of body modification. They often prefer natural jewelry materials to high-tech metals, and they pay tribute to their ancestors or different cultures through their adornments. Fakir's legacy lives on through the work of the Fakir Musafar Foundation in San Francisco, California, which offers some of the most respected piercing courses in the United States.

Piercing as an expression of rebellion and identity assumed a harsh manifestation when the punk movement of the late 1970s and 1980s embraced it. This faction was launched by working-class youth in Britain, and it quickly spread through the force and anger of punk rock music. Punk rockers shoved safety pins through their flesh to cause shock and disgust; their piercings and tattoos conveyed group solidarity, social discontent, and class angst. Like the sideshow performers of the past, they used self-injury as performance art. Punks raised public awareness of piercing and helped pave the way for its later popularity.

PLEASURE AND PAIN: THE GAUNTLET

The first groups to embrace body piercing as a contemporary lifestyle choice included gay men, BDSM practitioners, and others who used piercing as a profound means for expressing their alternative sexuality. Nipples and genitals were experimented upon with enthusiasm, and these piercings remain in demand to this day.

The field of modern piercing would be quite different, or perhaps nonexistent, without the involvement and commitment of a group of gay SM enthusiasts in California. These pioneers formed a network of men with a shared interest in piercing, spearheaded by the organizational and networking skills of Doug Malloy (see "The Legacy of Doug Malloy," page 15). Meeting informally, they helped to usher piercing into the United States.

One of the leaders of this group, Jim Ward, is regarded as the founding father of modern piercing. With Malloy's encouragement and financial backing, Ward started a small piercing business at his West Hollywood home in 1975. Inspired by too many late-night calls from piercing clients, and a desire to legitimize his work, Ward eventually moved to a storefront. In November 1978, Gauntlet Enterprises opened on Santa Monica Boulevard in West Hollywood—the first professional piercing specialty studio in America.

Gauntlet's initial clientele came from the local alternative communities and the "T&P" (tattooing and piercing) social club organized by Doug Malloy. Gradually public figures, including musicians, models, and actors, started to patronize the studio, followed by growing numbers of the general public. At first, Jim Ward made the jewelry himself on the premises, and the piercings had an element of trial and error. An "installation" was free with a jewelry purchase. The jewelry designs (including Ward's names for them), piercing techniques, and placements pioneered by Gauntlet established the foundation for today's piercing industry.

Jim Ward, along with Doug Malloy and Fakir Musafar, also produced the world's first professional publication dedicated to the subject, *Piercing Fans International Quarterly* (PFIQ). The inaugural edition of the magazine was published in 1977, and had a run of fifty issues before it succumbed to the unfortunate fate of Gauntlet itself in 1998. Despite having grown to encompass multiple retail branches, a jewelry manufacturing department, corporate offices, and a mail-order division, Gauntlet went out of business. After twenty years in operation, a series of bad business decisions necessitated an infusion of outside capital. Subsequently, a hostile takeover led to Chapter 7 bankruptcy and permanent closure.

I received the first honorary "Master Piercer" certificate that Jim Ward bestowed, and I was the first to present an enthusiastic female face to the world as a piercing advocate. As the book *Modern Primitives* gained recognition, the press began to seek out professional piercers. As vice president of the original Gauntlet branch in Los Angeles in the late 1980s and early 1990s, I was in the right place at the right time to participate in a flurry of media exposure that helped to broaden the appeal of piercing in the United States.

Body piercing is a distinctly sexual form of self-expression for many piercees, and at times, this aspect of piercing has overshadowed its broader meanings and popularity. During the 1987 police raids in Britain referred to as Operation Spanner, sixteen men were arrested and charged with assault for private, consensual gay sex and activities, which included piercing. One of these "Spanner Men" was Alan Oversby, also known as Mr. Sebastian, who is considered to be the father of European piercing. An influential British tattooist and piercer, he was largely self-taught, and like Jim Ward, he received some instruction from Doug Malloy. The authorities arrested Oversby for performing a genital piercing on a client and sentenced him on the charge of "assault occasioning actual bodily harm." The courts refused to hear the defense that the activity was consensual, saying, "Pleasure derived from the infliction of pain is an evil thing,"[22] illustrating the bias against alternative sexuality and piercing. The legal decisions from this court case have long impacted UK law as it applies to body piercing.

THE LEGACY OF DOUG MALLOY

If you have ever heard that the Prince Albert piercing was named after the one worn by Queen Victoria's consort, or that Roman centurions attached capes to their pierced nipples, you have been visited by the spirit of Doug Malloy. This name was the pseudonym used by Richard Simonton, a wealthy businessman who concealed his passion for piercing and his life as a gay SM practitioner from his family and professional associates. His profound enthusiasm for piercing as a sexual behavior has had a lasting effect on the development of the industry.

Malloy created two informal underground publications about piercing. One was a fictionalized autobiography that was available briefly as a booklet in the 1970s. The other, which has had an astoundingly enduring influence, was a leaflet titled "Body Piercing in Brief." It contained descriptions of a dozen piercings—including their fabricated histories—with drawings by Jim Ward. This sheet aroused substantial interest in piercing and was widely disseminated by Gauntlet for many years. In spite of the problems Malloy's inventive stories have caused for researchers, Jim Ward emphasizes their importance: "I sometimes wonder if people into piercing today have any deep appreciation of the tremendous impact Doug Malloy has had on their lives. . . . What was it that made him the center from which the whole modern piercing movement sprang? . . . No one before him had ever presented such a broad palette of piercing possibilities complete with history and lore. It didn't matter that he probably made up a lot of it. . . . it was a message a lot of people were waiting to hear, whether they realized it or not."

THE MEDIA BRINGS THE MESSAGE

By the late twentieth century, the time was ripe for piercing to escalate in popularity and availability. As it became more prevalent with alternative groups in the 1980s, the press took notice, which led to even greater media attention. By the mid-1990s, widespread publicity in print publications, television talk shows, news programs, and sitcoms fed the interest in the subject, and pierced celebrities put the cherry on the top. Piercing became part of our modern world; people were getting new holes poked all over the place.

Rock stars have had some of the greatest impact in bringing an awareness of piercing to the public. A defining event in the popularity of piercings was the 1993 launch of a rock music video by the band Aerosmith. The video for "Cryin'," which won an MTV Music Video of the Year award, featured actress Alicia Silverstone getting a navel piercing. According to my former apprentice Paul King, who portrayed the piercer in the video, the procedure was staged using a body double because the actress was still a minor. Ironically, she described navel piercing as "gross" during the video shoot.

After this dramatic musical introduction, hordes of young women across the country sought to follow the new trend. The immense demand for piercing, however, occurred before a ready supply of skilled piercing professionals was available to do the job. With nowhere better to turn, would-be piercees swarmed tattoo studios. Although people might perceive different types of body modification as similar activities, piercing was not universally accepted in the tattoo world. Since the late 1970s, the tattoo community had pushed for mainstream acceptance of their art. A few influential figures, however, decided that the media's portrayals of piercing hurt the tattoo community's public image, regardless of tattooists' and enthusiasts' personal views on the subject. Public displays of piercings were prohibited in tattoo contests, and professional piercers were barred from events for about a decade. This created an artificial schism with persisting repercussions.

But in the early 1990s, after an army of gals had approached tattooists inquiring, "Do you do belly piercings?" they started replying, "Well . . . yes!" even though they did not possess the appropriate training, skill, or passion. Those young women essentially inspired the creation of piercing as a full-fledged industry. Driven by desire, the art was ushered into the Western world through brazen experimentation.

Throughout the 1990s and into the new millennium, navel piercing maintained its widespread popularity, and other piercings have followed suit, becoming acceptable with ever-broadening segments of the population.[23] Many people began to emulate popular fashion models, actors, musicians, sports figures, and social media influencers by wearing visible piercings, and middle-aged professionals and parents have joined the ranks of the pierced, though not always as openly.

MTV and tabloids were responsible for much of the exposure in the early days of piercing's introduction to the general public. In more recent times, social media has proved to be a significant bottom-up force driving popular piercing styles and jewelry trends. An image of a triple forward helix (ear cartilage) piercing was posted on Pinterest, which caused an all-out mania for the attractive but challenging jewelry arrangement. Facebook, Instagram, and other social media outlets are also responsible for the vastly increased demand for high-quality branded body jewelry—even in markets that had been resistant to change.

When the general public was first introduced to body piercings, it was aghast—even appalled. Nowadays, those same people seldom give piercings a second glance, and some of them have piercings of their own.

MEDIA IMPACT

In 1990 the *National Enquirer* ran a story about piercing with the humorous headline, "Bizarre New Fashion Fad Turns Folks into Human Pincushions." A photo showing my septum and tongue piercings was among those printed with the commentary.

Surely most readers of that article must have believed that piercing would be a short-lived craze, as reported. But the depth of attraction to body adornment proved far stronger than anybody might have imagined. This wacky article actually instigated the popularity of tongue piercings!

THE NEW MILLENNIUM AND BEYOND

By the turn of the century, modern piercing had shed much of its shock value, and it continued to gain acceptance and lose its radical edge during the first decade of the millennium. Piercing finally became widespread enough to be considered a potential career path. But it was not unusual for aspiring professionals to be warned by their loved ones, "Don't base your livelihood on a passing fad!" The last twenty years have clearly demonstrated that piercing is anything but a temporary trend. Instead, it has permeated mainstream Western society from street style to haute couture. It isn't out of the ordinary to see a pop star with a septum ring, a grandmother with a nostril piercing, or a doctor with a highly ornamented ear. Piercing has become more and more ingrained in our contemporary culture, and it has never been more accepted than it is now.

PART 2

GROUNDWORK AND PRELIMINARY CONSIDERATIONS

RISKS, MYTHS, AND WARNINGS........ 20

IS PIERCING RIGHT FOR YOU? 30

IS PIERCING RIGHT FOR
YOUR CHILD? 36

YOU AND YOUR PIERCER................... 40

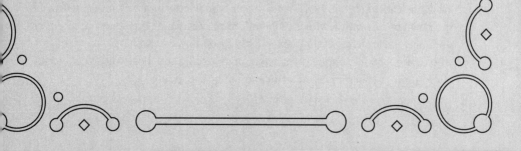

3

RISKS, MYTHS, AND WARNINGS

I see *so many* regretful individuals who have made poor choices from a lack of knowledge or failure to take piercing seriously. Some patronized incompetent practitioners, and others were punctured by a friend or self-pierced at home. Plenty purchased the cheapest jewelry available or tried wearing unsafe objects including safety pins. These and other errors in judgment have resulted in a great deal of suffering and countless fiascos and scars. There are real risks to piercings, but you can minimize them by becoming educated and making sound decisions.

IS PIERCING RISKY?

Over the years, a great deal of hype and hysteria about piercing was perpetuated by the media and by conservative religious, medical, and educational communities. They described piercing as a highly dangerous behavior related to everything from juvenile delinquency to cancer and death. Fortunately, this has subsided in today's more piercing-friendly climate.

Even professional piercings performed according to accepted practices can end up experiencing complications, and a poorly done one is quite likely to have problems. Educate yourself before getting pierced to diminish the dangers and prepare to deal with any issues that do occur. The most common piercing risks are introduced here. In-depth information on identifying and troubleshooting these and other complications is presented in chapter 16.

PIERCING: NOT A DO-IT-YOURSELF (DIY) HOBBY

At the beginning of the modern piercing movement, few skilled practitioners were available. Lacking professional help, people who felt the urge for a piercing lanced their own bodies with sewing needles or ordinary earrings. Even today, amateur or unethical hack piercers will pierce anything on anyone, *badly*. Young teenagers who cannot obtain parental permission for a piercing and those who cannot easily afford professional services in a studio often go this route.

Many online vendors sell piercing kits, which advertise that they come with "complete instructions" and are "easy to use." Wrong! These are no safer than a home root canal kit, and you must avoid them. A DIY piercing is often poorly placed and has a significantly increased risk of infection and other problems. Quality body art studios are prevalent now, so there is no excuse for shoddy piercings.

PIERCING GUNS

In an optimal procedure, a highly trained professional gently creates a piercing with sterile equipment and inserts quality body jewelry suited to the client's unique anatomy. The guns used to pierce earlobes, ear cartilage, and sometimes nostrils or other body parts do not meet these standards, so you should avoid them. Jewelry retailers use stud-gun piercing as a sales incentive: "Free Piercing with Purchase of Jewelry." The devices are also available directly to consumers over the internet and in beauty supply stores. They may appear to be a cheap, convenient option, but several factors make piercing guns unsafe and inappropriate for body—and ear—piercings.

Stud guns (whether spring-loaded or hand-operated) force a pointy earring through the skin. This causes *more* tissue trauma and discomfort than the razor-sharp needles used by body piercers. The one-size post length does not "fit all" and cannot accommodate a plump earlobe or any swelling; it is certainly not long enough to be worn in a body piercing. Stud earrings typically employ a butterfly-style clasp that is not suggested for wear in any fresh piercings. This jewelry design can inhibit the healing process and increase the risk of infection by compressing the tissue, limiting circulation, and trapping secretions and bacteria. A stud-gun nostril jewelry design is meant to be worn without a backing. Its exposed sharp point creates obvious dangers for the nasal septum inside the nose.

Blood from a piercee can *aerosolize* (become airborne in microscopic particles) and contaminate the inside of a reusable gun. These surfaces could come into contact with the next client's tissue, and it is possible to transmit disease in this way. Sometimes guns are "sanitized" between uses with alcohol or other disinfectants, but this does not kill all surface microbes. One outbreak of severe infections that caused several piercees to be hospitalized was attributed to a contaminated spray that "cleaned" the gun between customers.[1] Most of these ear-piercing guns contain plastic parts that melt, so they cannot be processed in an *autoclave* (a machine that sterilizes equipment using heat and pressure) between clients. The gun manufacturers have attempted to address this issue by producing "one use" cartridges that contain the jewelry. However, when these cartridges are inserted into a reusable device, they still pose a higher risk of infection than piercing with a sterile, disposable needle.

Other problems sometimes occur: the stud fails to go through the skin on the first try, or the earring doesn't discharge from the gun, leaving the device stuck to the piercing. These situations require handling the tissue, and gun operators frequently do not wear (or even have access to) medical gloves. Many are teenagers who are not well trained in proper procedure, placement, or sanitation techniques.

INFECTION

Infection is one of the most frightening and potentially grave dangers associated with piercing, especially as bacterial resistance to antibiotics becomes increasingly common. Two distinct phases are of concern. If you get pierced in unsanitary conditions, or with unsterile implements or jewelry, an infection can be transmitted *during* the piercing. Or, if you fail to care for the wound properly throughout its healing period, you can get an infection *after* the piercing is done.[2] Studies show that these risks increase when either the piercer's technique or the aftercare is poor.[3]

None of the published statistics I've seen on piercing complications remotely reflect my professional experience, in which infections—even minor ones—are rare. In any case, the true incidence of infectious complications is difficult to calculate because there is no reliable information about how many piercings are being performed.

Our world is full of *microorganisms* (germs, including bacteria, fungi, and viruses). Many of these are harmless—or even beneficial—to us, but some are *pathogenic* (capable of causing infection or disease). We are all routinely exposed to countless germs, but many complex factors impact how they affect us, including the potency and number of microorganisms entering the body, and how they get in, as well as the strength of a person's immune system.

The viruses hepatitis B and C and HIV are examples of *bloodborne pathogens* (microorganisms that can cause disease when present in the blood). They are of particular concern, because if the needles or jewelry are not sterile, there is potential for these serious bloodborne diseases to be transmitted during piercing.

HIV, the virus that causes AIDS, is quite fragile, and becomes inactive relatively quickly when exposed to air. There have been *no* documented cases of HIV transmission through piercing.[4] The hepatitis virus, however, is easier to transmit because it is quite hardy. Studies show that hepatitis B can live outside the body and remain infectious for at least seven days![5] Even though the virus is robust, professionally performed body art does not have a high incidence of hepatitis transmissions.[6]

Microbial contamination can cause a range of issues, from minor skin eruptions to deadly infections in the brain or the lining of the heart. Never ignore a suspected infection; left untreated, certain kinds that begin as trivial can become lethal. *Localized cellulitis* (a bacterial infection at the site of a piercing) is the most common sort; deeper, more extensive invasions, or systemic syndromes in healthy piercees, are rare.[7]

The medical field has developed specific infection-control practices, called *Standard Precautions* (formerly *Universal Precautions*), for dealing with blood or other potentially infectious body fluids and any equipment that could be contaminated with them. Safe piercers are educated about these procedures and adhere to them meticulously, to protect themselves and their clientele.

HEALTH CONDITIONS AND PIERCINGS

Some medical conditions make piercings riskier, and in some cases, inadvisable. Bleeding disorders have obvious ramifications. Health problems that weaken your infection-fighting defenses, including diabetes, lupus, HIV/AIDS, and other immune system disorders, can slow healing. You might be more vulnerable to infection, and if you do develop one, it could be more severe and harder to cure.

Some heart conditions make you susceptible to *infective endocarditis* (a potentially deadly infection of the lining of the heart or heart valves, previously referred to as *bacterial endocarditis*). If you've had this illness or have a history of a severe cardiac issue like a valve replacement, an ethical piercer will require proof that you have consulted with your doctor before proceeding. If you ordinarily must take antibiotic *prophylaxis* (preventive treatment) before dental or medical procedures, your physician may recommend this before piercing. Cardiac ailments are among the few preexisting conditions that can increase the risk of a fatal outcome: if a doctor advises you against piercing due to your health, heed them!

Rashes such as eczema or psoriasis and other skin abnormalities can be less critical health issues, but compromised skin should not be pierced. If you are considering a piercing in an area affected by one of these conditions, seek an evaluation by an experienced piercer and a piercing-friendly doctor.

Some states have regulations requiring piercers to ask clients specific health-history questions on a release form before a piercing, whereas others have laws prohibiting piercers from asking certain health questions. Be honest and informative about your medical history, and respect a piercer who has the principles to decline to pierce you if the risk is unacceptable.

ALLERGIES AND SKIN PROBLEMS

All sorts of bumps, lumps, and skin irritations can crop up around a piercing, coming and going during healing and occasionally remaining permanently. Some of these are caused by mechanical friction against the area; others are caused by a cleaning product or jewelry material. Skin disorders can be challenging to diagnose, even for dermatologists, so trial and error is sometimes necessary to identify and correct a problem. Conditions can also have a combination of causes, which further complicates diagnosis and treatment.

Jewelry made of inferior metals can trigger allergies and sensitivities. This type of reaction can be severe and irreversible, which is one reason it is critical to wear only high-quality, inert jewelry (see "Jewelry Materials for Initial Piercings," page 91).

MIGRATION AND REJECTION

Two distinctive piercing complications that can occur are *migration* (when the piercing moves from its initial placement, then settles and heals in a new location) and *rejection* (when the body expels the jewelry completely). Migration is likely to happen when unsuitable or insufficient tissue is pierced, or if your jewelry is too small in diameter, thin in gauge, or of poor quality. Inexperienced, careless, or untrained piercers often make these errors.

Migration and rejection can also result from using a harsh aftercare product, having poor health habits, or experiencing excessive physical trauma or emotional stress during the healing period. And, unfortunately, even when everything is done according to accepted practices, a piercing will sometimes migrate or reject for no known reason. This is simply one of the risks of placing a foreign object through your skin: it may not stay in the desired position.

SCARRING AND PERMANENT PHYSICAL CHANGES

A piercing has the potential to be a temporary adornment (especially when compared to a tattoo) because the jewelry can easily be taken out. However, there is the risk of irreversible changes to the body, including discoloration, a scar, bump, dimple, or permanent hole.

Many piercings shrink or close incredibly quickly, but some remain open indefinitely, even if left empty. The placement of the hole, the *gauge* (thickness) of the jewelry, and the length of time you wore it, plus your individual tissue, all impact whether or not your piercing stays viable following jewelry removal.

Piercings that are stretched to large dimensions sometimes leave significant voids that could be considered disfiguring. Plastic surgery is required if you wish to restore the area to a more normal appearance. Stretching too rapidly or attempting to expand unsuitably thin tissue leads to problems. One potential consequence of overzealous enlargement is a *blowout* (part of the interior channel pushes out, leaving an unsightly lip of flesh on one side of the piercing). This distortion will usually be a lasting reminder of your hasty actions, unless it is surgically removed. Overstretching can also lead to thinning skin that does not regrow. A worst-case scenario is tissue *necrosis* (death), and the loss of the piercing and some adjacent flesh. Jewelry that exerts excessive pressure against underlying bone could potentially cause bone necrosis.

Certain piercings tend to effect changes such as a hardening or thickening of the tissue surrounding the openings, which can be irreversible. For example, nipple piercings sometimes cause permanent enlargement, primarily in small builds. Specifics are covered in chapters 11–14.

Scarring and tissue discoloration at the piercing site are relatively common occurrences, especially if you have a history of hyperpigmented (darkened) scars. This can happen even when a piercing is performed appropriately and heals uneventfully. Avoid tanning and sun exposure on healing piercings to minimize this possibility. Migration often leaves a small scarring track or discoloration from where the piercing was initially placed. Rejection frequently results in a split scar. Ear cartilage is prone to disfigurement and collapse, causing a "cauliflower ear" appearance if a severe piercing infection develops.[8]

Excessive scarring sometimes occurs in reaction to piercing, and it can be very challenging to resolve. If you have a history of problems with scarring or *keloids* (large growths of fibrous tissue), piercing is generally inadvisable. For more on this topic, see "Excessive Scarring" (page 256) and the subsequent sections in chapter 16.

UNFORTUNATE EVENTS

Accidents happen, and it is possible to catch your jewelry on something and tear your piercing. An act as simple as taking off your shirt can be dangerous if you have a ring or bar on your torso, face, or ear. Strenuous workouts, airbags, pets, children—even sexual activities—can potentially cause ripping or splitting. Piercings that are healing are more delicate and susceptible to injury, but older ones are still vulnerable.

Stay aware of your jewelry and movements, protect your piercing, and avoid activities that could lead to such accidents. If you engage in sports or other behaviors that pose a risk to your piercings, wear protective gear. See "Protective Patch," page 231, for details.

Jewelry that is too thin can carve through flesh like a wire slicing a wedge of cheddar; hence, I coined the term *cheese-cutter effect* to describe this unpleasant (and preventable) occurrence. Wearing charms or heavy weights on thin-gauge wires makes this type of problem likely.

Somewhat less predictable incidents can occur when jewelry in oral or nasal piercings is swallowed or, far more alarming, inhaled. The best way to prevent this is by wearing quality jewelry of the proper fit and ensuring the closure (bead or ornament) is affixed securely.

DANGEROUS PIERCING PLACEMENTS

Certain piercings are inherently hazardous or rarely heal; you can view scores of photos of unquestionably dangerous placements online. Simply because someone is willing to do a piercing on you or has done it on others doesn't mean it is safe or advisable. Preferring to err on the side of caution, I suggest avoiding the piercings listed in the following chart due to their risky nature.

RISKY PIERCINGS

LOCATION	RISK
Face and Mouth	
Eyelid	Scratched and scarred cornea, dry eye, blindness
Chin surface	Migration, rejection, scarring
Horizontal (transverse) tongue and "snake eyes" horizontal tongue tip	Hemorrhage, nerve damage, tooth injury, gum injury
Tongue surface "scoop"	Rejection, scarring
Cheek (beyond the first molar)	Punctured parotid duct or gland, saliva leakage; see "The Worst Piercing Story," page 150
Lowbret and vertical lowbret (between cheek and gumline inside)	Gum and bone erosion, scarring
Mandible (below the tongue through soft palate to underside of chin)	Gum and bone erosion, saliva leakage, scarring
Gums	Gum, bone, and tooth loss
Torso	
"Outie" navel	Herniation, peritonitis
Subclavicular (underneath the collarbone)	Hemorrhage, nerve damage, potentially life-threatening risk of pneumothorax (collapsed lung)
Vulva	
Isabella (deep clitoral shaft piercing from bottom of the clitoris to the top of the hood)	Hemorrhage, nerve damage
Deep VCH piercing (from under the hood but passing through excessive tissue)	Hemorrhage, nerve damage
Penis and Scrotum	
Deep penile shaft piercing or trans-scrotal piercing	Hemorrhage, nerve damage
Additional Areas of Concern	
Uvula (soft, fleshy extension that hangs at the back of the throat)	Loss of jewelry or needle (caught in throat or aspirated into lungs)
Piercing close to the surface through a small amount of tissue	Migration, rejection, scarring
Piercing behind bone, tendon, or other anatomical structure	Hemorrhage, nerve damage, loss of function
Anal piercing	Infection, hemorrhage
Hand web, all *interdigital spaces* (between fingers or toes), anywhere on feet or hands	Infection (high risk), migration, rejection, scarring

LESS OBVIOUS RISKS

It's easy to understand that a piercing could become infected or snag on something and get torn, but some risks are subtler. Though body art is more accepted than it used to be, a person with abundant facial piercings could still experience disapproval. This might be minor, such as dirty looks or comments, or more extreme, like problems with school, family, or employment. These consequences deserve consideration if they are relevant to you; for example, if you're reliant on your parents for tuition or other support. Piercings can also cause relationship problems if your genital jewelry is not enjoyable for your lover.

MYTHS AND MISCONCEPTIONS

One frequent (and sometimes disastrous) misconception is that any piercer who posts a license or certificate must have some training or skill. You can find out much more about piercers in chapter 6, "You and Your Piercer."

Luckily, most stories about uncontrolled bleeding or post-piercing paralysis are fabrications. Of course, *some* bleeding is a normal consequence of any piercing, though many do not bleed at all. There is no "special nerve" a piercer can hit to cause paralysis from any traditional piercing. Nor is there any major artery located in the pathway of the most popular piercing sites.

Piercers routinely puncture the smallest and most peripheral of the vessels and nerves with no ill effect whatsoever. Piercing through capillaries, *venules* (small veins), and *arterioles* (tiny arteries) is an unavoidable part of the process. See "What to Expect," page 225.

One misunderstanding that remains widespread, even in the health care realm, is that piercings always create a pathway to the interior of the body. This is untrue! A healed piercing is a sealed channel of tissue from end to end (in medical terms, a *fistula*), and only when a piercing is healing, injured, or experiencing a flare-up is it an open wound, or pathway into the body. See "The Wound-Healing Process," page 224, for details.

The information throughout this book will clear up numerous fictions, falsehoods, and mistaken beliefs about piercings, such as:

o Many people think that sterling silver is a good metal for new piercings, and gold is a bad one, but that's backward. See chapter 10, "Jewelry 101: Sizes, Shapes, and Materials," especially the "Gold" section on page 94.

o You should not twist or move your jewelry to prevent it from getting stuck, nor should you use antibacterial soap, alcohol, peroxide, or ointment during healing. See chapter 15, "Essential Guide to Healing and Aftercare," for instructions.

o   Oral and genital piercings do not get infected more readily than other areas. Similarly, they are not always more painful or harder to heal. In fact, some of the piercings in both of these areas are just the opposite. See chapters 12 and 14.

o   Piercings do not always set off the buzzers in airport checkpoints. See "Metal Detectors and Security," page 307.

o   Body jewelry can sometimes be left in for X-rays, MRIs, and medical examinations and procedures. See "Medical and Dental Emergencies and Appointments," page 303.

o   Nipple piercings do not normally preclude nursing a baby. See "Nipple Piercing and Breastfeeding," page 309.

PIERCINGS AS MEDICAL TREATMENTS

An unfortunate urban myth has led people to get pierced for the wrong reasons. There is no sound medical basis to the belief that daith piercings can cure migraines, tragus piercings can lead to weight loss, or helix piercings can reduce anxiety. Nor are there other piercings likely to resolve any issues or health conditions.

The underlying theory that these piercings work by passing through acupuncture points is erroneous. The daith is nowhere near the auriculotherapy (ear acupuncture) locations for treating headaches; it pierces the points for the mouth and anus. Further, even if the right acupuncture points are pierced, leaving jewelry in continuously would likely cease to be effective in a matter of weeks. (Acupuncture traditionally stimulates a point to activate it, then the stimulus is removed to constitute a treatment.)

Even *if* medical evidence showed that these piercings had therapeutic or curative effects, piercers making such claims are working outside the scope of their profession, and could potentially be charged with practicing medicine without a license. They either don't know any better or don't care that they're doing something illegal. Neither is a good quality in a piercer!

PIERCING AND ACUPUNCTURE

I have worked closely with several licensed practitioners of traditional Chinese medicine and acupuncture. They feel that piercing through an acupuncture point might briefly treat or impact a condition associated with that specific spot. But after continuous stimulation, the point would cease to be affected. They postulate that the acupuncture point then relocates near the piercing site but is not obliterated. Other acupuncturists also subscribe to this theory.[9]

MINIMIZING RISKS

You greatly diminish the hazards of piercing by becoming an educated consumer. Severe complications are extremely unlikely if:

- You are in good health
- You get pierced by a qualified practitioner who follows all hygiene precautions
- You wear quality jewelry of an appropriate material, size, and style
- You consistently follow sensible cleaning and care procedures

THE POINT

Living is dangerous, and none of us gets out of this alive, so enjoying your journey is essential. If you want a piercing, learn all the facts, evaluate your health and other personal considerations, and weigh the risks. If you do go for it, get the job done properly and chances are you and your piercing will be just fine.

4

IS PIERCING RIGHT FOR YOU?

If you want to experiment with your appearance, piercing can be a suitable option because it isn't as drastic or lasting as a tattoo. Piercings might intrigue you, but you may not feel sure you should actually take the plunge. You could be fearful of needles, worried about experiencing pain, or anxious about taking off your clothes in front of a stranger. The suitability of piercings for your lifestyle or health status is a reasonable concern. If you are attracted to piercings but hesitate out of fear or perceived obstacles, this chapter will help you form realistic expectations, minimize unfounded worries, and encourage you to think carefully before making a final decision.

RESPONSIBILITY AND COMMITMENT

Getting a piercing is kind of like adopting a pet: maturity and patience are required to deal with it. Even the most resolute of piercees can feel challenged by the need to consistently follow all post-piercing requirements. Do you have the fortitude to wait many weeks or months before changing your jewelry, going swimming, or touching your piercing with unwashed hands?

If you are lax about your health or hygiene, you are not a suitable candidate for piercing. You must support the healing process by taking care of yourself and keeping your environment—including your clothes and linens—clean. A nonstop party lifestyle, poor eating habits, or a lack of sleep can severely inhibit your body's ability to heal.

A level of financial solvency is also necessary, because quality body jewelry can be expensive. If the piece you are wearing causes irritation, you lose a part, or some other emergency comes up, you may have to purchase new jewelry without advance notice. You must have the means to buy the best products and not borrow used jewelry from a friend (danger!) or pick up a cut-rate item at a novelty store.

Finally, emotional maturity and poise are needed to deal with any negative reactions. Will your feelings be hurt if your relatives, friends, or coworkers don't approve?

EAR PIERCINGS ≠ ALL PIERCINGS

The earlobe seems destined for piercing. Throughout history, humans have adorned that humble bit of flesh with plugs, rings, and dangles. It is perfectly positioned for ornamenting the face without any troublesome veins or nerves getting in the way. The earlobe usually heals readily and tolerates most jewelry without complaint.

You may believe that the same trouble-free conditions apply to all piercings, but you are likely to run into problems (and be disappointed) if you have these unrealistic expectations. Having pierced earlobes won't prepare you for the challenges of most other piercings. The lobe can heal in as little as a month, but few spots take so little time. Many require two to three months or more to heal, and some, such as navel or surface piercings, take six to nine months or longer (see the "Minimum Healing Times Chart" on page 333 for a complete listing).

Many piercings are unsuited to frequent jewelry changes. Some placements and jewelry closures can be difficult to deal with on your own, and you can end up damaging your tissue if you try. Once healed, earlobe piercings usually stay open well, but most other areas do not. The majority of placements (including the ear cartilage) are different from earlobe piercings in many ways.

HEALTHY BODIES HEAL BETTER

The healthier you are, the faster and easier you will heal. Remember: *your body* handles the healing process—not some magic lotion or potion you put on the piercing. Therefore, you should make an extra effort to pay attention to your health habits when getting pierced. Piercing is generally inadvisable in any of the following situations:

- You are sick or run down (especially if you are taking antibiotics or steroids)
- You have sensitive skin or are prone to scarring
- You are under an unusual amount of physical or emotional stress
- You are already healing from other piercings or wounds
- You plan to have surgery or a significant medical or dental procedure

LIFESTYLE CONSIDERATIONS

Before getting pierced, think carefully about your lifestyle and circumstances. It is best to delay or forgo piercing if your current situation makes it apparent that you would have trouble healing.

- **Season/weather:** Wearing heavy clothing over a piercing during cold weather can cause discomfort and complications. Pools, salt water, sand, and sunscreen all have the potential to irritate or infect. Swimming would expose your piercing to microbes or chlorine and other harsh chemicals, and must be avoided while healing.

- **Physical activities:** Participation in contact sports makes it challenging to heal a piercing due to friction, sweat, and trauma. Although it is possible to combine piercings with an active lifestyle, it is generally not a good idea to get pierced if you are a dedicated athlete, training for an event, or engaging in rigorous sports that could pose a physical danger to your piercing. Schools usually prohibit piercings for student athletes due to safety concerns.

- **Pending plans:** Traveling to places where water quality is poor (or simply different from what your body is accustomed to) or upcoming activities that would necessitate removing your jewelry are valid reasons for postponing a piercing.

- **Career path:** Whether your job is blue collar, white collar, or no collar, consider how piercings fit in with your livelihood. Construction workers, cooks, mechanics, and others whose employment routinely involves sweat and grime may have problems healing due to unhygienic workplace conditions. The risk of snagging your jewelry is a safety concern for a variety of jobs. In professional realms, employers may still frown on visible piercings. Conservative fields such as law and medicine have a history of being especially unwelcoming to the visibly pierced. However, attitudes continue to shift, and employers are more receptive in certain regions. There are significant differences in the acceptability of piercings in the workplace, depending on geographic location, so you'll need to consider the prevailing viewpoint in your area. If you are a student contemplating a particular career or an employee interested in changing your current position, ask yourself if the piercing you desire could be an issue.

CONCEALMENT AND REMOVAL

Sometimes people get a new piercing and plan to take the jewelry out for certain activities or to conceal it at school, home, or work. Popping your jewelry in and out may sound simple, but it irritates delicate cells. Such abuse of the area will result in complications like scar tissue formation and migration. Touching your fresh piercing and jewelry during removal and reinsertion increases your chance of infection, too. Because piercing was prohibited by his coach, one young man took his nipple ring out every day before football practice and then pushed it back in afterward. No wonder he suffered from problems including pain and delayed healing!

Retainers and various jewelry alternatives are available to camouflage piercings, though some spots can be disguised more readily than others. Unfortunately, the most invisible retainers are unsafe to wear until after you have healed. Concealment issues are addressed in a separate section under each piercing, where applicable, and retainers are covered in chapter 19 on page 305.

OBSTACLES

People who are interested in getting pierced may perceive other impediments. "I'm too old" and "I'm too fat" are two common concerns. Age and weight can affect healing, but most often, these are emotional barriers that do not preclude getting pierced. This kind of negative self-image can be disheartening and difficult to overcome. Therefore, a little reassurance may be in order.

Unless advanced years cause health problems and slow healing, age is not a barrier at all. In fact, people in their sixties and seventies are among my clientele; they're getting genital and nipple piercings! You may feel concerned about looking foolish if you are older, thinking body art is reserved for the young. Rest assured, many mature adults have and enjoy piercings.

Extreme obesity or emaciation can affect your health and, therefore, your ability to heal. Poor circulation, compromised immune function, and other medical problems related to excess weight are sound reasons to forgo piercing. You could still be a candidate if you are healthy, committed to taking proper care of your piercing, and a competent practitioner deems your anatomy pierceable. One area of exceptional concern is the navel. If you are overweight, the *avascularity* (lack of blood supply) in this area is even worse than usual, and the configuration of a large midsection is often unsuited to piercing.

Below-the-neck placements require disrobing and revealing specific parts of your anatomy, so piercers routinely see bodies of all shapes and sizes. Whether you are fat, thin, or in between, and even if you are modest by nature, a piercer worth their salt will put you at ease by acting in a manner that is professional and compassionate.

EXCESSIVE ANXIETY

If you feel unduly anxious about your piercing, the anticipation can be the worst part of the whole experience. Rest assured: your imagination is probably much worse than the reality. But your apprehension can make getting pierced far more harrowing than it needs to be. If you are excessively nervous or needle-phobic, prepare yourself by learning ways to deal with your fears. It will make your visit to the studio more tolerable. Practice the "Breathing and Relaxation Techniques" on page 65 before and during your appointment.

Seek a piercer who will be supportive of your decision to conquer your fears and who will take you through the process with sensitivity. A good piercer will have a wealth of patience and understanding; however, they're not a therapist. There is a limit to how much time and energy they can spend with you during a single session.

Your piercer will be able to do a better job if you are not an emotional wreck requiring extensive support and reassurance. When they have to devote themselves to consoling you, they're less able to focus on the technical aspects of the job. If you are so anxiety-ridden that you panic and interrupt the procedure (ask the piercer to stop, or grab at their hands), you make the situation worse and can cause a needlestick accident. If you cannot rein in your emotions so the piercing can be accomplished safely, your piercer should ask you to return at another time when you are composed and ready.

Expectation plays a role in the perception of pain and the experience of the piercing.[1] Prepare yourself by forming realistic expectations of the sensations associated with piercing.[2]

RELATIVE PAIN LEVELS AND SENSATIONS

Below is a general comparison of pain levels according to feedback from approximately 50,000 piercees—my customers. These describe *relative* intensity as perceived by the majority of my clients, but sensitivity levels vary.

- *Easy:* Earlobe, eyebrow, tongue, navel, fourchette
- *Easy to medium:* Bridge, nasal septum, teardrop, most labrets, most surface piercings (on flat areas that lack a defined fold, lip, or protrusion of tissue), Prince Albert, guiche, scrotum, foreskin, lorum, frenum, pubic, vertical clitoral hood, horizontal clitoral hood, inner labia, Princess Albertina
- *Medium:* All ear cartilage, nostril, philtrum (upper lip center), tongue tip or sides, outer labia, Christina
- *Medium to intense:* Triangle, nipple
- *Intense:* Ampallang, apadravya, reverse Prince Albert, dydoe, clitoris

Almost everyone I've pierced has remarked, "It wasn't nearly as bad as I expected!"

I have worked diligently to become proficient at piercing swiftly and smoothly, factors that are largely responsible for the perceptions of my clients. Only when your piercer is skillful can you expect the sensations to be minimal.

"DOESN'T THAT HURT?"

Pain is a very charged topic, and because it is subjective, even the most in-depth discussion leaves much to the imagination. Some people are concerned about being able to tolerate the pain they expect to feel during a piercing. This dread is a reason people may decide against getting one, even when they genuinely want it.

Some areas of the body are more sensitive, and certain piercings are generally accepted as being more intense than others. For instance, nipples are frequently described as tender, though usually more for men than for women. Then again, some piercees *enjoy* getting nipple piercings and do not find the procedure to be painful at all.

It is much easier to endure a quick, smooth procedure than a bumbling one that continues for an extended period. The brief sensation experienced as a "pinch" can turn into "stabbed by an ice pick" at the hands of a less skillful piercer, so choose wisely!

The sensations should begin to fade as soon as your jewelry is in place. For a few minutes afterward, you might experience tenderness, stinging, or warmth.

> **"I absolutely LOVE my VCH piercing! I haven't felt any discomfort or pain since the split-second poke from the piercing (lol) . . . no joke, the piercing was really like a split second, honestly! If I didn't know better, I would forget it was pierced—that's how normal and comfortable it feels!"—T.**

NEEDLE PHOBIA

Statistics show that approximately 20 percent of the population is needle phobic.[3] Even so, plenty of piercees are included in this number.

The fact that tattoos, scarification, and piercing all involve some degree of pain or discomfort demonstrates that a person is capable of enduring it. Without it, there would be little difference between these types of body art and dyeing your hair. It is part of what sets modified people apart.

Though modern body piercing has roots in the BDSM community, few people get pierced because they want to be hurt. Even those who engage in consensual masochistic practices don't usually want to receive excessive pain from a piercer; they prefer it within the context of a relationship. Besides, the procedure should be so brief as to disappoint the rare pain-seeker who tries to satisfy their desires in a piercing studio.

Many people admit that they do enjoy the rush of endorphins and adrenaline that are released when getting pierced. Some piercees relish the anticipation and excitement leading up to the event. Others derive a form of pleasure from the *sensation* of the act; even if it is intense, it might not be perceived as "pain." This is a subtle but real distinction. Many enthusiasts describe a sense of relaxation and release afterward. These are natural highs that you can achieve by getting pierced.

THE POINT

Now you can make a realistic assessment about whether piercing is right for you. Fortunately, many obstacles are perceived rather than genuine. If a hurdle is truly insurmountable, however, you must accept that reality. Consult your doctor if you have health concerns, or a qualified piercer if you have questions.

5

IS PIERCING RIGHT FOR YOUR CHILD?

There are some extra considerations when it comes to the piercing of minors. These include legal and policy matters, philosophical viewpoints, and practical aspects. Piercing isn't right for all adults, and it certainly isn't suitable for every child—but it can be for some.

KIDS VS. PARENTS

Because parental consent should be required for all professional piercing of minors, families sometimes have disagreements over the subject. Kids who want to get pierced may perceive their parents as too strict, while parents might be concerned that piercings could get infected or just be a passing whim. Parental attitudes vary, but even if you have piercings yourself, you may not be ready to give your child permission to get one.

Piercees must be responsible and disciplined, but many young people lack these qualities, especially when faced with an extended healing time. There is no specific age that always indicates readiness for an ear or other piercing, but a below-the-neck adornment should wait until the body is fully developed. A piercing could end up in an undesirable location by the time the child has finished growing—and leave a mark if abandoned later. The navel is the only traditional body piercing placement that might be acceptable for some minors, and I would decline to pierce this area on anyone under sixteen years of age.

A piercer willing to work on the nipples or genitals of your minor child (under age eighteen) has terrible judgment, poor ethics, and risks being charged with sexual assault of a minor. Moreover, signing a consent form for your underage offspring to get an adult piercing could result in charges against you for child endangerment.

Laws vary by region on aspects such as minimum age requirements, the extent of parental involvement, and which piercings are sanctioned for minors. Studio policies also differ depending on the principles and preferences of the piercer. Some will not perform certain piercings on children, even if the law permits it.

Good piercers have strict and scrupulous identification requirements, so always check with the studio before going in.

PRACTICAL ADVICE FOR PARENTS

Maybe a desire to get pierced *is* a phase your child is going through—some young people *do* grow out of their early interests—but try not to be judgmental. Piercings can fulfill the normal urge youth have to adopt a style that is different from yours and fit in with their friends. Think of the bright side: you might be able to negotiate, using a piercing as a reward for good grades or other desirable behavior.

In some cultures, getting a piercing or tattoo is an essential step into adulthood and acts to bind a family together. If you support your kid's choice to get pierced, it might bring you closer. And when you help your child find a competent piercer, you prevent the consequences of a do-it-yourself or hack job, which could result in unsightly permanent scars or expensive medical bills.

PRACTICAL ADVICE FOR YOUNG PEOPLE

If you sneak around behind your parents' backs to get pierced, you are proving that you cannot be trusted. It is against piercer ethics—and usually the law—for a minor to get pierced without the permission of a parent or legal guardian (not another relative or a friend's mom or dad, *yours*).

If your parents refuse to consent and you attempt to pierce yourself or have a buddy do it, there is a very high risk of infection. You will get a terrible piercing that will cause you endless trouble. Don't count on being able to hide it, either— fresh piercings are difficult to conceal. Your parents *will* find out. Show them you are patient to help earn their respect.

INFANT AND CHILD EAR PIERCING

The debate about piercing the ears of infants and young children has two principal elements: philosophical considerations including ideas about cultural identity and ownership of the body, and practical aspects. As examples of different viewpoints about body modification, Western parents readily subject their children to metal bands that painfully force their teeth into new positions. But they may shudder to see the youth of the Matsés tribe of the Amazon sporting sticks through their pierced lips. Similarly, some people think nothing of circumcising an infant's penis but condemn practices like *female genital cutting,* or *female circumcision,* in which the external female genitalia is altered or partially or entirely removed, for cultural or religious reasons.

Every society has its particular customs, standards of beauty, and marks of identity; they are part of the glue that holds groups together. Parents naturally want to adhere to established norms and raise their offspring in their image. Piercing the ears of young girls is a relatively established practice in the Western world, and some piercers are amenable—but no ethical practitioner would consider piercing any other part of a youngster.

If you are interested in having your child's ears pierced, consider the following practical matters:

- The risk of infection is high when a piercee is not old enough to refrain from touching the area, either because they are too young to understand the instructions or lack the self-discipline.

- A piercing positioned in the center of your baby's earlobes sometimes ends up being too low or close to their face when they're grown.

- Established earlobe piercings seldom close entirely, and they do leave a permanent mark (however small) if abandoned later.

- Doctors blame the rise in nickel allergies on the popularity of ear piercings done with inferior-quality jewelry.[1] Once they have developed, these allergies may be severe and lifelong. For more information, see "Contact Dermatitis," page 260.

If you decide to proceed with piercing, it is sensible to bring your child to a reputable body art studio. Children's immune systems are not fully mature, so it is essential to do everything as hygienically and safely as possible. Fortunately, many parents are now savvy enough to know that piercing guns are dangerous and should be avoided. See "Piercing Guns," page 21. Some piercers require a consultation first to meet you and the child, familiarize you with the studio, and explain what to expect during the process. They might also go over jewelry options, and then they'll schedule piercing for another day. For pertinent details, see "Earlobe Piercing" and subsequent sections on page 102.

Fewer than 10 percent of piercers surveyed would pierce the ears of an infant in their first year of life, though nearly half would do so once the child is a year old. My professional boundary was to pierce only the earlobes of children old enough to request and consent to the act. They had to comprehend the need to keep dirty fingers away and promise to abide by my aftercare instructions during healing, usually with a parent's help. Obviously, this includes declining to pierce babies or toddlers who were too young to grasp the situation. Some of my colleagues are more accommodating, and others even stricter.

One practical consideration is finding a local piercer who is qualified and willing to do the job. If you are unable to, the best option may be to travel. Alternatively, seek a sympathetic pediatrician or dermatologist who is trained in ear piercing and uses appropriate sterile equipment and jewelry. Beware: some doctors charge a small fortune for piercing with the same problematic stud guns that are used at the mall!

THE POINT

As a parent or legal guardian, it is especially critical to be informed, conscientious, and deliberate in your decisions when it comes to the piercing of a minor because of the additional factors involved.

6

YOU AND YOUR PIERCER

Many consumers will drop by the nearest studio and get pierced by whoever is on duty at the time. Although this method is convenient, you cannot be assured of getting a safe piercing without learning some facts about the piercer's abilities and hygiene practices. This chapter details exactly how to evaluate piercers and studios so you can make a sound decision.

PIERCER SKILLS

There can't be that much difference between one professional piercer and another, can there? If they work in a licensed studio, and charge money to do the job, they must know what they're doing. Right?

Wrong!

A license or permit does not mean that a piercer is competent. In some cases, obtaining one merely requires paying a fee to a city or state agency. Such a document does not guarantee that the piercer has received adequate training to perform the job. Even in regions with the most stringent regulations, almost none require any evaluation of a piercer's skills.

Your experience and the outcome (how well your piercing heals) are highly dependent on the proficiency of the person wielding the needle. Piercing is a hands-on profession that must be learned through practical experience. It can then be mastered only through practice, which commonly involves trial *and* error. No courses of study (not a single one!) are available from any accredited institution to confer a degree or adequately prepare someone to work in the field. Sound instruction ideally involves a lengthy apprenticeship with a qualified mentor, but such opportunities for aspiring piercers are rare. Watch out for certificates that look impressive, because they do not always represent much formal instruction. See "Piercer Training" on page 325 to learn about piercer education.

Many so-called "professional piercers" have never had any relevant training, and plenty are utterly indifferent and sloppy. Some lack passion or aptitude, and others have immature or inappropriate motivations. Without specialized knowledge, a piercer is a menace; and without considerable savvy to evaluate prospective practitioners, you will not be a safe consumer.

"I didn't know the quality of a good piercer till I actually went to one. I got my helix [ear cartilage piercing] at my old tattoo parlor, and I'm pretty sure none of them were piercers so much as tattoo artists with piercing needles. It hurt like a bitch, he stopped halfway into it, and then almost tore it out trying to close the ring, *and* dropped the ball on the floor but still put it in my ear . . . When I considered getting my next piercing I was skeptical because of the last experience. I looked up as much as I could about piercers in the area. I came across [a piercer who] was great . . . made me comfortable; very informative; great experience, turned me on to a life of future piercings."—R.

SKILL-LEVEL SCALE

Imagine a scale from one to ten. At level one or level two, the piercer is a beginner. They may have pierced some friends, taken a brief course, or watched some "how-to-pierce" videos. Getting pierced by someone this inexperienced is no bargain, even if the cost is cheap. They will take considerably longer to perform the procedure and cause you far more pain than necessary. Novices often don't know the best size or style of jewelry for you, or the optimal placement to suit your anatomy. This affects not only the aesthetics of the piercing but also your ability to heal. Neophytes frequently have trouble inserting the jewelry once they make the perforation. This causes undue tissue trauma, which further disrupts your healing, and it is also *terribly* painful. Finally, but importantly, piercers at this beginning level are less able to help you if troubleshooting becomes necessary later—and it probably will.

Further up the scale, a piercer has more skill. A professional at level five has sufficient training and ability to accomplish the job adequately. This piercer may have completed an apprenticeship and gained some experience, yet they are still relatively unseasoned. There are finer points they have yet to learn and situations they may not be able to handle, depending on the difficulty of the piercing and challenges presented by your anatomy. This piercer can do a decent job, but they are not the best you can get.

A pro at level nine or ten is a true master. A specialist with this superior ability pierces almost like a magic trick in which the hands move faster than the eye. They perform the act gently and place the piercing perfectly for your anatomy. This is art and science combined. A piercing by this expert is easy to tolerate, and you may even describe it as a pleasant experience. Should you require help during healing, they are versed in all there is to know, and you can rely on them to assist you. The best among them is always available and eager to help.

In general, your pain level is inverse to the piercer's ability: the lower the skill level of your technician, the greater your discomfort or pain, and vice versa. Similarly, your likelihood of having a successful experience and outcome goes up with the proficiency of your piercer.

Many piercers have years or even decades of experience, yet they fail to pierce at a high level. They may not be applying themselves or could suffer from a lack of aptitude. Just because a piercer has been working at their job for a long time does not ensure that they are competent; some piercers are doing the same bungling job as always, many years later.

Although this numbered skill-level scale is not a convention used within the industry, it helps to illustrate how expertise differs substantially from one piercer to the next.

ATTITUDE AND ETHICS

A suitable attitude includes being professional, pleasant, and patient. Sometimes piercers fail to grasp that they are performing a service for you, not a favor! Your potential piercer must earn your trust by demonstrating knowledge and competency. Don't settle for someone who does not fully answer your questions; if they are annoyed by your inquiries or exude a "too cool" attitude, they are a poor choice.

Before taking your money, a piercer should be willing to provide a consultation to inspect your anatomy, discuss jewelry selection, the procedure, potential risks and complications, the healing course, and aftercare guidelines. If a piercer cannot be bothered to attend to you politely before a piercing, it is even less likely they will be there for you if you need assistance later.

A poor attitude also prevents a piercer from gaining true mastery in the field. The professional who takes their craft seriously is going to work harder to do a good job. The know-it-all, on the other hand, will not attempt to enrich their education or improve performance.

If you are unimpressed by your local piercers, you may have to search in a broader geographical area. Consider the following experience from a piercee in Arizona:

> "I was a little disappointed with my piercing experience. . . . I went in the shop with an excited, happy frame of mind. The guy who did it was not the one who normally did the piercings. . . . He called [the girl who was] on the phone right from the front counter and told her she had a piercing; obviously the conversation didn't go well, because he just hung up and was *obviously* very irritated. He had me come around to the chair, marked my belly with a pen, and *wham!* just did it. I was expecting him to at least explain what he was going to do, talk to me for a minute, explain the different choices of jewelry . . . *something*. After he did it, I got up, he gave a *brief* aftercare speech, and sent me on my way . . . I knew I needed more aftercare info. If I ever go to get anything else pierced, I'm going to find a different shop."—A.

As well she should.

A piercer with sound ethics is committed to honing their skills and keeping their studio clean and equipment sterile. Their actions are guided by honorable principles and a strong conscience, not the almighty dollar or an inflated ego. A professional with proper standards will refuse to bring out a needle any time it is inappropriate. Respect a piercer for declining to pierce you when they shouldn't; that's the kind you should return to when circumstances are right.

STUDIO STANDARDS AND EQUIPMENT HANDLING

Even the best piercer cannot do a good job without a studio that is appropriately set up and maintained for this specialized task. Professionals do not pierce out of a smoky nightclub, a friend's car, or their home.

You have every right to inspect the environment and be assured of suitable *aseptic* (free of disease-causing microorganisms) conditions and hygienic practices before you have someone break your skin. If you're unsure, make a preliminary visit to check out the studio before getting pierced. This gives you time to evaluate the piercer and the premises thoroughly and helps to alleviate any nervousness that could cloud your judgment.

The way the piercer handles equipment in the studio is critical, because if it is not done correctly, there is a risk of disease transmission.

DIRTY DEED

I once visited a studio where I observed a piercer accept cash payment for a job and then stuff the filthy bills into the drawer with her "sterile" piercing equipment. She appeared completely unaware of the fact that she had done something disgustingly dirty and incredibly dangerous.

Learn what to look for, because some mistakes are more noticeable than others. Use the list below to make an effective appraisal.

SETUP AND SANITATION CHECKLIST

- ☐ Posting of state or local license(s). Check with your health department or other governing agencies to determine what kind of permit is required for piercing in your area, if any.

- ☐ Printed handouts containing detailed aftercare guidelines.

- ☐ A selection of body jewelry. A studio carrying only a handful of styles and sizes will be unable to meet the needs presented by the wide range of human anatomy.

☐ Cleanliness throughout! The premises and staff should be pristine. Smoking or drinking alcohol should never take place there.

☐ If studio policy permits customers to try on piercing jewelry—*run*.

☐ A public bathroom that is never used for cleaning contaminated piercing equipment.

☐ A hand-washing sink for the piercer stocked with liquid soap and paper towels.

☐ A separate room for piercing that has bright lighting and proper ventilation. This room should not be used for tattooing, haircutting, or anything except piercing.

☐ A *sterilization room* (separate enclosure with no public access, for processing contaminated tools and equipment). This room may not be required in a disposable studio, depending on local regulations.

DISPOSABLE OR SINGLE-USE STUDIOS

Any instruments on the premises are discarded after use, including forceps, hemostats, insertion tapers, or other tools. When everything is disposable, a separate sterilization room is unnecessary. There is no chance of an error or failure in the instrument reprocessing procedures, and one of the staff's riskiest duties is eliminated. More studios are opting to work in this fashion, and other piercers aspire to it.

VITAL EQUIPMENT: STERILIZERS AND ULTRASONICS

An autoclave sterilizer is required equipment in *every* piercing studio. Autoclaves are extremely expensive, but for sterilizing piercing equipment and body jewelry, there is no acceptable alternative. Boiling in water, soaking in alcohol, or passing over an open flame definitely does not accomplish the job. Hospital-strength liquid disinfectants that reduce the number of microorganisms and chemical cold-sterilant solutions are not suitable substitutes for sterilization equipment. Of course, *having* an autoclave is not enough: it must be operated and maintained in strict accordance with the manufacturer's instructions.

There must also be proof that the machinery is functioning correctly, which is the purpose of *spore tests* or *biological indicators* (test strips containing heat-resistant spores). These are run through an autoclave sterilization cycle and then mailed away for laboratory evaluation to determine whether all the spores were destroyed. The results (pass or fail) are provided to the studio. A printout should be available for any prospective customer to see upon request. A piercer without knowledge of spore tests or proof of results (at least monthly) is one you must avoid. The system in Europe is different, so you may not find spore tests there.

A "Class S" cassette sterilizer is a faster type of autoclave that is a popular alternative to the larger and slower traditional models. Sixty-one percent of piercers surveyed use this kind of machine. The most common unit used by piercers in the United States is called a StatIM. In Europe, they commonly use vacuum "Class B" sterilizers. These are convenient because they have a briefer cycle than traditional autoclaves (less than ten minutes versus over half an hour).

Some piercers work primarily with prepackaged sterile tools and jewelry and use the Class S unit only for display items and special circumstances. Others do not keep any packaged sterile piercing equipment or jewelry on hand. These piercers place everything into the cassette and sterilize it just before performing a piercing. This system is called "point of process" sterilization. Your piercer may work directly from the cassette but must not put used items back into it. This machine must also be spore tested. A good piercer will not be annoyed if you are informed and concerned enough to ask about test results.

An autoclave must be used, even in disposable studios. Needles and jewelry shipped in bulk must *always* be sterilized before use. Additionally, piercers should not simply trust claims by body art industry suppliers that "presterilized" needles or body jewelry are ready to use. A supplier must be able to provide certification that the items are commercially sterilized, packaged, and stored according to the medical field's stringent requirements, or they must be autoclaved before use.[1] Nearly a quarter of piercers surveyed use such equipment, likely without the extra precautions.

Another essential piece of equipment is the ultrasonic unit (a machine that removes debris using agitation from sonic waves in liquid). Used piercing tools are run through a cycle before autoclaving. Some piercers claim to sterilize using an ultrasonic unit, but this appliance is not a substitute for an autoclave, so don't believe it!

New jewelry should be put in an ultrasonic unit to remove any polishing compound before sterilization, but it must not be the same machine that processes contaminated equipment. If the studio also uses an ultrasonic unit for tattooing, it must be solely for use with tattoo equipment.

The ultrasonic machine has a high potential for environmental cross-contamination, particularly if it is operated uncovered. It must *never* be located inside the piercing room or in a break room where food is prepared or eaten.

This brief introduction is meant to familiarize you with the equipment that should be in a piercing studio. It does not contain enough information for you to perform sterilization procedures—only to evaluate if the proper equipment is present and basic processes are being followed.

EQUIPMENT CHECKLIST

☐ An autoclave sterilizer *and* current spore tests for it.

☐ Ultrasonic unit(s) sufficient to satisfy the needs of the studio. A steam cleaner is also suitable for removing polishing compound from new jewelry. Some shops use a machine called an automated medical instrument washer, which is a safe and effective alternative to the ultrasonic unit, though vastly more expensive.

☐ A *sharps disposal* (a special container for safely discarding used piercing needles). If they don't have one, leave. They either reuse needles or fail to dispose of them appropriately. Both are unacceptable, unethical, and in some places illegal. Needles *must* be used on only one client and then carefully deposited in an approved container.

EQUIPMENT HANDLING AND HYGIENE PROCEDURES

Piercers must follow specific protocols to keep a studio hygienic enough to break your skin safely. Even if the autoclave is functioning, many potential pitfalls in equipment handling procedures could put you at risk.

In the traditional system, new piercing needles, tools, and jewelry are individually sealed into special pouches before the sterilization cycle. One side of the pouch will usually be transparent plastic, so the contents are visible, and the other side will be medical-grade paper. Sterile packs should be handled only with clean or gloved hands once removed from the autoclave to preserve their germ-free condition. They should be kept in a closed sanitary location until used, such as a piercing room cabinet. Nearly 70 percent of piercers surveyed follow this process for at least some of their equipment.

Regulations sometimes mandate resterilization of any unused equipment one month after processing, and this date must be marked on or in the sterilization pouch. If this is not required, an "event-based" sterilization practice may be used, like in the medical field. If the autoclave bags are intact, and items are handled and stored correctly, the contents are considered sterile regardless of the processing date.

Before touching any equipment, your piercer must first wash their hands. They should carefully peel the packages open to expose the sterile contents, and must put on or change gloves before touching the item within. When donning gloves, the exterior should be handled only by the cuffs (to avoid transferring any germs remaining on the hands to the outside surface of the gloves). In the point-of-process system, after opening the exterior cassette, fresh gloves must be put on before contact with the sterile contents.

Piercers need focus and training to adhere to these protocols consistently; even a small lapse can spread germs throughout the studio. Most piercers with a

YOU AND YOUR PIERCER

minimum of education are not aware of all the necessary precautions, and, unfortunately, neither are many experienced practitioners. To protect your health, select a professional who properly maintains the cleanliness of their studio.

FINDING A PIERCER

How do you locate a good piercer? Looking online for local studios and checking reviews is a logical first step. It is also a good idea to talk to people who have piercings and ask them if they can recommend a piercer (or if they know of one you should avoid). Word-of-mouth referrals are standard in the body art field. Getting a reference from a friend who has had a good experience is an excellent starting point. Still, even a sterling recommendation is no substitute for personally assessing a piercer.

> **"I went to this piercer, and he was really nice and everything, and he did an awesome job. But he had some trouble getting the jewelry through, so he had to pierce me twice. And, well, the piercing turned out crooked and then it rejected. He told me to use alcohol on it. But really, he's a great piercer!"—J.**

ONLINE RESOURCES

When reviewing websites, look for a studio with ethical shop policies, a photo gallery of nice-looking work, and sensible advice on post-piercing care. Steer clear of any establishment that posts images of tattoos and no piercings! Clearly, piercing is an afterthought there. Generally speaking, piercing-only businesses are a better option, as they focus specifically on just one form of body art.

Social media is a great place to see pictures of piercers' handiwork. Notice whether they promote only the wild and unusual, or if they show the standards, too. Take time to evaluate the images, especially of the placement you're considering. This graphic representation of a piercer's aesthetic reveals how you might expect your piercing to look. Try to determine if pictures of clients with healed work are shown, particularly if you are considering a challenging or rare piercing.

Scrutinize photos for apparent legitimacy. Odd cropping could indicate removing someone else's watermarks, and devious people can alter pictures of unhealthy piercings, or even add body jewelry onto an image of an unpierced person.

Unfortunately, pictures alone will not give you much information about other aspects of their professionalism. Reviews on Yelp, Google, Facebook, and other sites will allow you to see what prior clients have to say, and if a prospective piercer has a good reputation. Videos will show a piercer in action, so you can see if they appear adept, informative, and caring. Unless you're genuinely impressed, keep looking.

ASK TO WATCH

Some piercers and piercees are open to having a spectator present during piercing—even a stranger—so it doesn't hurt to ask. If you wish to observe, the studio may ask you to sign a waiver to protect them from liability. This may seem strange, but it is an accepted practice. Occasionally, the piercee feels just fine, but the onlooker passes out!

Notice whether the piercer appears confident and composed. Do they perform the piercing rapidly with steady hands, or are they slow and fumbling? Also, consider whether they have a comforting bedside manner. This demonstration reveals the experience you can expect for yourself, so be sure you like what you see. Learn about handwashing and piercing room protocols and procedures in chapter 9 to make a more comprehensive evaluation.

MEDICAL PROFESSIONALS AS PIERCERS

Piercing is similar to certain medical practices, but simply because an individual is licensed to provide health care services does not mean they are capable of performing piercings. There may be an overlap of skill sets, and knowledge of anatomy, *venipuncture* (drawing blood or inserting an intravenous line), and infection control is relevant to both endeavors. But you would never consider visiting a chiropractor to treat your toothache or a gynecologist for an ingrown toenail. Similarly, it doesn't make sense to go to a nurse, chiropractor, dentist, EMT, or any other medical professional for a piercing unless they have received *specific* instruction in the particulars.

Any health care professional who feels confident to perform a piercing based on medical training alone demonstrates how little they actually know about piercing. Even a surgeon is unsuited to the task if they don't have knowledge of jewelry sizes and styles, placements, and piercing techniques.

Doctors do not ordinarily make an effort to learn about standard piercing practices or equipment. Some use injectable anesthetics to numb the area, but this increases the potential for complications and is not necessary when a piercer is skillful. Physicians will sometimes pierce the skin, remove the needle, and then attempt to force the jewelry through the fresh channel because they are not familiar with piercing needles, which facilitate jewelry transfers. If you get pierced badly by a novice *or* a doctor, excess tissue trauma will make the aftermath more painful and healing more difficult, and the placement of the hole will seldom be optimal. Finally, medical practitioners are often unaware of industry standards for piercing aftercare and may advise using products that are not optimal for healing this unique type of wound.

There are good piercers who are also medical personnel; however, these individuals have sought information and instruction on piercing as practiced by professionals in the industry.

THE ASSOCIATION OF PROFESSIONAL PIERCERS

The Association of Professional Piercers (APP) is an international nonprofit health, safety, and education organization. Piercers who are "Professional Business Members" meet specific personal and environmental criteria. They adhere to a safety agreement that encompasses minimum standards for using quality jewelry, maintaining cleanliness, and behaving professionally. The APP's website, www .safepiercing.org, includes information about piercing and member listings.

The APP is a respected and reliable resource. Anything described in this book as "industry standard" refers to the APP's guidelines and requirements. The organization, however, does not monitor the "artistic merit" of piercers. This means that you can be confident that members maintain an acceptable level of hygiene and use quality jewelry, but no claims are made about the technical skills of the piercer. Still, APP members have at least one year of professional experience, and they are clearly among the most conscientious piercers.

It is reasonable to ask any piercer who is not a member of the APP, "Why not?" Do they fail to come up to the organization's standards, are they unfamiliar with their own industry's professional association, or are they apathetic? Those are all flawed characteristics in a piercer.

Note that this association is not a certifying agency. Any piercer who is promoting themselves as "APP certified" is making an illegitimate claim.

TRUST YOUR INSTINCTS

Your instincts are a valuable tool, and you should listen to them when selecting a piercer. Still, you have to distinguish between any apprehension you may have about getting pierced and a feeling of mistrust about a piercer. If you're especially anxious, this is an excellent reason to visit the studio before scheduling your piercing.

If you encounter a piercer who acts unethically or makes you uncomfortable in any way, you have the right to say "Stop." You can leave. Trust your intuition, and *never* stay in a situation that feels wrong. This isn't a haircut. Your health is at stake. Any of the following should cause warning bells to clang and are reasons to call off your piercing:

- You don't feel safe or comfortable
- The piercer touches sterile or used piercing equipment without wearing gloves
- The studio does not have up-to-date spore tests, and nobody there knows what they are

- A piercer or other staff member makes sexual innuendos or behaves unprofessionally
- The piercer reeks of liquor or allows (or drinks!) it in the studio, or you spot active track marks or other signs of drug abuse

PRICEY HACK JOB

A mother took her teenage daughter to one of the most respected dermatologists in her state to get a navel piercing. The teen brought her own jewelry, which the doctor swabbed briefly with alcohol instead of autoclaving it to ensure sterility. After piercing her, the doctor dropped the jewelry-closure ball on the ground, picked it up, wiped it again with alcohol, and put it onto the ring in her fresh piercing. He advised her to use hydrogen peroxide and antibiotic ointment for aftercare and keep a bandage on it for five days. *None* of this is accepted practice in the piercing industry. He charged $120 for this service, which didn't even include the jewelry. This girl knew that the doctor did not adhere to professional piercing standards, but her mother refused to listen because, she felt, "doctors know best."

THE POINT

A good piercer can be an inspiration and a tremendous resource, but a bad one can cause you agony and infection. Don't settle for a less-than-competent practitioner, an impatient piercer with a condescending attitude, or a so-called professional who doesn't adhere to appropriate hygiene protocols. You must be confident that your piercer is safe and qualified in every aspect.

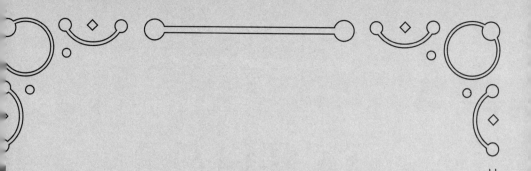

PART 3

PIERCING PREPARATION

PICKING AND PREPARING 54

AT THE STUDIO 59

PIERCING PROCEDURES 68

JEWELRY 101: SIZES, SHAPES,
AND MATERIALS 78

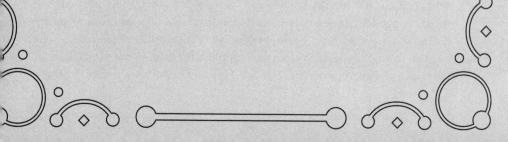

7

PICKING AND PREPARING

Deciding on a new piercing can be fun and exciting. And preparing for the procedure—both mentally and physically—can help assure the best possible outcome, especially for novice piercees.

DECISIONS, DECISIONS

Deeper motivations aside, most people choose to get a piercing because they like the way it looks. You may be inspired by photos of extraordinary piercings, but could be unaware that they're digitally altered images. You may not know that some placements and jewelry are downright hazardous. The piercing your friend wears, or that you saw in the latest social media blitz, might not work for your unique body. These are some of the reasons it is necessary to consult a professional to assist you with safe and suitable piercing placement.

Anatomy (physical structure) and *aesthetics* (physical appearance—especially when considered pleasing) are the two most critical issues when deciding on placement. The primary practical consideration is whether you have suitable tissue to support a specific piercing. You can attempt a preliminary evaluation for yourself, but your piercer will ultimately determine how appropriate the piercing you desire is for your body. The other matter is far more subjective: will it suit your appearance? If your piercer gives you the go-ahead based on your anatomy and even gives you a thumbs-up as their personal opinion, you will still be the one to decide on the aesthetics for yourself.

ANATOMY

People and their pierceable body parts come in a tremendous range of shapes and sizes. Examine the ears of a few friends to see how different they are from one side to the other and from person to person. Anatomical variations may be subtle, but the distinctions are vital when it comes to the safety and success of piercings. A few areas are universally pierceable, but even spots like the daith, eyebrow, and navel are not safe or possible for everyone. Try not to get your heart set on a precise placement until you consult with a piercer. Be open to alternatives they may suggest based on your anatomy if your configuration is not suited to the spot you have in mind.

AESTHETICS

Jewelry will bring attention to the area in which it is worn. If your ears resemble those of Dumbo the Flying Elephant, you might not want all eyes drawn to them with conspicuous jewelry. (Or maybe you do!) Perhaps an eyebrow piercing to bring the focus away from your large ears would be preferable? Conversely, if you have never liked your nose's shape or size, you might consider customizing your nostril or septum with jewelry to make it more pleasing to you. Then again, if you have a lovely nose, why not embellish it with a glimmering jewel? Whether used to downplay, modify, or highlight a particular feature, your piercing can be personally empowering and gratifying.

Symmetry is another matter to contemplate. You may prefer *midline* (in the center) placements like traditional navel or tongue piercings. If you got only one nipple pierced, you might feel lopsided. You could have a fondness for an asymmetrical style or an inclination toward balanced asymmetry in which you have multiple smaller piercings on one side, and a single stretched hole on the other, for example.

Envision how the piercing and jewelry will look and what overall effect you wish to achieve. Does a subtle ornament suit you, or would a bold adornment look better? These are merely personal preferences. Other than the anatomical and practical considerations, there isn't one correct way to place your piercings. If you have doubts or concerns, ask some trusted friends for their opinions. A professional piercer is also a useful resource, but ultimately *you* must be pleased with the appearance.

The placement should be your primary focus and the jewelry secondary. The ornament can be changed, but the location of a hole can't—at least not without getting another piercing. Don't forget that leaving some unpierced *negative space* (an area in between) usually looks best.

HOW MUCH IS TOO MUCH?

Opinions on this range from one extreme to the other, and what is too much for one person will be not nearly enough for another. Only you can say what feels right for you. At what point do piercings become excessive? If they negatively affect function in any way—including your ability to be employed—that can reasonably be considered "too much."

Piercings tend to be most aesthetically pleasing, and more widely accepted, when placed with a focus on accent and enhancement. If your piercings begin to take over, it may be time to slow down and take a good look at your external appearance. And if you're getting lost in a sea of metal, perhaps some scrutiny of your motivations is warranted.

In addition to aesthetics and function, health considerations are also important. If you feel compelled to get one piercing after another regardless of your
ability to heal or a medical condition (mental or physical), this is also piercing
overkill. There is, however, no way to pin down a precise number that pushes
one over the edge to "excessively pierced."

THE CONSULTATION

A consultation with a piercer is helpful if you have questions about your suitability
for a piercing or can't make up your mind about which spot to choose. It's also an
excellent way to get acquainted with a piercer, evaluate their professionalism, and
see if you develop a comfortable rapport. An appointment might be required, or
you may be able to walk in without a prior arrangement.

A qualified professional will be able to evaluate your anatomy and make suggestions for piercings that will work with your body—and explain why any
requested spots might not. Your jewelry options can also be covered so you can get
a whole picture of how the piercing will look. Most shops do not charge a fee for
this service, but if a consultation is done separately from your piercing and takes
up a lot of the piercer's time, tipping is appropriate.

PREPARING FOR YOUR PIERCING

You've done your homework and made your decision to get pierced. You are
excited, but maybe a little apprehensive too. You might worry at least a bit: How
much will it really hurt? Is it going to look good on me?

There are a few extra things you can do to prepare. By readying yourself physically and mentally, and by gathering the supplies you'll need, you can play an
active role in making sure you have a great experience.

SUPPLIES

Some of these items may be provided free or sold by your piercer. Find out what
aftercare product(s) your piercer suggests and whether they are available at the
studio to determine what else you might need to purchase. Possibilities include:

- Juice to drink after the piercing to stabilize your blood sugar
- Panty liners or sanitary pads to contain bleeding after genital piercings (see chapter 14 for more information)
- Saline spray and gauze, or other supplies for compresses (see chapter 15 for complete aftercare guidelines)
- Paper towels, swabs, or other clean disposables for drying your piercing after bathing
- Shaved ice, freezer pops, or other frozen treats, if you're getting an oral piercing

THE PIERCING-READY BODY

Pay attention to your health and do what you can to enhance it prior to your piercing. It's prudent to avoid drinking alcohol the night before, as it could cause you to bleed excessively, and a hangover will surely intensify any discomfort you experience. For obvious reasons, do not take any medications that have a blood-thinning effect, such as aspirin, Advil (ibuprofen), or Aleve (naproxen). Avoid large doses of caffeine for several days before piercing. Vitamin E may also thin the blood. Know the properties of any herbs, supplements, or alternative remedies you're taking to avoid increasing your risk of bleeding. If possible, stop using anything questionable two weeks before your piercing. Herbs that have blood-thinning effects include chamomile, licorice root, ginkgo biloba, ginger, garlic, ginseng, goldenseal, and many others. Vitamin K supplements help to support optimal clotting. They are available at health food stores. Take them according to the package instructions for two weeks *before* the piercing unless it is inadvisable due to a health condition.

Have a dental exam and teeth cleaning in the weeks before getting an oral piercing. Your mouth will be sparkling fresh, and this can also help avoid a dental emergency during healing. The first few months (when the lining of the channel is forming) are critical.

You'll feel best if you are rested and clearheaded on the day of your piercing. Pay attention to your hygiene as a courtesy to your piercer and to safeguard your health. It is polite to avoid eating garlic and onions before an oral piercing and to brush your teeth shortly before entering the studio. Spend some extra time cleaning your ear, nose, or whatever area will be the focus of your visit. Unless you customarily do so, you may not *have* to shave the area to be pierced; however, doing so will facilitate the procedure in a hairy area.

Give some thought to the clothing you will wear to the studio if you have to disrobe. Dress for comfort and practicality; avoid clothes that would obscure or rub against your new jewelry. If you are getting an ear or facial piercing, put up long hair so that it doesn't get in the way.

HAVE A SNACK

To prepare yourself physically for your piercing, eat a light meal an hour or two before visiting the studio. This is one of the simplest yet most effective things you can do. This sustenance will help to assure stable blood sugar levels and provide your body with some fuel reserves to prevent lightheadedness. Even if you feel as though you are too nervous to eat, have a smoothie or small snack, but avoid eating heavily right before your piercing, or you could experience nausea or vomiting.

THE PIERCING-READY MIND

If you're feeling anxious, the following may help to minimize your apprehension during a visit to the studio:

- o Do something you find relaxing in the hour before your appointment.
- o Be confident of your decision to get pierced and your choice of piercer.
- o Remind yourself that a piercing takes only a few moments of your life; it will pass quickly.
- o Practice breathing and relaxation techniques (page 65) to use during your piercing.

THE POINT

You have done your research and selected a piercer and a spot to adorn. By preparing yourself mentally and physically, you've moved a step closer to the event. Next, you will learn all about what takes place in the studio before a piercing, during the process, and through its aftermath.

8

AT THE STUDIO

When the time finally arrives, piercing day is an exciting one. No matter how well prepared you are, feeling at least a little bit anxious is normal. But a good piercer will do everything possible to put you at ease and make your experience at the studio a positive one. This chapter covers the piercing process from your point of view as the piercee.

MORAL SUPPORT

Feel free to have a friend or family member join you at the studio for support and possibly to drive you home if you have any concerns about operating heavy machinery afterward. You should ask about the studio's policies, however, if you want to bring your whole bowling team or have someone join you in the room during your procedure. Some piercers have rules against admitting visitors.

Children tend to be distracting for both you and your piercer. They are best left at home or in the retail area with a friend or relative for supervision. The procedure room is not a suitable environment for a young child unless they're the piercee. Sterile equipment is present and must not be played with or touched. Used tools, a sharps container, and a biohazard waste bin are also standard items in the piercing room. These are potentially dangerous areas for a child—especially when the adults are focused on other matters.

HOW TO BE A GOOD PIERCEE

Piercers justifiably expect appropriate behavior from their customers. When visiting a piercing studio, you should show respect to your piercer by:

- Demonstrating a commitment to caring for yourself and your piercing
- Being educated about the process, sober, and mentally prepared—not unduly anxious or hysterical
- Understanding that piercing is highly individual and the jewelry or placement that worked for your friend may not be right for you
- Arriving on time if you have an appointment
- Being conscious about what you touch to avoid contaminating the premises

Though piercing can be an expression of personal choice and autonomy, it is important to accept and appreciate the boundaries of others, including your piercer. If they decline a request or politely refuse service for any reason, you must respect their professional decision.

HOW MUCH DOES IT COST?

The cost will depend on the difficulty of the placement, experience of the piercer, jewelry material and style, store policies, and customary fees in your geographic area, which can have a wide range. The piercing, jewelry, aftercare product(s), and a tip all factor into the total expense.

Check with local shops to get an idea of the average price for the piercing you are considering. The cost should never be the sole determining factor for selecting a studio. You will be paying someone to put a needle through your body—go for verifiable expertise, not the cheapest rate! Similarly, a high price doesn't guarantee superiority; overcharging is sometimes done to cover up substandard abilities and junk jewelry.

Fees for the piercing service (not including jewelry) are usually for each hole, rather than a pair. A small discount might be offered if you get multiple piercings done in the same session. Don't be surprised if earlobe piercings run the same as other parts, or if the charge is higher for children's ears. Above-the-neck piercings might cost less than those on the body, but not always. Genital piercings and surface work are commonly pricier. Studios stocking a wide jewelry assortment generally charge separately for the piercing fee and ornament, because different styles and materials vary in cost. About a quarter of the shops surveyed offer package-deal pricing for the piercing, basic jewelry, and sometimes an aftercare product.

Avoid a piercer who charges an exorbitant fee for penis piercings and a pittance for vulva piercings, or vice versa, because something is amiss! The cost should be approximately the same for all genders. Think twice about any piercer who charges excessively high prices (for example, $100 *extra*) for genital piercings. This is often done because the piercer doesn't like to do them or is unskilled, which are good reasons to go elsewhere.

If you wish to purchase jewelry from another source or bring in your own, you will need to have the piercer's prior approval. Many studios have rules against using so-called "outside" jewelry for initial piercings; this reasonable policy helps to assure that your piece will fit properly, and allows for control over quality, sterility, and condition. Fresh, unworn jewelry won't have nicks, scratches, or residual proteins from previous wear to damage your delicate new piercing or your health.

Apprentices do not provide the same level of service as experienced professionals. So, if you get pierced by a novice, you should not be charged the same fee as for a pro. Otherwise, you are paying with your cash (and body) to train a student. That shouldn't be your burden unless you make an informed decision to participate in a piercer's education—and if you do, a break on the price is absolutely appropriate.

TIPS AND OTHER FEES

Many shops charge a minimal fee to sterilize jewelry purchased elsewhere, change your jewelry, or do a consultation. Some of these services might be provided for free, especially when you buy something, get a piercing, or schedule an appointment for one. Whether or not payment is requested for such assistance, it is courteous to give the piercer a tip if they spend a lot of time attending to you.

If you are pleased with your piercing experience, tipping your piercer is appropriate unless the establishment has a policy against it. Signs to that effect or tip jars may be in evidence to guide you. If you aren't certain about the prevailing custom in your area, you can ask whether tips are accepted. If you don't have cash, nearly half of piercers surveyed take credit card tips. Piercers perform a personal service similar to those provided in salons and spas, and they are usually happy to receive a token of your appreciation. Although tipping is not as common in Europe, if you reside in North America, you can apply the same guidelines you use for tipping in restaurants, though anything short of pocket change is courteous. If you are low on funds or tipping is not standard where you live, you can always return later with some cookies or other small gift if you feel inspired to express your sentiments. A good piercer will always do their best whether a tip is forthcoming or not. A great way to show that you are pleased is by posting positive reviews and spreading the word about your great piercer to your friends and associates.

PIERCING AS RITUAL

Getting a piercing can be an intensely altering experience that echoes the ancient traditions of indigenous societies—or not. But a piercing does change you. When you come out of a studio with a new piercing, you emerge a different person, with an altered body. You are not the same as when you entered. The way your modification affects you and any meaning you impart to it is entirely up to you.

Today, piercing often functions as an observable means of cutting the apron strings that connect child and parent. As a youth enters adulthood, they can take ownership of their own body by receiving a piercing without involving their parents. This rite of passage is practiced—consciously or not—by many of today's young piercees.

You can use your piercing as a sacred celebration of a joyous occasion like a birth or marriage or as a solemn commemoration of a death. Your ceremony may draw upon the customs of your ancestors or other cultures, but it need not have historical precedence to be filled with special meaning. Merely connecting your intentions to the transformative nature of the event can bring a profound sense of value and importance to your piercing.

Some piercers are amenable to incorporating personal rites into the piercing encounter, provided their clients discuss it with them first. A good piercer will act as a facilitator without imposing their agenda on the process, leaving room for you to create your own significance. Your experience does not have to include elaborate actions or words. An act as simple as reciting something during your piercing—aloud or in meditative silence—can have a powerful and lasting impact.

STUDIO PRELIMINARIES

Be mindful of what you touch while in the studio to avoid contaminating yourself or the premises. To maintain rigorous hygiene, every shop should have a strict zero-tolerance policy on customers handling any piercings or worn body jewelry. Any piercing, regardless of age, can secrete potentially infectious matter or fluids. This discharge can be transferred to your hands, and then to surfaces in the studio. Someone with a fresh piercing (or a cut finger) can encounter the contaminated spot. This represents a possibility for the transmission of disease-causing microorganisms. Do not be offended if you are asked to stop handling your piercing or jewelry and to wipe down or wash your hands. Don't be insulted if a piercer puts on gloves to handle jewelry that has been in your body, even if you haven't worn it lately. The worst-case scenario is that nobody working in the studio seems to care what anybody touches, because this is an indication of potentially perilous ignorance or indifference.

When you arrive, inform the person at the counter that you are planning to get pierced or have an appointment to do so. Let them know which piercing is of interest. If you haven't had one already, you might be given a brief consultation to check your suitability and determine jewelry size. Some shops have dedicated counter staff to assist you; in others, a piercer will guide your jewelry selection. In a well-stocked studio, you may be shown a selection of possibilities. Jewelry should be chosen for your anatomy and placement and should never be based solely on whatever is left in stock. In the best studios, you will get detailed descriptions of the material and design features of the suitable jewelry options plus a demonstration of how each piece opens and closes. Be suspicious if you are permitted to choose jewelry without any guidance, because size and style are crucial aspects for successful healing.

Unpackaged display jewelry is not sterile. If you select an item that is taken directly from the showcase, it must be run through a sterilizer before being inserted into your new piercing. If the studio does not have a short-cycle cassette autoclave such as a StatIM, this will delay your piercing for thirty minutes or longer. Pick up suggested care products if they don't come with your piercing and you didn't stock up in advance. The piercer or shop personnel may discuss the aftercare guidelines with you and request payment in advance (or this might take place after the piercing).

DO LITTLE HARM

When selecting your jewelry, remember this vital principle: to do a minimum of damage and preserve the maximum number of nerve fibers, start your piercing with the thinnest appropriate gauge. The smaller and more sensitive your anatomy, the more critical this advice is. I perform piercings no larger than 10 gauge, though many piercers make holes that are much bigger, or use the pierce-and-stretch method (see page 280). However, the same results are achievable with much less risk if you can be patient and stretch over time.

SIGN ON THE DOTTED LINE

Before your piercing, you can expect to fill out a waiver or release form and present valid identification for proof of age. Ethical piercers are unwavering in their demand for the proper documentation. Even if you are a senior citizen, it is common for piercers to look at your ID and to copy it onto your form, which is mandated by law in some areas. Check with the studio for specific requirements if you are underage. Your parent or guardian should also be required to present identification to prove the relationship. If a minor and accompanying adult do not have the same last name, records may be requested such as guardianship papers, a divorce decree, or proof of a legal name change. Certain IDs, including those from the US military, cannot legally be copied or photographed. Make sure you have a form of identification that can be copied, if that is required by the studio's policy.

The paperwork you encounter will depend on the studio's policies and local regulations. You may be asked what you've most recently eaten and when, and if you've ingested any prescription medications, supplements, recreational drugs, or alcohol. Disclose pertinent medical history that could affect your piercing experience or healing course. If you have sensitivities or allergies, especially to skin antiseptics, certain metals, or latex, call attention to this verbally and note it on your release form. Then your piercer will be sure to make any necessary jewelry suggestions and product substitutions. These forms are essential for protecting both you and your piercer. Any studio that does not require this type of paperwork is a fly-by-night operation. You should take flight in the other direction!

You may have to wait for the piercer to prepare the cleaning and marking supplies, sterile instruments, and jewelry that you will be wearing. Some piercers invite you in to observe, while others prefer to use this time to focus and prime themselves for your procedure.

FOLLOW ME, PLEASE

Next, you will be taken to the piercing room. It may resemble a medical office with a massage table, dentist's chair, or doctor's examination table (with or without stirrups). Don't be put off if this area seems a little cold or sterile—it's appropriate for a clean room to look that way. A piercing room could have an earthier ambiance, but it must have surfaces that can be disinfected and are easy to keep clean.

Your piercer should show you where to place your personal belongings. Be careful not to plop your sunglasses or bag onto a sterile tray or contaminated surface such as the biohazard trashcan. To avoid causing a distraction during your procedure, turn off your phone unless you discuss this with your piercer.

If necessary, you'll remove or adjust your clothing to expose the area for cleaning and marking. Your piercer will indicate where and how you should position yourself. You may need to change positions several times. Depending on the piercing placement, you might, for example, be marked while you are standing and pierced while you are seated or reclining. A good piercer will guide you along; you won't have to wonder what is about to happen. Tell them if you have a preference for more information or less.

Piercers, like health care personnel, should have a professional demeanor when dealing with unclad bodies. Your piercer should not make you feel self-conscious or uncomfortable by staring or acting improperly while you are undressing. Many studios have a policy against leaving clients unattended in the procedure room, so you may not be permitted total seclusion while you undress. However, you should have relative privacy and be well away from other customers and staff.

YOU WANT IT WHERE?

Now is the time to reiterate the placement you have in mind and the effect you wish to achieve with your piercing. Mention any ideas you have for stretching or adding more piercings in the area. Future modification plans often affect the best location for the current hole.

Your piercer will mark the prospective spot after cleaning the tissue. Take your time to consider the marked placement carefully; envision how your jewelry will look. Bring in a friend for another viewpoint if you need help, and it is permitted. Don't be afraid to ask your piercer why they selected that spot. A skilled pro can always explain why they chose a particular location—and why the one you requested is not optimal.

For precision, I mark with dots the same size as the jewelry gauge I will be inserting. Some piercers draw lines or crosses instead of dots or make reference marks in the area. Almost a third of piercers surveyed use a pressure mark. If you can't tell where the proposed site is, ask for clarification and make sure the piercer seems equally clear on the agreed-upon location if a distinct mark is not evident.

Once you are both pleased with the proposed spot for the jewelry, your piercer will begin the procedure. After marking, they may prep the skin with a topical antiseptic, soap, or surgical scrub and apply a sterile drape around the area with a moisture-repellent material called *CSR wrap*. This helps to protect and isolate the site and maintain asepsis. Gauze might be used, but this inferior substitute gives the piercer a false sense of security because moisture passes through it. Your piercer should put on fresh gloves just before touching the sterile instruments. Depending on the placement, they may use fingers or a tool to support the tissue for piercing.

BREATHING AND RELAXATION TECHNIQUES

The conscious use of breath is a simple, time-honored technique for managing stress, pain, and anxiety.[1] Most piercers will at least instruct you to take a deep breath right before inserting the needle and have you exhale as they perform the actual piercing. If they fail to coach you, do this for yourself as the procedure commences: Inhale through your nose slowly and deeply, filling your lungs. Exhale through your mouth even more slowly; completely empty your lungs. Try to let all your muscles loosen and relax as you maintain your attention on each calming breath. Keep your breathing slow, controlled, and deep until your jewelry is secured in place—don't hyperventilate.

Visualization or distraction can also help. Close your eyes and picture yourself walking on the beach. Enjoy the warm afternoon sun heating your skin and the gentle breezes caressing your hair. Hear the waves breaking on the shore nearby and imagine smelling and tasting the salty sea air. Use any pleasant scenario you like and engage as many senses as possible; stay focused on this throughout the procedure.

Another technique is to concentrate on an object or hold a friend's hand (if permitted) to help you transfer any tension elsewhere.

ANESTHETICS

In most parts of the world, injectable anesthetics may be administered only by a licensed medical professional. Over-the-counter topical numbing products may be available, but they can cause *edema* (fluid buildup) and other temporary tissue changes, which could affect the placement or procedure. Adding such substances also increases the risk of an adverse reaction or complication. When you visit a competent professional, the piercing is so momentary that anesthetics are not necessary.

A QUICK STICK

Next is the actual piercing. Some people prefer not to look at the needle; others feel it is essential to observe it to know what is happening and maintain a sense of control. Try your best to stay absolutely still.

Ow! The piercing should be a brief—though possibly sharp—sensation.

Okay, maybe it pinches or stings, but most (of my) piercees find the feeling is so fleeting that it is over before they even realized it was starting. Next, the piercer will insert your jewelry, pushing the needle out as they do so. A little maneuvering may be needed to get the jewelry in and securely fastened. This part of the procedure is sometimes more uncomfortable than the needle stick, especially if your piercer is not skillful. Try to breathe deeply and stay relaxed. As the adrenaline and endorphins pump through your system and then dissipate, it is not uncommon to get a little light-headed. Don't worry; it should pass quickly. Alternatively, enjoy the rush while it lasts. Your piercer will clean up the area and offer you a look in the mirror. Congratulations! You did it.

THE AFTERMATH

When the experience is over, your piercer may offer you a glass of water or some candy. It isn't a bad idea to accept. Or, if you brought juice, drink it now to stabilize your blood sugar. During the aftermath, you may perceive some sensations such as aching or stinging, though seldom much pain—or at least not for long. These feelings can remain or return intermittently throughout the rest of the day. Analgesics are not suggested before your piercing due to their tendency to increase bleeding, and afterward they are seldom necessary. If you experience discomfort, bleeding, and/or swelling, ice packs can be helpful. See "Running Cold and Hot," page 236. Ibuprofen and other over-the-counter nonsteroidal anti-inflammatories (NSAIDs) should be avoided since their use can impair wound healing.[2]

If your piercer did not already discuss aftercare, it should be covered at this point. Ask questions until you feel clear about how to take care of your piercing, what product(s) to use, and how often. Take as much time as you need in the studio to relax and recover. If you don't feel steady, be honest with yourself and your piercer. Arising before you are ready can result in a serious injury if you fall. Your piercer should be happy to let you remain for as long as necessary before you depart.

Understandably, you could be distracted during your visit to the studio and may not recall all the details of the aftercare instructions later, even if the piercer discussed them at length. When the excitement of the piercing has subsided, take out your copy of the printed care sheet, or go to the relevant page on the studio's website to review the post-piercing guidelines carefully.

MAKE A NOTE

While you are in the studio, ask your piercer the exact dimensions of your jewelry, and write them down. A lack of accurate information can present challenges down the road if you need to change your jewelry or buy replacement parts. For instance, if you lose a ball, you'll need to know what gauge you're wearing. It might also be beneficial to write down where you made your purchase or the brand. Not all parts are compatible, especially with threaded jewelry—though members of the Association of Professional Piercers carry interchangeable stock. If you need to adjust the fit of your original piece or you decide to change the style, it is helpful to know the size and other specifics.

Record everything you can: the gauge (thickness), length of the post (if it is bar-style jewelry) or inside diameter (for ring-style jewelry), the ball or ornament size, material, and the studio or piercer. Keeping notes about your healing course or trials with different care regimens can also be useful.

ENVIRONMENTAL IMPACT

Piercing is a particularly egregious profession when it comes to ecological matters. Though unavoidable for safety reasons, we discard an excess of single-use disposables, including paper towels, gloves, and many other items and materials. The mining of stones and metals for jewelry production involves the use of toxic substances and a host of environmentally destructive practices. The manufacturing processes for creating alloys and plastics are also damaging. Therefore, piercers are encouraged to be aware of conservation and engage in sustainable practices wherever they can. Earth-conscious piercees may want to purchase a certified carbon offset for the environment following piercings and jewelry purchases.[3]

THE POINT

Now that you know about the details involved in a visit to the studio, you are almost fully prepared to get pierced. However, we have touched only briefly on piercing procedures, so read on to learn about the tools and techniques piercers use.

9

PIERCING PROCEDURES

Once you've decided on the piercer and the placement, filled out the paperwork, and entered the piercing room, what will the piercer do? Although you don't need to know every detail, familiarity with the standard equipment and procedures can help you form realistic expectations and evaluate whether your piercer is working in a manner consistent with accepted practices. This chapter introduces you to the instruments and technical aspects of piercing; it is *not* an instructional manual. Always patronize a competent professional; *do not attempt to pierce yourself or anyone else without appropriate training.*

SETUP

Your piercer must thoroughly wash their hands with soap and water, dry them with disposable towels, and put on clean medical gloves before touching you or any sterile piercing equipment. A hands-free sink is best, but if they touch the faucet to turn on the water, then a paper towel or elbow—not their clean hands—should be used to turn it off. Next, the piercer should don a fresh pair of gloves.

Nearly all piercers surveyed (95 percent) use nitrile gloves or another latex substitute. But if you have a latex sensitivity or allergy, make sure to mention it to your piercer. One-third of practitioners in the survey wear sterile gloves to pierce. They are the safest type (when the piercer is trained in their use). However, as of this time, they are mandated by law in only a few places, and standard industry practice still deems exam gloves acceptable for performing piercings.

Once your piercer is gloved, they should handle only the piercing equipment (including cleaning and marking gear), and the area of your body that will be pierced. Gloves *must* be changed if they come into contact with anything else. To hygienically perform a piercing, at least three pairs are needed during the setup, piercing, and cleanup.

In the traditional process, your piercer should assemble all of the supplies on a clean tray. The tray should be single-use, autoclavable, or have a disposable plastic-backed paper liner, like those used in a dentist's office. They should work from a sterile field (such as the interior of an autoclaved package or sterile tray drape) placed on this surface. An alternative is the cassette autoclave setup described in "Vital Equipment: Sterilizers and Ultrasonics," page 44.

PIERCING TOOLS AND TECHNIQUES

The equipment and techniques used by your piercer will depend on their professional preferences and which piercing you're getting. One tool that all piercers must use is a piercing needle. In the United States, extremely sharp, beveled-tip hollow needles are manufactured expressly for the piercing industry. They're sometimes referred to as *needle blades*. Quality needles are razor-sharp; they penetrate most tissue with a minimum of force. The needle is usually held and pushed through by hand. Rarely do piercers use a needle holder or pusher. Good needles are crucial for a comfortable procedure. Piercers sometimes say "Your skin is really tough" to excuse a slow or botched piercing, but that is seldom the problem when they use top-of-the-line needles.

Piercing needles come in a range of sizes to suit piercer preferences; I favor a two-inch long straight needle. Body jewelry and needle thickness are sized by *gauge* (a numerical standard of measurement for the thickness of wire). The higher the number, the thinner the item (see "Gauge Measurements," page 81). It is standard practice to use the same gauge needle and jewelry for most piercings. Needles are also made in odd measurements, called *half-gauges*. Over 50 percent of piercers surveyed use them for specific techniques that are discussed later.

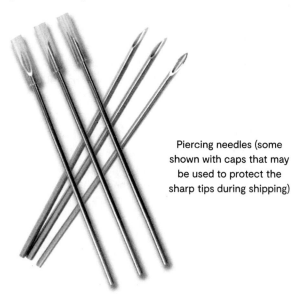

Piercing needles (some shown with caps that may be used to protect the sharp tips during shipping)

Curved needles are another commercially available item. Piercers use these in areas where a straight instrument does not conform well to the anatomy or surrounding area. More than two-thirds of piercers surveyed modify their own needles in some way, at least at times. Curved needles should have a smooth arc and no dings, burrs, or marks from pliers or other tools. *Chamfer* or *O-needles* have a flat end with a sharp circular bevel instead of a pointed tip. They are usually made only in the smaller sizes used for initial piercings. This alternative is sometimes used for cartilage piercings or surface work.

Like all instruments in the traditional piercing setup, sterile needles should be stored in individual packages. Just before use, the wrapping should be peeled open carefully to minimize the potential for contamination. The needle (and other equipment) will not usually be wrapped if it is sterilized in a cassette autoclave just before use.

Most people are not fond of needles, and many find them distressing, so I avoid calling attention to them in the studio. Instead, I use the abbreviation "P.N." for piercing needle, or simply refer to them as a "piercing instrument." Should you want to see or talk about it, I will certainly oblige, but any piercer who forces you to look at a needle against your wishes is treating you in an abusive manner. There is no reason that you must see the piercing instrument, and if you are needle-phobic, this would be unnecessarily traumatic.

Both the American-style needle and the cannula type (described next) can be safe for piercing when the technician is trained to use them correctly.

CANNULAS

Piercers outside the United States sometimes use a *cannula* or *catheter needle* (a solid needle covered with a flexible plastic sleeve). In certain countries, it is illegal for piercers to use American-style piercing needles because they are considered medical devices. The sharp tip of the cannula makes the piercing, and when the needle is withdrawn, it leaves the hollow casing in the piercing channel. If jewelry is to be inserted in the same direction the piercing was made, sterile scissors are normally used to cut off the attached hub (part of the equipment that is needed when the cannula is used for its intended medical purpose). A newer type has also been manufactured for piercers in which the hub can be disengaged easily without scissors. The jewelry is fed into the plastic casing inside the piercing channel, the sheath is then withdrawn, and the ornament is in place. Cannulas may cause a little more bleeding because the hole is slightly larger than the jewelry.

CORKS

Some piercers place a small sterile cork or rubber stopper on the exit side of the tissue for support during the piercing, and to receive the needle. As the industry's needles have gotten sharper, corks are used less, since they are not as necessary for support. Piercers may use corks to cap a needle carefully before a jewelry transfer or just prior to disposal.

FORCEPS

Piercers may use *forceps* (a medical grasping tool) to hold and support the tissue to assist in making a quick, safe, and accurate piercing. A variety of shapes, sizes, and styles are available, though forceps are not suited to all areas of the body. Nearly three-fourths of piercers surveyed make use of them for some procedures. *Pennington forceps* (a triangular-jaw clamp) and *Foerster sponge forceps* (a larger oval-headed model that is often preferred for tongue piercings) are the most common types found in body art studios.

Forceps secure and compact the skin but should never cause pain or undue tissue trauma. The tool should not leave scratches, deep grooves, or produce a contusion (though bruising in the pierced region can be a normal consequence of the piercing itself). The forceps are sometimes rumored to be "the worst part" of a piercing, but in the hands of a skilled technician, you will only feel some pinching. Clamps limit circulation, which may have a slightly numbing or distracting effect. When your piercer removes them, you may feel more sensation than when they are in place, and this is apt to occur if they are left on longer than usual. Tighter or denser tissue might feel more sensitive when clamped.

The piercer will carefully position the forceps on your tissue so that the marks for placement are aligned evenly. When they pierce with the needle square to the jaws of the forceps, they will hit the exit mark; your piercing will be in its intended position. A good piercer will get the forceps on and off quickly, leaving them as loose as possible while they are still secure. Manipulation of the tool after it is attached to you is unnecessarily painful and can be damaging, so it should be moved very little once it is clamped in place. I find that forceps with a relatively small head provide the best support for many piercings.

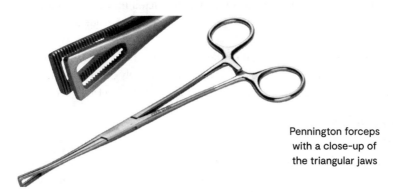

Pennington forceps
with a close-up of
the triangular jaws

Forceps are often left in place until the jewelry has been inserted into tongue and some labret (lip) piercings. The tool must have a large enough head for the barbell or labret stud ends to fit through, so the clamp can be removed. Otherwise, the forceps will be attached to your body by the jewelry. An alternative type that eliminates this issue is *slotted forceps*, which have a segment of the jaws removed so that they can be taken off after the jewelry is in place. However, if a piercee jumps or pulls back during a piercing, which happens occasionally, the forceps could slide off.

Traditional metal forceps are reusable following appropriate reprocessing (cleaning, decontamination, and sterilization). Various types of disposable clamps are also available.

NEEDLE RECEIVING TUBES (NRTs)

Needle receiving tubes serve a similar purpose as forceps but are used in areas where clamps don't fit or aren't practical. The NRT is a hollow tube with a *lumen* (space inside) large enough to accommodate the needle; it supports the tissue on the exit side during the piercing procedure. Some have flat or flared ends, and others are angled to better conform to the anatomy. Receiving tubes in metal, shatter-resistant glass, and disposable hard plastic come in various diameters, lengths, and shapes.

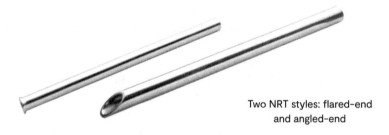

Two NRT styles: flared-end and angled-end

Piercers often use NRTs for various placements, including the septum, VCH, Prince Albert, and certain ear cartilage piercings, including the rook, daith, and forward helix. Some piercers use them for nipples, navels, or inside the nose when performing nostril piercings.

In addition to offering support, the tube also functions as a protective sheath by enclosing the sharp tip of the needle. An NRT can also safely cap the needle during a jewelry transfer, even if the tool isn't used for support during the procedure.

NEEDLE BLANKS

Needle blanks are versatile and affordable tools. These disposable tubes come in a wide range of sizes from 26 to 4 gauge. The thinnest (26–20) are ¾-inch straight pieces called *transfer pins*. Different sizes work with the various gauges of body jewelry, alone or in combination. For example, the straight 20-gauge needle blanks press-fit into the ends of internally threaded 14- and 12-gauge posts. The exposed portion of the transfer pin fits into the back end of the needle, keeping it connected to the jewelry to facilitate a smooth, secure transfer into the new piercing. When used in place of a taper, this avoids the need to pass a few extra inches of metal through freshly pierced tissue. In combination, an 18-gauge needle blank with a 26-gauge transfer pin bent gently inside it makes an excellent disposable taper to use with 18-gauge threadless jewelry.

The thicker gauges of needle blanks come in 2- and 3-inch lengths. They are inexpensive when compared to standard metal receiving tubes and are being used in their place as a disposable option. Even the larger needle blanks can be bent into different forms. A periscope shape is frequently used for tragus, forward helix, and other piercings. These are available premade, or the piercer may alter them in the studio. They can even be formed into a loop and used to support tissue for scapha and other ear piercings.

Piercers may use an array of other items to brace the skin, including sterile steel wire bent into certain shapes, *curettes* (medical tools with small loops on the ends), and cotton swabs.

TECHNIQUES

Depending on the area being pierced, and the style and skill of your piercer, you may experience some of the following techniques during your procedure.

FREEHAND PIERCING

Freehand piercing (done without tools other than a needle) is a common approach, and it is indispensable for specific procedures, including surface piercings and anchors. Instead of using forceps, a receiving tube, or another device, the piercer supports the area manually. Their fingers can be quite close to where the needle exits your tissue, so this method carries a heightened risk of the piercer getting stuck. The freehand technique is best left to experienced hands.

Historically, tools were used for most procedures, and it was believed that accuracy and speed might suffer when executing freehand piercings; however, many professionals have developed impressive skills. Some piercers find that this tool-free method allows them to feel the tissue they are piercing, which provides critical feedback that assists in guiding the needle through smoothly.

Unfortunately, some piercers perform freehand piercings due to a lack of instruction, a shortage of equipment, or reasons of ego. Some consider it a point of pride that they perform only freehand piercings. In reality, a piercer can work very quickly, gently, and safely whether using tools *or* performing a freehand procedure. It all comes down to training and expertise. About two-thirds of piercers surveyed employ all of the principal techniques: forceps, tubes, and freehand; just 6 percent solely use the latter.

The primary considerations of your piercer should be to use an approach that will provide a safe procedure for both parties, a pleasant (or at least tolerable) encounter for you, and a precisely placed piercing. Carefully interview a prospective piercer about their training, piercing philosophy, and level of proficiency if they perform freehand piercings exclusively. A piercer who believes that forceps always cause tissue damage never learned to use them properly. Make sure they are not self-taught or minimally experienced before you let them pierce you.

TISSUE MANIPULATION

Skin that is taut or inflexible can make the procedure more challenging for both you and your piercer. This simple but effective technique loosens and prepares your tissue to make the piercing as comfortable as possible.

For forceps or freehand: The piercer performs highly localized manipulation by gently lifting and rolling the flesh between their fingers for ten to thirty seconds. It might go on for a minute or longer if your tissue is especially dense or tight.

For NRTs: The area can be prepared with a form of tissue manipulation for any septum and ear cartilage piercings that use an NRT, though for a slightly different reason. This technique helps to compact the tissue and seat the end of the tube, so it does not slip during the procedure. The piercer places a sterile swab, insertion taper, or gloved fingertip at the point where the needle will enter and puts the tube into position at the exit; they gently apply pressure from both sides while massaging in a barely perceptible circular motion.

ILLUMINATION

Your piercer might illuminate certain areas with a penlight or other bright, focused beam to check for visible structures such as veins and arteries in the proposed pathway of the piercing. They may do this during marking, right before the stick, or both. The tissue might be adjusted to move a vessel aside; the placement might need to be altered if a problematic structure is in the way, or the piercing called off if it is unavoidable.

COMPRESSION TECHNIQUE

This technique is used for placements in the cartilage, including the ear (above the soft lobe) and the nostril. As soon as the piercing is done and the jewelry is in place, the piercer uses sterile gauze or cotton swabs to apply firm pressure on both sides of the piercing for fifteen seconds to a minute, as if attempting to stanch bleeding, even if no blood is present. This simple technique is intended to reattach the surface tissue to the cartilage underneath. It also helps reduce the likelihood of localized bumps during healing. This is suitable for all cartilage piercings covered in chapter 11. If your piercer is not familiar with this simple technique, describe the practice and ask them to perform it on you. However, if the angle of a cartilage piercing is too far off from perpendicular, bumps are likely regardless.

BASIC PIERCING PROCEDURE

Below are the fundamental steps your piercer should follow. Unfamiliar terms can be found in the Glossary and are discussed in detail later in the book.

- o **Clean the area to be pierced,** commonly with alcohol and/or Betadine (povidone iodine), or another surgical scrub. A germicidal mouth rinse may be used for oral piercings. Prepping inside and out is required for *orofacial* piercings such as the upper or lower lip. In the United States, alcohol is not generally used as a sole prep product for piercing, though it may be used before marking, and the skin antiseptic applied after. Betadine and other iodine products occasionally produce skin irritation reactions. However, the sensitivity is usually to other ingredients, and true iodine allergies are described in medical literature as a myth.[1] Also, contrary to popular lore, an allergy to shellfish or seafood does not increase the likelihood of sensitivity to iodine.[2] If you have a history of trouble with topical iodine, remind your piercer before they prep your skin, and they will use an alternative product. Single-serving packages for prep products are safer than bulk dispensers, which can become contaminated. Even so, 37 percent of piercers surveyed use the latter.

o **Mark the placement,** commonly with a single-use surgical marker or disposable items such as a sterile toothpick with a drop of *gentian violet* (the purple water-based fungicide also used in surgical markers). If your piercer marks you with a pen, they should give it to you or dispose of it; marking implements should not be reused. Almost one-third of piercers surveyed use pressure marks, which might be harder to see, and 10 percent do not create marks. Be sure to discuss placement carefully before proceeding with piercing.

   • This part of the process should never be rushed. Don't hesitate to ask questions or request adjustments until you and your piercer feel the proposed placement is perfect. For many piercings, it is common to mark both the entry and exit points.

o **Brace the tissue,** either with forceps, a receiving tube, fingers, or other support.

o **Pierce the skin** with a sterile, disposable piercing needle. Ideally, this should be a single motion that is swift and smooth. Stopping and starting or pausing partway through causes added discomfort.

o **Insert the jewelry,** pushing the needle out with the ornament. This should also be accomplished in one smooth movement. The needle should not come out of the tissue before the jewelry has passed through the channel.

o **Close the jewelry** with a captive bead, threaded ball, press-fit end, or other closure. Some styles, such as a nostril screw, do not require this step.

o **Clean up,** wiping with saline or water on a sterile pad or gauze to remove any blood and remaining iodine, which can irritate the tissue if left on for an extended period. Foil-wrapped saline towelettes are effective, non-irritating, and cooling. They instantly help to diminish the stinging sensations that often follow piercing. Alcohol should *not* be used; it is irritating and painful on a fresh wound.

- Your piercer should carefully dispose of the needle directly into the sharps disposal container as soon as possible following your procedure.
- Any reusable instruments, such as some metal forceps, should be placed into an appropriate storage container (often in an enzymatic foam) for subsequent reprocessing and sterilization.
- Paper and disposable items used in the procedure should be discarded in a covered waste can containing a plastic trash bag.
- Your piercer cannot clean the premises with the gloves worn during your procedure; they are considered contaminated. After your piercer discards the tray setup from your piercing, they must don a new pair for cleanup. The table or chair, tray, and other surfaces that were contacted but not autoclaved or disposed of should be cleaned with hospital-grade, hard-surface disinfectant.

PROCEED WITH CAUTION!

The following things should *never* happen during a piercing (and if they do, bolt!):

- Your piercer asks you or your friend to hold the forceps with unwashed, ungloved hands.
- The forceps are locked tightly onto your tissue.
- The forceps are left hanging from your body, even momentarily.
- The piercer drops something on the floor (such as a tool they are using, or your jewelry), then picks it up but does not change gloves and replace or resterilize the item.

OTHER TOOLS

A number of specialized tools are made to facilitate the insertion and removal of body jewelry, including pliers and hemostats. These metal instruments must be sterilized between clients. They also have the potential to scratch and damage jewelry or pinch tissue, so they must be used carefully. Because of this, piercers should use their fingers instead of these tools whenever possible. But for tasks that can't be done by hand, these implements work very well. For more information, see "Jewelry Tools," page 273.

INSERTION TAPERS

Also called *insertion pins*, or simply *tapers*, these tools are sometimes used to facilitate jewelry insertions and to stretch piercings to a thicker gauge (see "Insertion Tapers for Jewelry Changes," page 270, and "Stretching," page 276). They look similar to needles, but there are differences. Tapers are not sharp, though they may be pointy in the thinner sizes. Also, they are solid, not hollow like piercing needles. The back end is concave, convex, threaded, or another shape to fit with specific styles of jewelry. Using the right type is imperative to ensure the successful transfer of jewelry into a piercing. They come in every standard jewelry gauge and are sized by the measurement at the thicker end. The thinner tip is usually two gauges smaller than the larger end, to assure a smooth gradation over two inches or so of length. A tool that has an abrupt transition to the thicker gauge can cause tissue damage. Tapers are commonly made of implant-grade stainless steel or titanium, though other materials are also available.

Tapers can be used during the piercing process to insert particular styles of jewelry. If a piercing is made from front to back, but the jewelry must be inserted from the other direction (for a gem to face the right way, for example), a taper can be used. A lubricated taper pushes out the piercing needle, then helps to transfer the jewelry into the piercing so that the ornament is situated correctly.

In the unfortunate event that your piercer fails to get your jewelry all the way through during a jewelry transfer, a taper can sometimes locate the channel. It may be more effective for your piercer to first get a thinner taper in, then follow it with one that is the same gauge as your new piercing, and, finally, insert your jewelry.

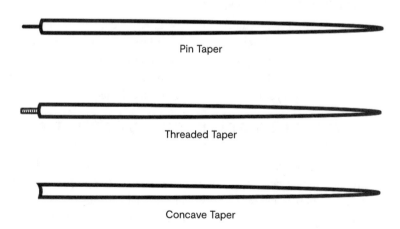

Pin Taper

Threaded Taper

Concave Taper

THE POINT

You now have an excellent idea of what to expect in the studio and throughout a piercing procedure. You are primed for a fantastic experience. Still, there is a great deal of valuable information about jewelry that has not yet been discussed. Round out your knowledge in the next chapter, and when the time comes to select body jewelry for a new or existing piercing, you will be versed in all the details.

10

JEWELRY 101: SIZES, SHAPES, AND MATERIALS

Much of the focus with piercing is on where and how to place the hole. But a vital factor for uneventful healing is wearing the right foreign object in your wound—the jewelry. The more you know about body jewelry, the better your chances of getting a suitable piece that will be safe for healing. Good quality is always essential, as cheap jewelry can wreak havoc, even on old piercings.

ALL THAT GLITTERS

From functional to flashy, the choices for body jewelry seem almost infinite. Only specific styles and types, however, are suitable for healing. Without knowing what to look for, you can easily be seduced into getting inappropriate (or even harmful) jewelry in a fresh piercing. Every element of the ornament—its size, design, material, *and* quality—affects your chances of having a healthy piercing.

EARRINGS, BODY JEWELRY—WHAT'S THE DIFFERENCE?

The traditional stud earrings and hoops you see at malls and in jewelry stores (even high-end pieces made of quality materials) are not appropriate for initial piercings. In addition to being too wiry, conventional earrings are often far too short for different areas of the body—including the ear. Additionally, the standard ear-piercing jewelry designs are unsuited to other areas of the body due to parts that could poke, irritate, or sink into the delicate healing tissue.

The piercing industry has developed safe, comfortable jewelry designs ranging from thinner pieces that are perfect for ears, nostrils, and certain other facial piercings, to the thicker options that are required for below-the-neck placements. We refer to the ornaments used in piercings as "body jewelry," whether located in the ear or somewhere lower. Good designs for fresh piercings are simple, of uniform thickness, and have secure closures, so they do not detach unintentionally during regular activities such as bathing and sleeping.

If you are not knowledgeable about body jewelry, you might buy whatever appeals to your fashion sense or fits your budget best, rather than what is optimal to wear in a new piercing. Some piercers are happy to sell you what you like rather than what you need, especially if you want a more expensive item than one that would be superior for healing.

Choosing jewelry for piercings is very different from shopping for a ring to wear on your finger. The appearance of the initial piece must always be secondary to safety aspects that affect compatibility with your body. There are countless options to wear after your piercing has healed, so you can change to a larger, smaller, or more elaborate ornament later. So why can't you pick just any piece of jewelry you like?

- The material may not be safe for a fresh piercing. It might not be able to withstand autoclave sterilization. It could also cause skin sensitivity, an allergy, or predispose you to infection due to incompatibility with your body.
- The design and/or manufacture may be flawed, leading to irritation of the fresh wound.
- Shoddy jewelry may have dysfunctional parts like balls that fall off easily, resulting in lost jewelry and accidental piercing closure.
- The size and shape may not be right for your anatomy, and ill-fitting jewelry can cause inflammation, embedding, migration, and other problems.

THE BODY JEWELRY BOOM

Many of the body jewelry styles we wear today have roots in the ornaments worn by indigenous people in their piercings. The designs were modified and modernized by Jim Ward, who introduced most of the basic pieces that remain in widespread use today.

In the past few decades, body jewelry has evolved into an enormous and profitable business. What was once made by only a handful of small companies is now mass-produced around the globe. With improvements such as the introduction of high-tech metals and advanced fabrication methods, the finest goods now approach aerospace precision in their quality.

Unfortunately, the explosive popularity of piercing has also brought on an epidemic of inexpensive, poorly made junk jewelry—much of it from overseas. A lot of the eye-catching novelty goods are made of inferior materials using substandard manufacturing processes. Uninformed or uncaring suppliers and piercers sell these shoddy items, unsafe designs, and low-cost knockoffs. Uneducated consumers purchase and wear them in their piercings, sometimes with regrettable consequences.

THE BASIC SHAPES

There are two basic shapes of body jewelry: the *ring* (a hoop) and the *bar* or *barbell* (a post with a ball, disc, or other closure on each end). Variations on these two forms comprise the most popular and functional styles that are suitable for the majority of fresh piercings.

There are two basic types of rings, though they are very similar in appearance:

- o Captive bead ring
- o Fixed bead ring

And there are two basic styles of bars:

- o Straight barbell
- o Curved barbell

A closed captive bead ring and an open fixed bead ring

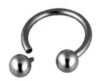

An unscrewed (open) circular barbell

A straight barbell and a curved barbell

Another standard style is essentially a combination of a ring and a bar; it is circular in shape, but the closures work like those on a barbell. For practical purposes, we'll include this with ring-style jewelry:

- o Circular barbell (sometimes called a "horseshoe")

Even though a studio's selection might be vast, the majority of items will be adaptations and modifications of these simple designs.

SIZES AND MEASUREMENTS

Body jewelry can be confusing because of the tremendous array of sizes, and the somewhat odd gauge system commonly used to measure the thickness. A clear, detailed ruler or *caliper* (measuring instrument) can be very handy.

Each piece of jewelry is measured using two dimensions:

- **Gauge** (thickness)
- **Length** (for the post of bars, curved barbells, nostril screws, and similar designs) or **inside diameter** (for ring-style jewelry)

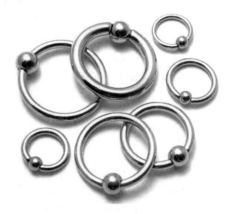

A selection of captive rings in a range of gauges and diameters

GAUGE MEASUREMENTS

The thickness of body jewelry made in the United States is measured using a system called *American Wire Gauge* (AWG) or *Brown & Sharpe*. (See "Gauge Conversion Chart," page 332.) In this system, the lower the number, the thicker the material. A 20 gauge is thin and wiry, whereas 4 gauge is very thick (and not a standard size for a new piercing). The thicker the gauge, the bigger the jumps between sizes. In practice, when we refer to a 14-gauge barbell, we mean the thickness of the metal that passes through your skin. Large ear jewelry like tunnels and plugs are sometimes referred to as "gauges," much to the chagrin of piercers. To us, *gauge* refers to a unit of measure, not an object.

Most conventional earrings are skinny, around 18 gauge or 20 gauge. The typical initial minimum for below-the-neck piercings is a little thicker: 14 gauge. Somewhat confusingly, the gauge sizing system for medical needles is not the same one used for piercing needles and jewelry. A 16-gauge medical needle and a 14-gauge piercing needle are equal in size. More sensibly, perhaps, outside the United States, everything is usually measured in millimeters.

DIAMETER OR LENGTH

In the United States, we generally size body jewelry using imperial units (fractions of an inch). Rings are measured across the inside diameter, at the widest part. Barbells are measured by the length of the bar, from one end of the post to the other. Balls or other ends are never included in the measurement.

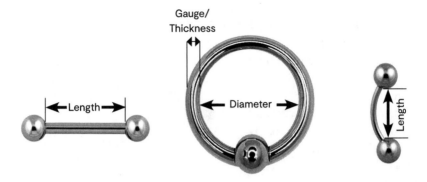

The length of a curved bar is measured straight across from one end of the post to the other. The extent of the curve is not taken into consideration; so a piece shaped with a deeper arc will have a little more room on it, but this is not reflected in its length measurement.

Barbell ends and captive beads are also measured by diameter at the widest point, in fractions of an inch or millimeters. Generally, the tinier the ring diameter, the smaller the ball, though some styles play with proportion to achieve different effects.

Ring diameters start at ¼ inch in the thinnest gauges, though hoops that tiny are not common. Due to practical factors and manufacturing limitations, a range of sizes is typically available in each gauge. For example, thin rings are wobbly and unstable in large diameters, and thick wire cannot be bent into tight hoops. However, a well-stocked studio has many sizes on hand to offer you the best possible fit for your anatomy and piercing placement.

Conscientious piercers carry barbells in increments of at least sixteenths of an inch for optimal fit. Typical ranges to accommodate a variety of piercing placements are from ³/₁₆ inch up to well over an inch. Some rings and posts are available in ⁷/₃₂, ⁹/₃₂, and ¹¹/₃₂-inch lengths or diameters for even better safety and aesthetics.

RING-STYLE JEWELRY

CAPTIVE BEAD RING

A popular style of basic body jewelry is the *captive bead ring* (CBR), also called a *captive, captive ring,* or *ball closure ring* (BCR). This metal hoop uses tension to hold a *captive ball* or *captive piece* (a removable bead or ornament) in a gap between its ends. This piece has dents or holes into which the ends of the ring are seated. The captive piece can be the same material as the ring or a

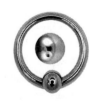

A captive bead ring with a close-up of a captive bead

contrasting one. There are thousands of different beads and other captive ornaments available in an array of colors, shapes, and designs. It may be possible to
interchange them safely during initial healing.

A well-made CBR has a smooth circular shape and ends that are convex to ease
insertion and hold the bead firmly. The tips should look even and finished—not
like someone filed them in a garage with a handheld rasp.

The captive ring opens by forcing the hoop to widen slightly, which releases the
tension on the bead, allowing it to come free. It closes by snapping the bead in
between the tips, engaging the spring tension of the ring. For this jewelry to be
fastened securely, the gap between the ends of the ring must be slightly narrower
than the captive piece it holds. When the metal is *annealed* (a process used to
improve a material's properties), the beads in average-sized rings can be removed
or changed without the use of tools (see "Annealing," page 97).

Use the following technique for changing the bead:

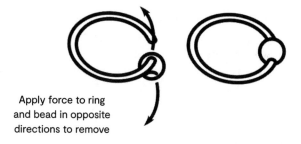

Apply force to ring
and bead in opposite
directions to remove

o **To remove the bead,** grasp the ring between the thumb and index finger
   of one hand (at three or nine o'clock, with the bead at twelve o'clock) and
   hold the bead between the thumb and index finger of the other hand. Draw
   the bead and ring in opposite directions (one toward you, the other away
   from you).

o **To insert a bead,** hold the jewelry the same way as for bead removal. Make
   sure that your fingers do not obscure the indentations on the bead. Start by
   seating the dent of the bead onto the side of the ring that you're not holding. It is usually best to do this by feel rather than trying to look at it. Use
   leverage on the ring via the seated side of the bead to ease the second side
   of the bead into place. It should "snap" into position, though the bead may
   still spin freely.

The gap may need to be wider than the one left by removing the bead to take the ring from your body without pinching the tissue. In this case, the hoop itself will need to be opened somewhat. To avoid warping your jewelry, it is generally best to twist the metal in a coil shape rather than simply pulling the hoop's ends apart. Except for swapping out a bead, seek professional assistance for any jewelry changes that become necessary during healing.

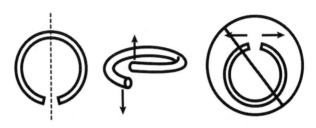

Twist the ring in a coil shape—
don't pull the ends apart

Before attempting to change your bead, practice with jewelry that you are not wearing. If you can't manage the job, you will need to get help from your piercer, or purchase some *ring opening pliers* (ROPs) (see "Jewelry Tools," page 273). You can chip beads made of fragile materials like natural stone or glass during insertion, so ROPs should be used to minimize the likelihood of breakage.

The CBR is a simple design that has several advantages: it is exceptionally versatile, secure *when properly fastened*, and easy to manufacture. One disadvantage is that the ball could fall out and become lost. The ring can follow, and your piercing might shrink—or even close. This type of ring can also be awkward for the uninitiated to handle and may take strength and dexterity to operate, depending on the gauge, diameter, and quality. The CBR comes in other shapes and forms (such as square, teardrop, triangle, D-ring, and so on), but these are generally best for healed piercings.

FIXED BEAD RING

The *fixed bead ring* (or *bead ring*) and the captive are almost identical in appearance, but, as indicated by its name, the ball is permanently attached to one end (see photo on page 80). A similar style without a bead is called a *seam ring*, which is better for healed piercings.

The jewelry twists open and closed for insertion and removal. The bead should be drilled so that the free end of the ring fits into it securely. When both ring and ball are the same material, you may not be able to tell the two styles apart without attempting to spin the bead. If it moves, it is a captive ring. Variations in this style include affixed gems and other ornamental designs instead of the ball.

Fixed bead rings lack versatility, but one advantage is that you can't possibly lose the bead. This is one reason they are popular in gold, which is pricey. This style is most common in the thinner gauges that are easier to manipulate for insertion and removal. Depending on its material, quality, and size, a fixed bead ring may require tools such as brass-jaw pliers for opening and closing. Another disadvantage is that such rings are unsuited to frequent changes. The metal can become disfigured from overuse, and excessive opening and closing will cause brittleness and, ultimately, breakage. For a fee, gold can be reannealed by a jeweler to restore it, but this must be done before the piece breaks. When your ring feels stiffer and more difficult to bend, you will know the time has come for a treatment.

After repeatedly bending a fixed bead ring, getting it to stay securely shut becomes challenging. The open end of the hoop may unfasten, pop out, and sit in front of (or behind) the bead. Also, you may see a small gap between the ring's end and the ball even when it is closed. To redistribute the tension properly, open the piece slightly, and carefully squeeze the ring together as if to make it smaller. Then, bend the ring as if to close it, but go further so that the open end passes over to the opposite side of the bead. (If the hoop's end sits in front of the ball, bend it to the back, or vice versa). You should then be able to close it tightly.

THREADED JEWELRY

The following sections introduce *threaded* jewelry styles, which have tiny *screw threads* on one side that fit into a hole that is *tapped* (drilled out) with the matching thread pattern on the other. The processes for creating these closures on high-quality barbells make manufacturing them—and other threaded jewelry—costly and complex, especially compared to captive rings. Threaded items tend to be either cheap junk or relatively expensive, well-made pieces.

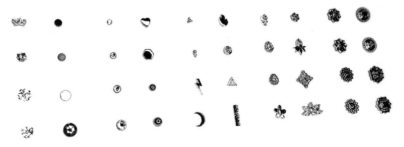

A selection of ornamental ends

An advantage of threaded jewelry is that you can interchange the ends. Balls are the most basic and standard option. An ellipsoidal piece called an M&M end (for its resemblance to the popular candy) is practical and comfortable for some areas, and flat discs are well suited to others. There is a genuine treasure trove of threaded jewels, geometric shapes, and other ornamental pieces available. Some manufacturers make jewelry with only one side that can be removed, but the sort with two interchangeable ends is more versatile. Threaded ends can be switched, possibly even while a piercing is healing.

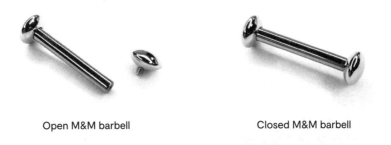

Open M&M barbell   Closed M&M barbell

A disadvantage of threaded jewelry is the possibility of an end unscrewing and the jewelry falling out. Wear quality products and regularly check the tightness of all threaded pieces to prevent this problem.

HANDY TIP

Your piercer should attach threaded jewelry ends securely, so they will not unscrew. Still, regularly checking is a good idea. Jewelry ends tighten clockwise. Remember: "righty-tighty, lefty-loosey." If you have ongoing issues with a piece unscrewing, you can try Loctite or another thread-locker product (available at hardware stores). After your piercing is healed, put a small dab on the threads, tighten the end in place, and carefully wipe away any excess. Use the regular strength product unless you never want to remove your jewelry.

CIRCULAR BARBELL OR HORSESHOE

This style functions the same way as a barbell—the end(s) screw off and on, but it is shaped into a hoop. (See photo on page 80.) A high-quality circular barbell is costly compared to a fixed or captive bead ring, due to the expense of machining the threading.

The circular barbell is simple to insert and remove because no bending or tools are needed. An additional benefit is that the inside diameter can be adjusted by spreading or narrowing the gap between the ends to best suit your anatomy. This is especially useful for areas that require a precise fit during healing. A more extreme version of this alteration is the "Customized Circular Barbell (C-Ring or U-Ring)," below.

The *captive circular barbell* is a useful style in which a captive bead is inserted to fill the gap between the two ends, forming a complete ring. This variation has three beads: two on the circular barbell, plus the captive in the center. The middle piece is secured by tension, the same way the ball is held in place on a captive ring. A bead of the right size that is inserted correctly will not fall out easily. By making it into a complete hoop, you reduce the possibility that your circular barbell will catch on clothing, a partner's jewelry, or other objects. A captive bead serves the added function of preventing the threaded ends of the circular barbell from unscrewing. However, it limits your ability to adjust the ring diameter, which becomes reliant upon the size of the captive bead.

Depending on your anatomy and the jewelry size, this style could get a little heavy for a fresh piercing. If it becomes uncomfortable, remove the middle bead during healing.

CUSTOMIZED CIRCULAR BARBELL (C-RING OR U-RING)

This modified circular barbell falls somewhere between ring- and bar-style jewelry. The base piece should be at least a diameter or two smaller than would be needed to accommodate the pierced tissue, depending on the ultimate jewelry size and shape. The piercer widens the gap between the threaded ends by spreading out the hoop using ring-opening pliers. This adjustment elongates the part that passes through the skin and fine-tunes the diameter. Jewelry can be made C-shaped or a low-rise U-shape to accommodate your build. I suggest this customized style as preferred initial jewelry for several piercings, including horizontal clitoral hood (HCH), triangle, Prince Albert, and Reverse PA.

RING-STYLE JEWELRY: WHAT'S THE DIFFERENCE?

Other than the design features described, no practical distinctions exist between these different rings. They may be worn interchangeably on all piercings that use ring-style jewelry.

INTERNAL AND EXTERNAL THREADING

On *internally threaded* pieces, the part of the jewelry that passes through your skin is smooth, and the threads are on the removable end, such as a ball or gem. The end screws *into* a hole in the jewelry that has been drilled or *tapped* with the matching thread pattern to receive it. This means that smooth metal will safely and comfortably pass through your body when you take your jewelry in and out. The APP considers this such a critical safety issue that, according to their standards, body jewelry for initial piercings must have internal tapping (no threads on the posts).

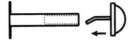 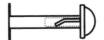 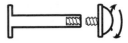

Threadless flatback open   Threadless flatback closed   Internally threaded flatback

Alternatively, *externally threaded* jewelry has the screw pattern cut onto the *post*, and this comparatively rough surface may be passed directly through the body. The removable end is tapped with a matching hole to receive the threaded post. With *step-down threading*, smaller threads fit inside a needle during piercing, and special tapers are sometimes used during jewelry changes to prevent threads from scratching the tissue. Without safeguards, inserting this style can be like running a small metal file through your body. It is more likely to cause discomfort and tissue damage, especially if the channel is tight.

Internally threaded jewelry is more difficult to manufacture. Machining the screws tiny enough to fit *inside* a 16- or 14-gauge post (and tapping it to receive them) is far more challenging than merely cutting screw threads onto the jewelry post, as with the external threading style. Therefore, quality internally threaded jewelry costs more, but it is worth the extra expense. Any jewelry in this style that seems extremely economical probably is substandard. Manufacturers who produce high-end internally threaded products are generally more likely than the bargain-basement guys to use implant-grade materials. For initial piercings, internally threaded jewelry avoids any possibility of scraping your piercing with screw threads.

BAR-STYLE JEWELRY

This basic jewelry style includes many straight and curved versions of a post with two ends.

BARBELL

Another standard body jewelry style is the barbell, along with its many variations. The basic barbell is shaped like the classic dumbbell found in a gym: a straight bar post with two spherical ends (see photo on page 80). Barbells are a good choice for piercings in areas where ring-style jewelry would be unwieldy, uncomfortable, or unsafe. Straight bars are suited to ear, tongue, nipple, and some genital piercings.

A barbell worn in a new piercing must be long enough to accommodate tissue changes such as swelling or *development* (see "Post-Piercing Nipple Development," page 162). A bar that is too short can cause discomfort, embedding, and healing problems. A post that is overly long can catch and cause trauma, which also leads to trouble. For certain piercings, a longer post is inserted initially, and then the jewelry is downsized to fit more snugly once swelling is gone or healing is complete.

The size of the barbell's balls or threaded ends is also critical to safety. They must be big enough to avoid becoming embedded, but not so large as to be irritating or to cause the jewelry to be pushed away from the tissue.

CURVED BARBELL

The terms *bent bar, curved barbell,* and *curve* all refer to a barbell shaped to form approximately one-fourth of a circle (see photo on page 80). It should be a manufactured piece with a smooth, consistent curve. This popular variation of the straight barbell is suited to areas like the navel and eyebrow, where a ring can be obtrusive, but a straight bar doesn't conform well.

JEWELED NAVEL CURVE (JNC)

This bejeweled variation is designed for vertical piercings. A set gem or stone is affixed to the bottom of the post so the ornament faces forward when the jewelry is in place. Only the top can be interchanged with a matching or contrasting stone, ball, or another threaded end. The version with very large gems is too hefty for healing.

Wearing top-quality jewelry is essential. If the stone falls out (a common problem with lower-end products), dirt and germs will lodge in the cavity left by the missing gem, increasing the risk of infection. You will need to replace the entire piece.

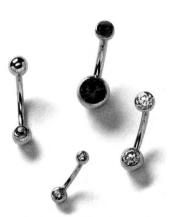

A selection of jeweled navel curves, a popular style for navel and VCH piercings

J-CURVE

Also called a *J-bar,* this style looks very much like a jeweled navel curve when it is worn, and it is suited to the same areas. Generally, both ends are threaded, so it is more versatile. The *J* shape projects the lower end of the jewelry forward, allowing the ornament on the bottom to be more visible, which is well-suited to some deep navels and hoods (for the VCH).

SURFACE BARS

This modified barbell is designed for piercings on flat areas of the body. It is shaped like an open staple, with a straight post between two short legs or uprights that are usually at right angles to the bar. The bar post should rest at a uniform depth under the surface with the uprights at 90-degree angles to the tissue. This reduces pressure, distortion, and irritation during healing. Bars used for some Christina piercings have only one upright leg. Threaded discs or flat gems can help to distribute pressure more evenly when used as the ends on a fresh surface piercing. An accurate fit is crucial; the jewelry must be the perfect length to encompass the tissue between the entry and exit of the piercing, and the barbell ends must not sink into the skin, nor

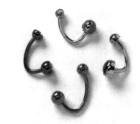

A selection of J-curves with gem, cabochon, and ball ends

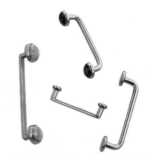

A selection of surface bars with flat discs and cabochon gem ends

should the legs protrude beyond the surface. The post may be slightly curved to conform better to the local anatomy. Some are made with a flat post portion to be less obtrusive under the tissue, though the standard variety may work better in areas where there's significant movement.

THREADLESS JEWELRY

Plenty of bar-style jewelry is threaded, but a popular alternative has a threadless push-pin closure. Over 90 percent of piercers surveyed use the threadless variety.

The removable end has a slightly bent pin that straightens out when inserted into the hole in a straight post. This spring-tension force holds the two pieces firmly together. Curved styles use a straight pin for tension. This type is available in many of the bar variations described above, including jewelry for nipples and navels.

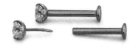

A threadless flatback post with prong-set gem (open and assembled)

In small gauges, threadless pieces are excellent for ear and facial piercings. One of the most prevalent styles is the *flatback* or *threadless labret*, which is widely used for ear and orofacial piercings. This short barbell has a flat disc attached to one end, which reduces contact with the teeth and gums in lip piercings. It is comfortable and safe for nostrils, earlobes, and many ear cartilage placements. Gemstone and geometric ornamental ends are wildly popular. Gold adornments may have pins of a different material for strength and durability.

Threaded jewelry is best for tongue piercings, which undergo stressors such as eating, and for heavy play with nipple piercings. Otherwise, both closure styles are usually acceptable when they are quality products. If a barbell doesn't unscrew, try pulling the end off instead.

ORNAMENTED CLICKER AND SEAM RINGS

These are hoops with an ornamental section that prevents the piece from turning in the piercing. The clicker is hinged, and the seam ring bends open and closed like a fixed bead ring. Jewelry with these closures used to be reserved for healed piercings, and still should be if there's any chance a seam could enter the tissue. They are primarily worn in certain cartilage and septum piercings.

A selection of ornamented clicker and seam rings

OTHER SHAPES

Although captive rings, barbells, and their variations are appropriate for the majority of piercings, certain areas of the body sometimes use jewelry designed or adapted for a specific part of the anatomy. One example is the *nostril screw*, a modified post style with a corkscrew tail that rests against the inside of the nostril (see photo, page 118). See chapters 11 through 14 for more details about anatomy-specific jewelry.

JEWELRY MATERIALS FOR INITIAL PIERCINGS

Relatively few materials are safe for wear in a fresh piercing, as the jewelry must withstand the heat and pressure of autoclave sterilization. Another crucial factor is *biocompatibility*: it must be well tolerated by the body and local tissues to avoid healing complications, allergy, irritation, and infection. Finally, the human body is a harsh host, so only highly corrosion-resistant materials fare well in the flesh.

For wear in initial piercings, the Association of Professional Piercers accepts jewelry that meets implantation standards for materials and quality by the American (now International) Society for Testing and Materials (ASTM) and/or the International Standards Organization (ISO). Examples with their numbered designation codes and the other APP-approved materials are listed below. See www.safepiercing.org for updates.

- Steel: ASTM F138 or ISO 5832-1, 10993-6, 10993-10, and/or 10993-11 compliant
- Unalloyed titanium (Ti): ASTM F67 or ISO 5832-2 compliant
- Alloyed titanium (Ti$_6$Al$_4$V ELI): ASTM F136 or ISO 5832-3 compliant; and (Ti$_6$Al$_7$Nb ELI): ASTM F1295, F1713, or ISO 5832-11 compliant
- Solid 14-karat or higher yellow, white, or rose gold that is nickel and cadmium free
- Solid unalloyed or alloyed platinum that is cadmium, nickel, and lead free
- Niobium (Nb): ASTM B392 compliant, including but not limited to commercial grade 2; and grade 4, which contains 1% zirconium
- Polytetrafluoroethylene (PTFE): ASTM F754 compliant
- Polymers or plastic materials: ISO 10993-6, 10993-10, and/or 10993-11 compliant and/or meet the United States Pharmacopeia (USP) Class VI material classification
- Glass that is lead free, including fused quartz, borosilicate, and soda-lime

All threaded or press-fit jewelry must have internal tapping (no threads on exterior of posts and barbells). Surfaces and ends must be smooth and free of any potentially harmful residues. Metals must have a consistent mirror finish.

METALS

The steel, titanium, and niobium grades listed above are highly biocompatible and very unlikely to irritate a piercing. However, making jewelry with them is challenging because the traditional techniques and tools for working gold and silver cannot be used. These harder metals must be machined with high-tech equipment rather than crafted by a jeweler's hand. They also require a great deal of polishing to be made smooth enough to wear in the body.

The implant-designation metals are used in medical devices such as bone pins and screws and joint replacements. They have been designed and tested for safe long-term wear in the body. Cheaper jewelry materials are frequently described as "surgical," but this is an intentionally misleading claim. You can't tell the metal grade just by looking, so how can you be sure?

Mill certificates, mill test certificates, or simply *mill certs* are documents that provide evidence of a specific grade of metal (with an ASTM or ISO code designation). By law, manufacturers of steel and titanium body jewelry must give these to their customers (for example, your piercer) upon request. Ask your piercer/jeweler about their metals and if they have copies of mill certs to demonstrate the grades. You don't need to understand exactly what the numbers signify, but mill certs should warrant that the steel or titanium is one of those in the APP's metals list. It is not possible to know whether the piece of jewelry you're buying is from the batch indicated on the paper, but the presence of a certificate showing a recent date and the appropriate material means you have at least a chance of getting the right metal.

Since you cannot be sure of the origin of any individual piece of jewelry, the best thing to do is shop with a reputable company and follow the guidelines presented in "What to Look for in Quality Body Jewelry," page 97.

IMPLANT-DESIGNATION STEEL

Steel was the most prevalent metal used for body jewelry in the United States for many years. Now, just over 50 percent of piercers surveyed are using implant-certified grades, but another 20 percent sell and insert steel that does not have an ASTM designation. Rumors that steel is not safe for piercings are untrue, *as long as the grade is appropriate*. Many types of steel do contain irritating components and have a high risk of causing problems, so only the particular alloys listed above should be used in body jewelry. Almost all piercees can tolerate them since the metal is chemically inert and created not to react with the surrounding tissues or immune system. Steel can be heavy in large sizes.

TITANIUM

Titanium has become the most popular body jewelry material by a large margin. Initial jewelry sizes are similar in price to steel. Almost all titanium body jewelry is made from implant-grade metal because of its frequent use in medical and dental applications. Titanium jewelry must have a high-polish mirror finish because the naturally porous surface can damage healing piercings.

Titanium is lightweight—about half the weight of steel—extremely strong, corrosion resistant, and durable. It can be beautifully colored using an *anodizing* process that changes the way the surface refracts light. In its natural, polished state, this metal appears similar to steel but is a bit darker in color. When anodized, it can range from a brownish shade to yellow, green, blue, purple, and even multicolored. The color may eventually fade depending on individual body chemistry, or if worn in a friction-prone area. This change is not harmful, but it could be disappointing. However, a studio with an on-site anodizing machine can recolor your jewelry.

Implant-certified titanium is considered the most inert of the metals used for piercings. This is an excellent choice for those concerned about nickel sensitivity, because none is present in the titanium alloys used for body jewelry.

NIOBIUM

Niobium is an inert, corrosion-resistant elemental metal in the same family as titanium. It can be anodized in subtle or vibrant colors in the same way. Niobium is the third most prevalent body jewelry metal after titanium and gold. Traditionally the piercing industry found the pure metal to be acceptable, but now only implant designation material should be used for all body jewelry, whether alloyed or not.

Niobium can be blackened through a heating and cooling process. The charcoal-colored finish is permanent; it will not fade like other colors of anodized titanium or niobium. Only high-polish niobium should be used for initial piercings; matte-finish pieces are rough and porous. Captive rings in niobium are readily available, but, oddly, balls cannot be formed from it. Cylinders of coiled niobium wire could be used as captive pieces, but otherwise, the beads and threaded ends on niobium barbells will be made of a different material.

GOLD

Gold has a long history of use within the body, and its applications in modern dentistry further attest to its safety. Still, specific implant designations for gold jewelry are not currently available. It comes in many different (often proprietary) alloys, so use caution when making a purchase, especially since gold is significantly more expensive than most other body jewelry materials. *Cheap gold is never good gold.* However, a high price tag alone does not guarantee quality or acceptability for wear in piercings.

The term *karat* refers to the purity of gold. Pure gold, or twenty-four karat gold (24k), is highly biocompatible, but it is too soft for body jewelry. It must be alloyed with other metals. Out of twenty-four parts of metal, eighteen karat (18k) indicates that eighteen parts are gold, and six are other elements (75 percent gold and 25 percent other elements).[1] Some piercers sell fourteen-karat (14k) gold, which is about 58 percent gold. Regardless of the percentage of gold, jewelry is safe to wear in the body when the alloy contains only inert components. If there is too much silver, copper, or other reactive material in the mixture, even eighteen karat gold can be problematic. Much of the white gold used for body jewelry is alloyed without nickel; for whiteness, it contains palladium, an inert element in the platinum family. Specialty colored golds could include irritating elements, though the rose shade has gained popularity and appears well-tolerated by piercees. According to the piercer survey, 14k and 18k white, yellow, and rose gold are the most prevalent body jewelry metals after titanium and niobium.

Moisture and various chemicals can react with certain alloys and cause a dark discoloration of the metal. Frequent use of a gold-polishing cloth will usually resolve this problem. Gold is durable, but excessive exposure to chlorine (in pools and hot tubs) can cause the metal to become brittle.

Some people are concerned that gold is unsafe for initial piercings, but when it is alloyed to wear in the body, it works very well. Because of its high cost, some studios do not stock all styles of body jewelry in gold, so you may need to place an advance order if you wish to start a piercing with it. Regular fine jewelers are often unfamiliar with the need for inert alloys, smooth surfaces, and safe closures. Consult a piercer about the exact requirements before you place an order or purchase gold jewelry.

PLATINUM
Platinum is an inert precious metal that is 60 percent heavier than gold. It is rare: ten tons of ore must be mined to obtain just a single ounce of platinum. It has a rich, bright white color and is very strong, but it is prohibitively expensive for most piercees. Platinum is difficult for jewelers to work with, in part due to the metal's extremely high melting point. When alloyed with inert elements, it is a safe choice for body jewelry. It is uncommon to find platinum inventory in a body art studio, so it would probably need to be custom ordered. Many piercers are unfamiliar with platinum, so you must find one with a lot of jewelry savvy to stock or obtain it.

NONTOXIC PLASTICS
Flexible synthetic polymers (plastics) are comfortable and can reduce stress on the body in areas with a lot of motion or changes in the size and/or shape of the anatomy. It can be safer to wear something softer than metal, especially in cases of pressure or friction from sports or other activities. One inert, high-tech plastic alternative to metal body jewelry is PTFE (polytetrafluoroethylene—a form of Teflon) if it is ASTM F754 compliant. Flexible plastics are economical, and can embody many characteristics that are excellent for piercings:
- Lightweight and not thermal reactive
- Adjustable cut-to-fit sizing in some styles
- Invisible on X-rays and other imaging tests
- Obviously nonmagnetic (quality metal body jewelry is too, but it can be tough to convince medical personnel, resulting in unnecessary jewelry removals)
- No issues with metal sensitivity or allergy

Though polymers lack the luster of body jewelry metals, the piercing field could use more chemically safe alternatives that meet industry standards for wear in fresh piercings. There are a few popular plastic product lines on the market, but the manufacturers have not provided documentation on the materials to prove that they meet implant-grade standards. These are more flexible than PTFE, and they're available in colors and shapes including curved bars, circular barbells, labret studs, septum retainers, and nostril screws. Plastic or metal barbell ends press-fit or self-thread onto the plastic posts. Unfortunately, they haven't been cleared by the APP for use in initial piercings.

JEWELRY TO AVOID IN FRESH PIERCINGS

Some common body jewelry materials are suitable for healed piercings, but you should avoid them in new ones. Other materials are unsafe and should be reserved for jewelry that is not worn through pierced tissue.

ACRYLIC

Acrylic is not suggested for wear in piercings. Though readily available in an array of inexpensive body jewelry, it poses safety risks, including allergic reactions and cytotoxic effects from chemicals leaching out, which can have local and systemic consequences.

GLASS

Certain types of glass are very inert and autoclavable; this jewelry *can* be suitable for wear in new piercings. The primary area of concern is the fragility of the material in small sizes. The sturdier tube or plug styles in 10 gauge or thicker are safe for some piercings.

NATURAL OR ORGANIC MATERIALS

Natural materials such as stone, horn, and wood have long been worn in piercings, but they are unable to withstand the heat, pressure, and moisture of an autoclave. They tend to be porous and cannot hold a finish smooth enough for exposure to open tissue, and in thin gauges, they are too fragile for safety. Though different cultures have historically used natural materials in the body, modern piercers must comply with the minimum safety standards of our time. You may find it appealing to reenact ancient rituals using natural materials, but today's piercees are advised to reserve them for healed piercings only. See "Natural Materials," page 285, for more information.

STERLING SILVER

Sterling silver is not suggested for use in fresh piercings or even healed ones other than the earlobes (if tolerated). It tends to tarnish, and this is an irritant to the body. The dark discoloration is a form of dirt, corrosion, and rust that can permanently stain the skin surrounding your piercing channel (see "Tarnish Tattoo," page 260).

GOLD-PLATED, GOLD-FILLED, GOLD-OVERLAY, VERMEIL, OR ROLLED GOLD

All of these techniques involve coating a base metal with a layer of gold to create an affordable piece of jewelry with the look of gold. The problem is that the gold surface (which is *very* thin—measured in millionths of an inch)[2] can wear or chip off, leaving the body exposed to an unsuitable metal underneath. Never wear any gold body jewelry that is touted as less than 14 karat *solid* gold. This isn't as critical when you are wearing a necklace or bracelet, but there is potential for severe consequences in a piercing.

FASHION AND NOVELTY JEWELRY

This inexpensive junk can be trendy or cute, but these poor quality pieces are machine-manufactured in massive quantities, and are not hand-finished or inspected. Novelty jewelry is sold in discount stores, kiosks, and shops that do not perform piercings. Avoid any piercers selling it because they either don't know enough to steer clear or have fallen prey to the lure of the dollar. You generally get what you pay for where body jewelry is concerned. Please don't go for the cheap stuff: it isn't worth the risk to your piercing and your health.

WHAT TO LOOK FOR IN QUALITY BODY JEWELRY

Quality jewelry differs significantly from cut-rate goods, but the products often look similar. The following explains how to identify safe jewelry.

FINISH AND POLISH

Metal body jewelry must have a *mirror finish*—a high-shine, super-smooth surface—to be safe for healing. Wearing a piece that has nicks, burrs, tooling marks, or scratches can cause severe complications. When your jewelry has an uneven surface, new cells that form during healing grow into the irregularities. Then, when the jewelry shifts or moves, these areas tear. As this cycle repeats, irritation, excess scar tissue formation, and delayed healing often result. A faulty finish can also introduce bacteria into the wound and lead to infection. A rough surface can cause grave issues, even with healed piercings.

ANNEALING

Annealing is a heating and cooling process that improves the properties of a material. In the case of body jewelry, it helps make metal pliable enough to bend reasonably easily. A jeweler can perform this procedure to refurbish gold rings that have become work hardened. They heat the material to specific temperatures and then cool it at particular intervals. Glass can also be annealed to improve its durability.

Cheap captive, fixed bead, and seam rings are not annealed. If you cannot bend a hoop (up to 14 gauge or so, in average diameters) with your fingers, then it is probably not annealed. It will be harder—or impossible—to insert and remove rings that are not annealed without tools.

BUYING BODY JEWELRY

Piercers typically require you to buy new jewelry for a fresh piercing from the studio, hopefully with guidance from the staff. This allows for appropriate control of size, style, quality, and sterility. Once healed, you can purchase jewelry online from reputable companies. However, body jewelry can be expensive and is not returnable due to sanitation issues, so be certain of what you need before ordering. A surer bet is to visit your local high-quality studio since they can help with the selection of suitable options and insert new jewelry for you.

YOUR BODY KNOWS THE DIFFERENCE

Body jewelry quality varies widely, from heirloom pieces of finely crafted gold with genuine diamonds and gemstones to inferior metals that can turn your skin green and infect you. Some of the cheap stuff is fashionable and attractive, but once you know the difference, do you *really* want that in your body? I remember the sign Jim Ward posted in the jewelry case at Gauntlet many years ago. It bore a sensible statement in calligraphy on parchment: "The bitterness of poor quality remains long after the sweetness of low price is forgotten."

THE POINT

Congratulations! You have amassed a great deal of knowledge about body jewelry styles, sizes, and materials. You are prepared both mentally and physically, and you know what to expect in the studio. The time has come to delve into a detailed discussion about each of the common piercings.

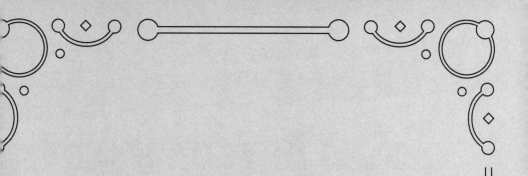

PART 4

THE HOLES

HOLES IN YOUR HEAD: EAR, NOSE,
AND FACIAL PIERCINGS...................102

KISS OF THE NEEDLE: TONGUE
AND ORAL PIERCINGS 132

TORSO PIERCINGS: NIPPLE
AND NAVEL PIERCINGS 151

BELOW THE BELT: GENITAL
PIERCINGS..166

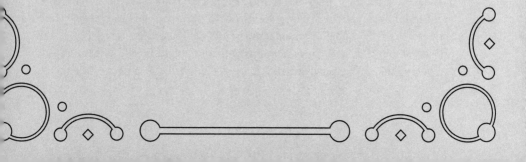

11

HOLES IN YOUR HEAD: EAR, NOSE, AND FACIAL PIERCINGS

The anatomy above the neck has a wealth of pierceable placements. Some, like the eyebrow piercing, are modern innovations. Many, however, have long histories in indigenous cultures, such as piercings of the lips, nose, and, of course, the ever-popular ears.

EARLOBE PIERCING

- o **Healing time:** 4 to 8 weeks
- o **Initial jewelry style:** Ring-style (fixed bead ring, captive bead ring, and circular barbell); bar-style (straight barbell, or flatback); or plug
- o **Initial jewelry gauge:** 18 to 10 gauge (some piercers will go thicker)
- o **Initial jewelry size:** From ¼-inch length for posts to ⅝-inch diameter for rings (rarely larger), depending on jewelry gauge and weight

Piercing of the *lobule* (the fleshy portion of the earlobe) has a rich tradition and lore that spans every inhabited continent. Ear piercings have achieved massive popularity and are worn by people from all walks of life, young and old alike. For considerations regarding piercing children, see "Infant and Child Ear Piercing," page 37. This universal ornamentation crosses gender barriers and can suit those who wish to celebrate femininity, masculinity, or nonbinary identities.

EARLOBE PIERCING: CHOICE OF JEWELRY
You have a vast choice of jewelry to wear in your ears, but one type is not recommended for fresh piercings: conventional earrings. For comfort and safety, quality body jewelry is far superior when compared to cheap costume jewelry and even pricey traditional-style earrings. Designs with straight posts tend to painfully jab you behind the ear, especially when you are sleeping or using a phone. The metals

in ordinary earrings are often substandard, potentially leading to sensitivities or allergies, and the posts are sometimes too short.

More sizes and styles of body jewelry are safe to wear in new earlobe piercings than any other placement. The main concern is to avoid excessively large or weighty pieces—especially in fine gauges—since they can cause delayed healing, migration, scarring, or thinning tissue.

EARLOBE PIERCING: PLACEMENT

The typical ear piercing is located in the center of the lobe. The angle can range from parallel to your face to perpendicular to your ear, depending on anatomy and preferences. It is wise to place the piercing *slightly* higher than the lobe's midpoint because the flesh is very soft, and the hole tends to settle a little lower over time, especially if you wear large or heavy jewelry. Still, the placement for earlobe piercings can be dictated almost entirely by aesthetics because there are few anatomical safety issues, unlike most other areas. Ears are prone to problems only when pierced in an extreme location. You could run into trouble piercing too low on your lobe, in too little tissue, or at the juncture of your earlobe and face, where a large artery is typically situated.

Let your piercer know before marking if you have a vision or concept, such as a plan to add multiples later, or an intention to stretch the hole after healing. They might want to adjust the placement depending on your goals. If multiple piercings are done on the same ear, they should be positioned at least ⅛ inch (3 mm) apart.

Placing a pair of earlobe piercings so that they appear symmetrical can be trickier than you might think; the left ear is often remarkably different from the right. Multiple lobe piercings along the rim of the ear are common. Further up, where the tissue becomes dense, you have cartilage, which is very different from the soft earlobe. The axiom, "The higher up you go, the more it hurts and the longer it takes to heal," is valid for many piercees. For more information about cartilage piercings, see the following section of this chapter.

EARLOBE PIERCING: PROCEDURE

Once the placement is marked and agreed upon, forceps may be used to secure the tissue for the piercing. Some piercers prefer a freehand or receiving tube method. This piercing can be made from front to back, or vice versa. There is seldom significant bleeding or discomfort, though a large-gauge earlobe piercing is more likely to feel tender and to bleed than a thinner one.

To avoid the potential for disease transmission and other problems, do not get your ears (or anything else) pierced with a gun. See "Piercing Guns," page 21, for more information about their dangers.

EARLOBE PIERCING: HYGIENE

Although earlobes generally heal quickly and easily, contact with dirty objects can cause an infection. Keep your phone and audio accessories clean while healing and avoid contact when possible. If you get only one ear pierced, use the other for the phone, and rest the unpierced side on your pillow if you do not sleep on your back. To keep your pillow clean, practice the "T-Shirt Trick," which is explained on page 229. Don't sleep with damp hair, which can lead to a "wet bump" on the back of a healing ear piercing.

The ear is not concealed or protected by clothing, so there is a chance you could touch the jewelry without even realizing it. You will have to avoid this for uneventful healing.

EARLOBE PIERCING: HEALING AND TROUBLESHOOTING

Ear piercings should be treated with the same aftercare suggested for body piercings. Even though a variety of products are marketed specifically for use on ear piercings, they are not among the top options. Learn why in "What Not to Use on Your Piercings," page 238. Four weeks is as fast as any piercing heals, so resist the temptation to change your jewelry prematurely.

The earlobe is the area of the body with the highest incidence of the "cheesecutter" effect. This undesirable vertical expansion of the hole can be triggered by a specific pulling incident or occur over time from excessively heavy jewelry worn on too thin a wire. Wearing a thick enough gauge will prevent this issue. If the hole hasn't migrated too close to the lobe's edge, ask your piercer about using an *eyelet* (hollow tube–style jewelry) to line the channel (see photo, page 296). This might allow you to wear dangling jewelry without further harm.

Unfortunately, plastic surgery is the only way to repair the damage. Due to the weakness of scar tissue, you must be careful when having these areas repierced. The new location should be slightly off to the side, rather than directly above an old hole, so it doesn't merge with the repaired skin. The area should heal from any surgical repair for a year or longer before repiercing.

EARLOBE PIERCING: CHANGING JEWELRY

Some styles must be inserted from back to front—but locating the hole in the back of your ear can be challenging when swapping jewelry. *Never* force anything through. If you have trouble changing your own jewelry, see your piercer for assistance.

If you need to camouflage earlobe piercings, you can use the suggestions for the nostril. See "Nostril Piercing: Concealment," page 121.

HAPPY SURPRISES

Reinsertion (inserting jewelry in a hole that was left empty) is almost always successful for an earlobe piercing if the channel was fully healed before it was abandoned. If I were the gambling sort, I would have won countless times by betting piercees that I could put in jewelry painlessly without repiercing, even when the client was convinced a hole had closed forever. I never did wager—but I'd have been a winner every time. I have seen plenty of surprised smiling faces, however, which is even more rewarding. Get help from a piercer or purchase an insertion taper, as you can cause injury by trying to force jewelry through a hole that has shrunk. See "Will It Close?" page 283, and "Repiercing after Loss," page 263, for more information.

EARLOBE PIERCING: STRETCHING

The earlobe is among the most easily stretched piercings on the body and the one that is expanded to the largest dimensions. You should be able to safely stretch up one gauge approximately four to six months after getting pierced if you have an uneventful healing period. Subsequent stretches in the smaller sizes may be possible after two to three months. For more information and instructions, see "Stretching," page 276.

EARLOBE PIERCING: RETIRING

At some point, you may consider *retiring* your piercing (removing the jewelry to abandon the hole). Once fully healed, the channel may shrink, but the vast majority of earlobe piercings will stay viable indefinitely without jewelry. Only the nasal septum, Prince Albert (penis piercing), and inner labia have an equal likelihood of remaining open.

THE CURATED EAR

A *curated ear* (sometimes called *constellation piercings*) refers to new piercing(s) and/or upgraded jewelry for existing holes that work with the individual anatomy to produce a unified, aesthetically pleasing look. Instead of focusing on each piercing as a separate entity, it involves viewing your entire ear and the ornaments for it as a cohesive creation. Upscale studios can customize jewelry in combination with earlobe and cartilage piercing variations, as described below, to suit your personal style and fashion sense. Innovative arrangements and gorgeous adornments (frequently in gold, often with gemstones) have elevated ear piercings to an elegant art form.

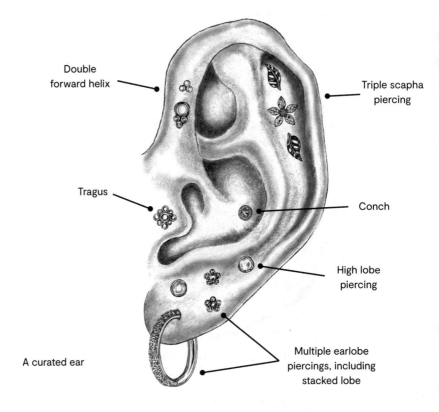

Double forward helix

Triple scapha piercing

Tragus

Conch

High lobe piercing

Multiple earlobe piercings, including stacked lobe

A curated ear

EAR CARTILAGE PIERCING (HELIX OR SCAPHA)

- **Healing time:** 6 to 9 months or longer
- **Initial jewelry style:** Flatback, straight barbell, or ring-style
- **Initial jewelry gauge:** Rarely 18 gauge, commonly 16 to 14 gauge, occasionally as thick as 12 or 10 gauge
- **Initial jewelry size:** 5/16- to 7/16-inch diameter ring-style jewelry; bar-style jewelry is anatomy-dependent (commonly with a post length of 1/4, 9/32, or 5/16 inch)

Like the earlobe, ear cartilage piercing has been practiced widely throughout history and around the planet. While still not quite as prevalent as the lobe, cartilage piercings have gained widespread popularity and acceptance in Western culture. Because the cartilage lacks *vascularity* (fluid and blood supply) of its own—circulation is in the surrounding tissues only—these piercings can be tricky to heal.

The contours of individual ear anatomy vary considerably, and so do the options for placing a cartilage piercing. Jewelry can be situated nearly anywhere along the rim, where the denser tissue begins, and higher—right up to the top of the ear. Aesthetics play a central role in selecting the placement.

The piercing can pass through your *helix* (the curled outer rim of the ear) if it is pronounced enough. Or you can pierce at the base of the helix where it joins the *scapha* (the flatter portion of the cartilage from which the helix curves). Depending on your anatomy, this sometimes allows a ring to rest parallel to your ear. If you pierce a little farther in on the smooth plane of the scapha (unsurprisingly called a *flat*), you can wear a stud there. Another possibility is a vertical helix placement at the top of the curve if you have sufficient definition. These locations are all in the realm of traditional ear cartilage piercing placements. See pages 109–115 for the array of variations.

Your piercer may use illumination to check your ear for visible blood vessels, which are usually easy to detect and avoid. Don't try to sidestep the cartilage by piercing a pinch of skin close to the edge. These tend to be unsuccessful because they are in too little tissue, and the pressure from hard cartilage behind them pushes the jewelry outward, so they migrate and reject. If your piercing is so superficial that a tiny ¼-inch diameter ring fits, or a bulge from the jewelry is visible beneath the tissue, the placement is too shallow. Ear cartilage has somewhat moveable skin over it, which creates challenges for your piercer. If the tissue shifts during the procedure and your skin gets "pinned" out of place by the piercing, it may ultimately fail.

EAR CARTILAGE PIERCING PROCEDURE

Forceps, a receiving tube, or a freehand procedure may be used to support the tissue for piercing. Many piercees find that ear cartilage piercings sting or pinch. Sensitivity varies; I've had some cartilage piercings that I would describe as tender and others that I barely felt.

DON'T SHOOT!
Piercing the ear cartilage with a stud gun is illegal in some regions.

EAR CARTILAGE PIERCING: WATCH OUT FOR BUMPS AHEAD

Cartilage piercings require gentle treatment and patience. This area tends to develop small bumps around one or both of the openings during healing. Generally, these are localized areas of inflamed excess scar formation, sometimes referred to as *irritation bumps* (see page 252). Piercings that are not perpendicular to the tissue or those that pin the surface skin out of its natural position over the cartilage have higher likelihoods of developing bumps. They can also form if the surface tissue is pushed away from the cartilage by the needle during piercing. If the exterior layer does not get pressed back into place, the body may fill in this space by producing excess cells. If your piercer practices the compression technique (see page 74) to reattach the tissue after piercing, this can reduce your chances of forming a bump.

EAR CARTILAGE PIERCING: GAUGE-UP PROCEDURE

When performing ear cartilage piercings, some piercers use a needle a half or full gauge larger than the jewelry. This technique is intended to promote the comfort and healing of the piercing by allowing your body to form a small cushion of scar tissue, so the theory goes. This may be more comfortable and make healing easier because the jewelry does not press directly against the dense cartilage. Your piercing may bleed a little more if a thicker needle is used. Over half of the piercers surveyed use this technique at least some of the time, though it may also be done to facilitate jewelry insertions.

EAR CARTILAGE PIERCING: HEALING AND TROUBLESHOOTING

You *must* minimize trauma and pressure to heal cartilage successfully. Try sleeping on a "doughnut" cushion, which has a hole in the center, or a soft pillow you can shape so that there is no direct contact with your ear. Snagging your jewelry on a brush or your hair will cause irritation. Avoid getting hair styling products on the area, as these can also cause trouble.

Healing ear cartilage takes time and patience, even when you take proper care of the piercing and wear high-quality jewelry. Your piercing may seem healed and then regress; this cycle often repeats for an extended period—sometimes a year or longer. Since cartilage can be challenging to heal under the best of circumstances, it is vital to make sure no aspect of your piercing is substandard. It is best to avoid healing more than two cartilage piercings at once, and it is often problematic to get them done on both ears at the same time.

EAR CARTILAGE PIERCING: PIERCING DRIFT AND DOWNSIZING

When post-style jewelry is worn, the length is a critical factor. If the bar is too short, the piece can become embedded. If too long, the piercing can migrate; it will drift from its original location and ruin an aesthetically pleasing angle. Your piercer may advise a follow-up visit to downsize your initial jewelry and prevent this. They will assess the post length after initial swelling has (mostly) subsided. Skipping this step can result in ruining a perfectly placed piercing!

EAR CARTILAGE PIERCING: CHANGING JEWELRY

Many piercees get help from a professional, especially for the first change. To swap out your own jewelry, support your tissue on the exit side as you transfer a new piece into place. Even fully healed cartilage piercings may respond poorly to frequent changes or attempts at introducing novelty jewelry.

EAR CARTILAGE PIERCING: STRETCHING
Ear cartilage is *not* pliable, so stretching a hole in it can be tricky and feel tender. It is imperative to wait until the initial healing is complete and the hole is fully settled before attempting to stretch. A large opening in the cartilage is quite challenging to achieve by traditional expansion methods; few piercees have the requisite patience or pain tolerance. See "The Dermal Punch," page 295, for information about an alternative tool that can create larger holes.

EAR CARTILAGE PIERCING: RETIRING
Ear cartilage piercings in average sizes usually leave a relatively inconspicuous mark when jewelry is removed, unless troubled healing caused excessive scarring. Most commonly, a small divot (*atrophic scar*—see page 256) will remain. Once established, some ear cartilage piercings will remain viable for an extended period without jewelry present. However, the hole usually shrinks, so it can be difficult and painful to reinsert jewelry. Sometimes the channel closes completely when a piercing is abandoned, even if you had it for a long time.

EAR CARTILAGE PIERCING VARIATIONS
The information above applies to all of the ear cartilage piercing placements described below. Details and differences are outlined for the most popular variations.

HOW MUCH DOES IT HURT?
Many piercees are especially anxious that a cartilage piercing such as a tragus, rook, or daith will be painful due to the relatively thick, dense tissue of those areas. However, some piercees report that these are *less* tender than a traditionally placed helix piercing. When performed by a capable practitioner, you may feel less of a sting (though perhaps more pressure) from some of the cartilage piercing variations. In any case, if you wish to wear a particular piercing, the brief procedure should not be your primary concern.

TECHNIQUES
Forceps, a receiving tube, or a freehand procedure are suitable for the various ear cartilage placements, depending on the specific location and the preference of your piercer. The gauge-up technique may be used for any of the different variations.

THE TRAGUS PIERCING

- **Description:** Frames the small protrusion of cartilage that juts out from the face in front of the ear canal's opening
- **Healing time:** 6 to 9 months or longer
- **Initial jewelry style:** Flatback, straight barbell, or ring-style
- **Initial jewelry gauge:** Sometimes 18 gauge, usually 16 gauge; possibly 14 gauge or larger for those with a substantial prominence
- **Initial jewelry size:** Posts start at 5/16 inch; rings are most commonly 3/8-inch diameter, though 5/16 inch or 7/16 inch is sometimes used.

TRAGUS PIERCING: PLACEMENT

Depending on the angle of your tragus, the piercing is usually placed relatively perpendicular to the tissue. It should be set at least 3 millimeters from the edge. If a bar is used, the angle at which a gem or ornament will sit should be considered.

If a ring is worn, it should rest comfortably in the *intertragus notch* (the groove above the earlobe at the bottom of the opening to the ear canal). An improper fit is not aesthetically pleasing and can cause irritation. Wearing ring-style jewelry will be problematic if your tragus is as wide as it is tall. Bars are best for a wedge-shaped tragus.

Note that the placement referred to as a "tragus surface" or "sideburn" piercing does not traverse the cartilage; it is a surface piercing. True vertical tragus piercings are rare because the cartilage there must be significantly more substantial and defined than the typical tragus.

TRAGUS PIERCING: PROCEDURE

Piercers use a wide variety of methods for tragus piercings, from freehand to supporting with a receiving tube (a periscope-shaped version is popular), to the forceps method. It might be pierced from the front or back with a needle that is curved or straight. Depending on jewelry style and the direction of the piercing, a taper may be used for the transfer.

THE CONCH PIERCING

- **Description:** Done in the deep bowl-shaped central shell of the ear
- **Healing time:** 6 to 9 months or longer
- **Initial jewelry style:** Flatback or barbell is preferred, though some piercers will use rings
- **Initial jewelry gauge:** Most commonly 16 and 14 gauge, with 12 and 10 gauge used less frequently

- o **Initial jewelry size:** Barbell length can be as short as 5/16 inch for thin cartilage, but some cartilage in this area is hefty enough to require a 7/16-inch post. A ring with a 1/2- to 5/8-inch diameter is usually suitable for a piercing placed an average distance from the edge of the ear.

A number of groups have practiced this piercing, including the Mangbetu tribe in Africa and a sect of Hindu yogis from India.

CONCH PIERCING: PLACEMENT

The *concha* (conch, or shell of the ear) is large enough that placements can be divided into lower (in modern history sometimes called *sadhus*, when large-gauge jewelry was worn), mid, and upper conch piercings. Piercers may separate them as *inner conch* (true conch piercings) and *outer conch* placements. The latter may refer to piercings of the scapha or antihelix. Some ears have sizable blood vessels in this region, and illumination can be used to identify and avoid them.

CONCH PIERCING: PROCEDURE

The conch piercing is generally performed with a receiving tube or the freehand method. Alternatively, septum forceps (described on page 125) can be used for this piercing, depending on your anatomy and the dimensions of the clamp.

THE ROOK PIERCING

- o **Description:** Placed in the small ridge of cartilage that originates near the face in the upper part of the ear
- o **Healing time:** 6 to 9 months or longer
- o **Initial jewelry style:** A ring, curved barbell, or mini barbell
- o **Initial jewelry gauge:** 18 gauge minimum, though 16 is more common; 14 gauge for a full build
- o **Initial jewelry size:** Rings or bars of 5/16- or 3/8-inch diameter

California piercer and innovator Erik Dakota is credited with pioneering this placement. It was publicized in Fakir Musafar's *Body Play* magazine in the early 1990s.

ROOK PIERCING: PLACEMENT

The rook is located in an area technically called the *inferior crus of the antihelix*. Some ears do not have a pronounced enough ridge. The piercing may be positioned vertically, or at a slightly outward-leaning angle. The jewelry can frame the center of that ridge or rest closer to your face. When you wear a curved bar, the piercing's angle must suit your anatomy and the shape of the jewelry. If not, the bottom end will press against your ear and cause discomfort, irritation, and healing problems.

ROOK PIERCING: PROCEDURE

A piercer must be skillful to get a well-placed piercing into this small, dense ridge of tissue. A needle receiving tube (NRT) with a flat or angled end can offer excellent support at the exit during the piercing. However, other techniques, including freehand, can also be successful, such as going from the bottom up with a curved needle.

ROOK PIERCING: HEALING

If you spend a lot of time with a phone or headset pressed against your ear, you will find the rook is not a practical or comfortable piercing. If the placement is too shallow, migration and rejection are common.

FAUX ROOK PIERCING

This alternative is positioned where the top of the rook would be situated. Instead of traversing the ridge of cartilage, it comes through behind the ear. A flatback is the jewelry of choice for this placement, which passes through less tissue than the traditional version. If the ear rests close to the head, there may not be room for the jewelry backing. This is not a good option if you tuck your hair behind your ears. Glasses can be problematic with this piercing as well.

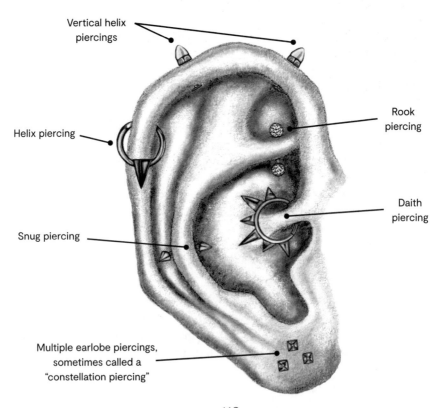

Vertical helix piercings

Helix piercing

Snug piercing

Multiple earlobe piercings, sometimes called a "constellation piercing"

Rook piercing

Daith piercing

THE DAITH PIERCING

- o **Description:** Placed in the cartilage adjacent to the face at the inner origin of the helix
- o **Healing time:** 6 to 9 months or longer
- o **Initial jewelry style:** Ring-style preferred, but some will use a curved bar
- o **Initial jewelry gauge:** 16 and 14 gauge, rarely thicker
- o **Initial jewelry size:** ⅜, ⁷⁄₁₆, or ½ inch

This innovation is also credited to Erik Dakota. The name *daith* (rhymes with *moth*) reportedly comes from the ancient Hebrew word *da'at*, meaning "knowledge." If your motivation for this piercing is to cure migraines, you probably shouldn't get one. See "Piercings as Medical Treatments," page 28.

DAITH PIERCING: PLACEMENT

This piercing rests deep in the ear's shell at the root of the *helix crus* (the ridge of cartilage just above the ear canal that fades down into the conch). Most anatomy is configured with a pierceable crest at this location. The daith is a subtle but attractive piercing because of its concentric appearance; the jewelry frames the tissue, and in turn, the ear frames the jewelry. When appropriately placed (according to Dakota), the lower part of a ring seems to come directly out of the ear canal.

DAITH PIERCING: PROCEDURE

The daith is tricky to perform due to its almost-internal placement. A straight or angled receiving tube might be used, though a short or bent tube and/or curved needle may fit better in the limited space. Hemostats can help with jewelry insertion and closure, especially if the piercer has large fingers.

DAITH PIERCING: HEALING

Compared to other cartilage piercings, the daith can be an easy one to heal because the surrounding anatomy protects it. You must still keep dirty phones away and avoid sleeping on a healing daith piercing if you experience discomfort or irritation. Bumps are likely to form if the jewelry is too small.

THE FORWARD HELIX PIERCING

- o **Description:** Placed in the front of the helix, at the upper juncture of the ear near the head
- o **Healing time:** 6 to 9 months or longer
- o **Initial jewelry style:** Flatback, ring-style, or barbell
- o **Initial jewelry gauge:** 18 to 14 gauge; 16 is the most common
- o **Initial jewelry size:** ⁵⁄₁₆- to ⅜-inch ring diameter, although a ¼-inch post may fit slim anatomy

FORWARD HELIX PIERCING: PLACEMENT

This piercing is placed in the relatively thin cartilage near the *helix root* (the juncture of the helix and head). It is usually angled reasonably parallel to the face, so the end of a short barbell can be displayed nicely. The post and backing tuck into the curl at the front of the ear, where the helix forms from the face. Or, a ring can frame the area. Multiples are common here, but not all anatomy is suited.

A small percentage of people have a divot called a *preauricular pit* (a natural channel that can have some depth) in this region. It is safest to avoid this spot, even if you have no history of local drainage, swelling, or infection. Most piercers will refuse to put jewelry through a preauricular pit. Show your piercer where eyeglasses or sunglasses rest over your ears to assist in appropriate placement during marking.

FORWARD HELIX PIERCING: PROCEDURE

As with many of the other ear cartilage variations, a receiving tube technique is prevalent. An angled tube often conforms well to the anatomy in this region, though a freehand method is also an option.

THE ANTITRAGUS PIERCING

- o **Description:** Placed through the small, relatively vertical lip of cartilage above the lobe formed by the lower front rim of the conch
- o **Healing time:** 6 to 9 months or longer
- o **Initial jewelry style:** Curved bar or barbell; ring-style jewelry may be an option
- o **Initial jewelry gauge:** 16 or 14 gauge; 12 gauge for fuller builds
- o **Initial jewelry size:** Minimum length of 5/16 or 3/8 inch, but 7/16 inch is sometimes needed for thick cartilage

ANTITRAGUS PIERCING: PLACEMENT

Anatomy varies in this region, but many ears have a pierceable protrusion in this cartilaginous rise opposite the tragus, framing the intertragus notch. The piercing should encompass the solid ridge of cartilage. If it is placed too deep, it can unintentionally pass through to the back of the ear, which will cause problems healing. If the area is small and undefined, it is best left unpierced. The angle must be considered in relation to your placement and jewelry selection. The tissue is vertical; therefore, ring-style jewelry will rest toward either the tragus or the edge of the ear. Most of the piercers surveyed perform these (87 percent).

ANTITRAGUS PIERCING: PROCEDURE

This piercing can be performed using forceps to support the tissue, or with a freehand technique, or needle receiving tube. A curved needle might be used, but isn't required.

THE SNUG PIERCING

- **Description:** A horizontal piercing that frames a vertical protrusion of cartilage called the *antihelix*
- **Healing time:** 6 to 9 months or longer
- **Initial jewelry style:** Usually a curved barbell, occasionally a straight bar
- **Initial jewelry gauge:** 16 or 14 gauge
- **Initial jewelry size:** If the tissue protrudes with substantial height but is narrow, a ⅜ inch could be safe

SNUG PIERCING: PLACEMENT

This piercing goes through the same anatomical ridge where a rook is placed, but farther from the face where the antihelix is vertical—usually across from the tragus. Many people do not have an outcropping to their cartilage in this location. Even if the tissue does protrude, it must be solid, or the piercing will come through behind the ear. In suitable candidates, the cartilage is generally quite thick. Therefore, it can be more tender than most other cartilage piercings and take longer to heal. The snug is not a phone- or pillow-friendly adornment. Just over three-quarters of piercers surveyed offer this placement.

SNUG PIERCING: PROCEDURE

This piercing is generally performed with a receiving tube or freehand technique. It might also be done with forceps. Whether forceps are used or not, if you do not have a tall enough ridge of tissue to clamp, then you are not a suitable candidate for this placement.

FAUX SNUG PIERCING

Relatively few ears have a sufficiently tall, defined, and unencumbered rise of cartilage for the snug piercing. Many ears are better suited to a "faux snug," which simulates the look with two separate piercings framing the ridge. One is made through the conch, and its companion is placed low on the helix to create the same appearance without passing through the thick nub of cartilage.

NOSE PIERCINGS

Two popular, time-honored piercings are done in the nose: the nostril (on the side) and the septum (in the center).

Before visiting the studio, give your nose a proper blowing with a tissue or two. Breathe through your mouth during skin prep if you find the cleaning product smells too strong. After the piercing, some tearing of your eyes, sneezing, or bleeding is perfectly normal, so if your piercer doesn't provide a clean tissue for you to hold, ask for one. Do not touch your face with your fingers after your piercer prepares the area; if your nose tickles or itches, use the tissue, but do not touch the prepped region at all.

You must postpone a nose piercing if you have a sinus infection or respiratory illness. However, if you suffer from sinus allergies, you might still be able to get a nose piercing, because normal nasal mucus is not harmful to an open wound. In fact, it is part of the immune system, and contains protective proteins and antibodies.[1] Trauma is problematic during healing, so you must be gentle when you blow your nose. Maintain hygiene by touching the area only with clean hands and disposable tissues, not reusable hankies. Once you are healed, blow your nose at will. Just wipe off your jewelry as well.

The nose functions as a filter, which is obvious if you've ever blown your nose and seen black contents in your tissue afterward. Avoid exhaling smoke through your nose and French inhaling while healing a piercing in this area. If you spend a lot of time in dusty or dirty environments, healing a nose piercing might be challenging.

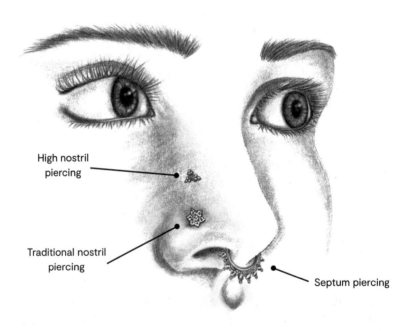

High nostril piercing

Traditional nostril piercing

Septum piercing

> ## A CLASSIC
> Curious onlooker: "Say, how do you blow your nose with that jewelry in it?"
> Piercee: "Very carefully."

THE NOSTRIL PIERCING
- **Description:** Placed on the side of the nose, traditionally seated in a niche called the *supra-alar crease* (where the nostril naturally flares)
- **Healing time:** 4 to 6 months or longer
- **Initial jewelry style:** Flatback or nostril screw; some piercers use rings
- **Initial jewelry gauge:** In 18 and 16 gauge, flatbacks are very common. Rings in 18 gauge or thicker, up to 12 gauge for a large piercing, or nostril screws in 18 gauge
- **Initial jewelry size:** Length on post-style jewelry is anatomy dependent and must leave room for some swelling; usually no shorter than 9/32 or 5/16 inch; ring diameters 5/16 to 7/16 inch

Nostril piercings are second in popularity only to ear piercings. Many indigenous populations in the Americas, Africa, and India have worn nostril piercings throughout the ages. In Western culture, the nostril piercing is primarily an aesthetic placement and does not ordinarily indicate marital, financial, or any other status, as it often does in other regions.

NOSTRIL PIERCING: ALL ABOUT JEWELRY
The traditional straight-post earring with a butterfly backing is dangerous if worn in the nostril because its sharp end can damage the inside of your nose if bumped. That style of clasp can harbor bacteria and secretions from both your nose and the piercing, which increases your risk of infection. Stud earring backings are often visible inside your nose, but the posts fall out easily if worn without the bulky closures.

Several jewelry styles are far better suited to the nostril, and each has its pros and cons. The way jewelry rests on the nose is closely connected to the placement and the angle of the piercing. Set gemstones and geometric or curvilinear shapes in various metals are extremely popular ornaments for this area. Many of these are flat in the back, where they attach to the post. For the jewelry to sit correctly, this must be factored in with the piercing's angle and the shape of your anatomy. On some noses, the same piercing angle may work for both a ring and a stud. On others, a single preferred jewelry style must be selected, and the piercing angled to suit it.

NOSTRIL PIERCING: THE NOSTRIL SCREW

The nostril screw is a stud modeled after a traditional East Indian design. The ornament displayed on the exterior rests atop a straight wire post that passes through the piercing; the tail terminates in a curl that rests flat against the interior of your nostril. This keeps the jewelry in place without requiring a backing. When properly sized and shaped to fit you, the jewelry is comfortable and is not visible inside your nose.

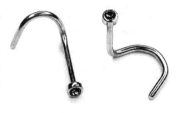

Nostril screws with bezel-set gems

Pre-bent nostril screws do not take into consideration whether the jewelry will be worn on your left or right side, or the individual thickness and shape of your nose. Ill-fitting nostril screws can cause severe problems, including embedding, tissue damage, and substantial discomfort. Your jewelry should be bent or adjusted to your anatomy.

NOSTRIL PIERCING: THE FLATBACK

A flat disc backing is attached to the post, which minimizes the amount of jewelry inside the nose, and eliminates the need to bend or adjust its contours. This press-fit style is versatile, as countless different gems, shapes, and other ornaments can be interchanged. This excellent option is wildly popular, and it is also extensively used for ears. Your piercer should initially insert a longer post to accommodate the expected amount of swelling. They should advise you to return for a swap to a shorter piece once it subsides, usually four to eight weeks after piercing. Ninety percent of piercers surveyed use this style of jewelry.

NOSTRIL PIERCING: THE L-BEND STYLE

Some piercees prefer a modified nostril screw, the *L-bend*, which lacks the curl on the inside portion of the wire. This makes the jewelry easier to insert (which is convenient if you change yours frequently), but it is also more likely to fall out. After you are healed, this style can work well if you are careful not to dislodge it. A standard earring post won't be long enough to form into an L-bend; specialized jewelry is still required. About one-third of piercers surveyed use these regularly.

NOSTRIL PIERCING: THE NOSE BONE STYLE

The *nose bone* is a short, straight post that consists of a gem or other ornament worn on the exterior and a small ball (approximately one-half to a full gauge thicker than the post) on the inside. This requires you to stretch the piercing somewhat to insert and remove the jewelry, which has the potential to damage your tissue. They work in healed piercings only if your skin is pliable. If not, changing them can damage your piercing. The nose bone is not a suitable design for initial jewelry.

NOSTRIL PIERCING: THE RING

Half of the piercers surveyed won't use rings initially, as it can be harder to heal with them, especially if you have a thicker nostril. The higher the piercing is situated on your nose, the larger the ring must be to fit. A ⅜-inch ring is an average diameter for this area; to wear it, your piercing must be placed just shy of that distance from the edge of your nostril—unless the channel angles downward a little on the inside. If the slant is overly steep, a ring will stick out too far from your nose. If you start with a stud but want the option to wear ring-style jewelry later, carefully plan the height and angle of the placement with your piercer.

NOSTRIL PIERCING: PLACEMENT

The traditional placement for a nostril piercing is just below the crease line on the side of the nose. A big smile accentuates this feature to help pinpoint the spot. This area is often thinner than the rest of the nose, so it may heal faster and feel less tender when pierced. The jewelry will rest in a natural niche, where it nestles most gracefully. It tends to be aesthetically pleasing when the placement of the piercing forms a relatively equilateral triangular shape with the opening of your nostril from end to end.

Depending on your preferences, other placements are also possible: higher or lower, closer to the tip of your nose or to your face. The backing of a nostril screw or flatback will be visible if the piercing is too low, even with appropriately sized jewelry. Multiple nostril piercings are another possibility. Due to space constraints, you will achieve the most attractive, comfortable results if you decide on an overall plan before your first piercing is made.

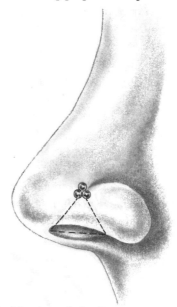

Traditional nostril piercing placement with the "pleasing triangle"

ALTERNATIVE NOSTRIL PIERCING PLACEMENT: HIGH NOSTRIL

This variation is placed much higher on the nose in the softest, thinnest part of the upper cartilage—but must not rest right against the bone. Matched pairs are typical. The piercings must sit at a 90-degree angle to the tissue. Scrunching up your nose can show your piercer the lowest-motion spot, which will be easiest to heal. Nevertheless, healing here is still likely to take longer than in the traditional nostril piercing region. Bring any eyewear to the studio to make sure glasses won't be in the way. They can irritate these piercings and make them very difficult to heal. Flatbacks are the jewelry of choice; a ring is not an option for this placement. Slightly thicker jewelry (16 or 14 gauge) may be preferable in this placement.

Some initial bleeding is possible, and more swelling than with traditional nostril piercings should be expected. You will likely experience a rocky healing course if you mistreat these piercings at all. A little over three-quarters of piercers surveyed offer this placement.

ALTERNATIVE NOSTRIL PIERCING PLACEMENT: FORWARD-FACING

Also called *front-facing nostril piercing*, or *mantis*, these are rare compared to other placements. They are done in pairs toward the tip of the nose. A 16-gauge bar of 5/16-inch or 3/8-inch length is the usual jewelry, with a small disc or ball on the inside. Depending on a person's anatomy, the appearance of symmetry can be tricky to achieve in this location. Extra swelling is possible in this area as well. Seek a top-notch pro for either of these alternative nostril-piercing placements, because they are especially challenging.

NOSTRIL PIERCING: PROCEDURE

The process could make your eye water—usually the one on the same side as the piercing. A small percentage of nostril piercings bleed freely for several minutes, though many bleed a single drop, and others not at all.

One method is to brace the tissue with a receiving tube or other support inside the nostril and pierce from the outside. Alternatively, it may be done with a freehand technique, often piercing from the inside. Some piercers use forceps, but the tool should not be clamped tightly onto the dense tissue. Optimally, your piercer will perform the compression technique (see page 74) to reattach your tissue, help prevent bumps, and stop any bleeding.

NOSTRIL PIERCING: HEALING AND TROUBLESHOOTING

The dense tissue takes months to heal, but the nose is less subject to trauma than some other pierced areas. Keep eyewear clean and don't let glasses rest on the jewelry. Avoid getting makeup, lotion, and other skin care products in your piercing.

Some localized redness or swelling is common during initial healing. If your jewelry fits correctly, it will accommodate a normal amount of inflammation. If the end appears to be sinking into your tissue, see a piercer as soon as possible to avoid embedding, which can require surgical removal! If you can't get in right away, try using a tiny piece of Micropore paper tape (available at drug stores) to keep the head of the ornament propped above the surface. Use a disinfected hole punch or scissors to cut a small circle in the tape. Snip a slit to the center and slide the piece around the post; then stick it down to cover the tissue. If this method proves helpful, change the tape daily until the swelling subsides and the skin has shrunk back sufficiently to prevent a recurrence.

If your jewelry has made a substantial hole by sinking well into your skin, you may have to wear a large flat end for the remainder of your healing. If switching to a stud with a longer post, a bigger head, or both does not resolve the issue, you'll need to wear a ring until the crater is gone.

NOSTRIL PIERCING: CHANGING JEWELRY

Once your piercing has fully healed, with a little patience and practice, you may be able to change your nostril jewelry yourself. However, many piercees prefer to get professional assistance at a studio. A nostril screw must be twisted *and* pulled to remove it, following the curve of the corkscrew. Most nostril screws are tiny and can be tricky to handle, especially at first. The hard part can be passing the tail all the way through the channel before it curves. Swapping the ornament on a flat-back post may be preferable since the jewelry doesn't need to come out of the hole, but this can be somewhat challenging to do on yourself.

NOSTRIL PIERCING: STRETCHING

Nostril piercings are challenging to stretch, but most wearers are happy with a small hole. If you have plans for a large one, take your time, and be aware that the lack of elasticity in this dense tissue may make the enlargement permanent. The comments in "Ear Cartilage Piercing: Stretching," page 109, also apply to the nostril.

NOSTRIL PIERCING: CONCEALMENT

There is no safe initial jewelry that will be completely invisible in a nostril piercing. Some options are very discreet, however. A tiny, flat, matte-finish disc can look like a freckle or blend in with your skin, depending on your complexion. Clear and skin-tone glass and quartz nostril screws are available for concealment, but they are not typically worn in healing piercings, since the size and shape cannot be customized. Use caution even when trying them in healed piercings, as they can be fragile and could irritate if they don't fit well.

Silicone retainers in an array of flesh tones are also an option for post-healing concealment. Since they are quite soft and more forgiving than the harder materials, they can also be worn for safety during activities with a risk of impact to the area.

NOSTRIL PIERCING: RETIRING

Many piercees find that nostril piercings do not stay open without jewelry in place. The hole can shrink in the time it takes you to remove, wash, and dry your jewelry and try to put it back in place. If you like the piercing, leave jewelry in at all times.

An abandoned nostril piercing should have minimal scarring if you wore the usual small-gauge jewelry and your healing was uneventful. The residual mark ordinarily resembles an enlarged pore. Troubled healing could leave substantial scarring.

THE SEPTUM PIERCING

- **Description:** Placed in the tissue that divides the nostrils
- **Healing time:** 4 to 8 weeks or longer
- **Initial jewelry style:** Ring-style, including a clicker or seam-ring variation, or a circular barbell or septum retainer
- **Initial jewelry gauge:** 16 and 14 gauge are popular, 12 gauge is suitable, and 10 gauge only for large anatomy
- **Initial jewelry size:** A 5/16-inch ring diameter is common, but 3/8 inch is needed for some noses; 7/16 inch may be an option, depending on anatomy and aesthetic preferences.

Historically, the nasal septum piercing was associated with aboriginal peoples who sported bones or feathers from the center of the nose. When modern piercing began in the West, septum jewelry was worn by leather-clad punks, radicals, and eccentrics. More recently, the septum piercing has turned the corner from counterculture to haute couture.

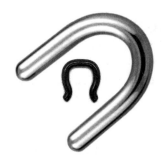

The best part? The jewelry can virtually disappear while you're at work, school, or other places it isn't acceptable. The remarkable secret of the septum piercing is that—on most people—it can be concealed inside your nose with a retainer so that only your dentist knows about it. (If someone looks up your nose in bright light, the jewelry will be visible.)

Two styles of septum retainers; the small one is actual size

SEPTUM PIERCING: PLACEMENT AND JEWELRY

A traditionally placed septum piercing is not in the cartilage that divides the nostrils. Instead, it is in a *sweet spot* (optimal location) in the soft, membranous tissue just below the cartilage but above the skin. On most people, this will be well up into the nose, toward the tip. This placement passes through minimal tissue; in fact, it is some of the body's thinnest pierceable skin. Piercing in the correct location allows for comfort (both during the procedure and for the wearing of jewelry), aesthetics, ease of healing, and maximal concealment.

The size of the septum's sweet spot does not necessarily correlate with the overall dimensions of the area; a large nose can have a small pierceable zone. Rely on your piercer for input about the initial jewelry gauge.

Unfortunately, not all piercers are aware of the ideal site or the technique needed to pierce it. Even slight asymmetry can make it very difficult to achieve a straight piercing. The proper position for the piercing is very specific, and on some individuals, it is extremely small. The piercing goes into the hidden recesses of the nose, so it is tricky for your piercer to see what they are doing. Even accomplished professionals sometimes find that the desired results are elusive. Seek an expert if you want a well-placed, aesthetically pleasing septum piercing.

If you can openly wear facial jewelry, a captive or fixed bead ring is suitable, as are certain ornamented seam rings or clickers. They must be designed so that a seam or hinge can't rotate into the piercing channel. The size should be proportionate to your nose and not so large as to interfere with eating and drinking. A ½-inch diameter is a reasonable maximum for most people. A very large, heavy ring could be dangerous to your front teeth when you run or jump!

A septum retainer is effective for concealment because the U-shaped piece of metal flips up inside your nostrils. A retainer is not the best initial jewelry because it can get knocked out during bathing, nose-blowing, or sleeping. Short plugs with O-rings or barbells with tiny ends are sometimes used as retainers, but these are difficult to clean and aren't as concealing, so they are not among the top options.

The circular barbell is functional and versatile because it can be hidden like a septum retainer if you are not always free to reveal your piercing. It is also attractive when you want to put your jewelry on display. A small diameter (usually 5/16- or 3/8-inch) circular barbell is superior for concealment, comfort, and safety. The gap between the two balls or ornamental ends allows you to flip up your ring and hide it in your nose, but an overly large diameter will distort your nostrils from the inside. On most people, a circular barbell will be as hidden as a septum retainer; however, if your nostrils flare higher than your septum, some metal will show. If you require maximum concealment, charcoal-colored niobium is best, because it is darker and less reflective than shiny steel or titanium.

Your piercer can adjust the gap on your circular barbell so you can flip the jewelry up with the ends still in place. It should have a snug fit when inside your nose, so it won't slip down at inopportune moments, though this makes it a little challenging to change its position.

SEPTUM PIERCING: ANATOMICAL ISSUES

A *deviated septum* is a common condition of displaced tissue between the nostrils. There is often a raised ridge on one side and a concave crease on the other, and this may be right in the area where the piercing should be worn. It might not be impossible to get a straight piercing if this is the shape of your anatomy, but it is a lot more challenging. The jewelry tends to sit further into the crease, and the other side rides up on the ridge so that the ring rests askew. Whether you have a deviated septum or the piercing simply turns out crooked, using intentional migration, you may be able to coax it straight—if it was placed in the sweet spot. During the first few weeks of healing, use clean or gloved fingers to twist the jewelry in the desired direction ten to twenty times a day. The opposite can also happen, so don't sleep with your nose pressed into a pillow during healing, or you can turn a perfect piercing crooked!

If you have had an injury, cosmetic surgery, or other alteration to your anatomy, let your piercer know. Excess bleeding is sometimes a consequence of piercing post-surgical nasal anatomy. If you have a deviated septum, an asymmetrical nose, or otherwise challenging anatomy, this piercing might still be worth a try. If your piercer is willing, you trust them, and you *really* want the piercing, go ahead; it won't leave a visible mark. The worst-case scenario is that you'll end up taking it out afterward. Perhaps you can negotiate with your piercer for a refund if the results aren't satisfactory. If an expert believes you are anatomically unsuited to a septum piercing and an acceptable outcome cannot be achieved, consider a different placement.

SEPTUM PIERCING: PROCEDURE

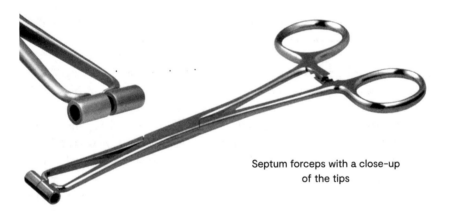

Septum forceps with a close-up
of the tips

After cleaning, your piercer may mark a guideline on your nose's undersurface to help them visualize the correct location during the procedure. At the very least, they will need to put gloved fingers or tools like a tube, insertion taper, and/or swab(s) into your nose to feel the septum for the proper spot to pierce.

For the procedure, you may be positioned anywhere from seated upright to a *supine* position (on your back) on a table. You might be asked to hang your head back over the edge of the table. It is not particularly comfortable to hyperextend your neck this way, but it provides an excellent view of the area from above and behind you—and you shouldn't be kept that way for long.

Some piercers use an NRT for septum piercings, and others work freehand. Tissue manipulation can be invaluable, especially if there is any irregularity in the area. The nasal septum has a soft tissue membrane on each side, and this structure is quite mobile. If the tools aren't seated securely, they can slip during the procedure, causing a crooked piercing.

Another option is *septum forceps,* which have a short piece of receiving tube soldered onto each end; these clamp onto the area. Precise positioning of this tool is crucial for a well-placed piercing. Regular Pennington forceps are not suited to the septum because they painfully crush the skin in the center of the nose.

When positioned in the sweet spot, piercees seldom describe septum piercings as intense, and often report feeling little more than pressure. However, if your local tissue is thicker than average, you have altered or challenging anatomy, or your piercing is placed incorrectly, it could feel much more tender.

SEPTUM PIERCING: HEALING AND TROUBLESHOOTING

Your eyes may water, and your nose may run for several minutes following the piercing. Some piercees describe feeling the urge to sneeze, but they seldom do. Of course, bleeding is possible, too, but it rarely lasts longer than your visit to the studio.

If your piercing comes out crooked and intentional migration doesn't seem feasible to straighten it, your piercer may offer to remove the jewelry and pierce you again. It is advisable to be repierced right away only if the first placement was very far from where it should have been. Otherwise, a redo in the same session is apt to go right back in the same place, unless the entry and exit sides are swapped.

SEPTUM PIERCING: SEPTUM STENCH

After the first month or two, you may encounter *septum stench* (the pungent, rotten odor from the sebum that accumulates in piercing channels). It is found in healed piercings (and hair follicles) throughout the body (see "Normal Piercing Secretions," page 224). However, because your septum piercing is inside your nose, the distinctive aroma is noticeable when sebum is present. Don't worry, only you can smell it!

The regular use of soap and water will help to diminish the smell. Wash and rinse the jewelry as you rotate it under running water. Some piercees find natural materials such as wood or horn are superior for minimizing odor.

SEPTUM PIERCING: CHANGING JEWELRY

Following the initial eight weeks, septum piercings are usually well healed, and the jewelry can be changed. The main challenge of swapping septum jewelry is that you cannot readily see where the piercing is situated; therefore, it is done mostly by feel. Since the channel is short, once you find the entrance, the exit is generally easy to locate.

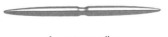

A septum spike

A *septum spike* is a fun and dramatic alternative jewelry style. It is a straight piece with tapered ends that comes in different lengths and materials. Clicker rings are an excellent option for healed septum piercings since they're easier to open and close than captive rings or threaded pieces. They're suitable for frequent jewelry changes, but any jewelry that you must bend for insertion and removal (such as a *seam ring* style) should be worn only if you can leave the jewelry in for long periods.

SEPTUM PIERCING: STRETCHING

Septum piercings are much easier to stretch if the hole isn't located in the cartilage or too low in the surface skin. The septum can routinely be enlarged safely by one gauge as early as four months following piercing. With a little patience, you can usually expand these piercings by several sizes. But, following a few stretches, you may reach a point where the space between the cartilage and the surface tissue is filled. Any subsequent expansion will become considerably more challenging. You might easily get to 6 or 4 gauge before running into this difficulty. When you stretch a septum piercing to these dimensions, your profile may be permanently altered by a visible hole. This is likely when you enlarge too quickly and lose tissue elasticity.

When your piercing is improperly placed, enlarging it can be problematic. If it is located in the cartilage, stretching will be very difficult. If the piercing is in your nose's surface tissue, stretching can cause rejection and leave an unsightly split in your skin.

SEPTUM PIERCING: RETIRING

The septum is one of few piercings that does not leave a visible mark if abandoned unless it was improperly positioned or stretched to jumbo size. If you remove your jewelry after healing, the channel is likely to remain open. Though, as usual, there is a tendency for the hole to shrink somewhat. There is no harm in having a septum piercing that remains viable but empty. Some people insert jewelry occasionally and are able to maintain the piercing without regularly wearing anything in it.

ALTERNATIVE NOSE PIERCING PLACEMENTS

There are a few rare piercings of the nose. The *septril* puts a single ornament along the midline, anywhere from the tip of the nose to its underside, between the nostrils. Having a large, stretched septum piercing is a prerequisite because the backing of a bar post rests inside it. It is the least risky since it is not a surface piercing. The next two are, so they're not highly recommended. If healing issues occur, permanent, disfiguring scarring of the nose is possible. One is the *Austin bar*, which looks like forward-facing nostril piercings, but is actually a horizontal surface piercing at the tip of the nose. The vertical version in this region is called a *rhino piercing*. Curved bars are the usual jewelry for both variations. Finally, the *nasallang* is a horizontal piercing across the nose. It passes through both nostrils and the cartilage of the septum. A barbell connects the three structures together, which might curtail certain facial expressions. It can be difficult to access inside, especially when the placement is high on the nose, so extra diligence is required for cleaning and maintenance. A pair of nostril piercings is much safer.

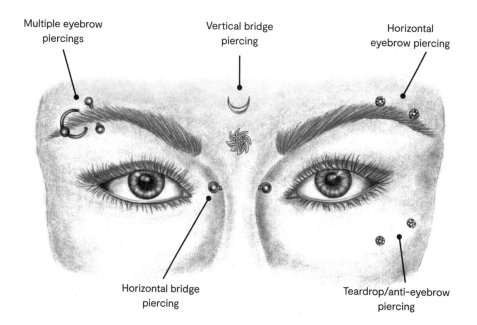

Multiple eyebrow piercings

Vertical bridge piercing

Horizontal eyebrow piercing

Horizontal bridge piercing

Teardrop/anti-eyebrow piercing

THE EYEBROW PIERCING

- Healing time: 6 to 8 weeks
- Initial jewelry style: Curved barbell, mini curved bar, or ring-style
- Initial jewelry gauge: 18 gauge minimum, but 16 gauge is most common; 14 gauge for full builds
- Initial jewelry size: Minimum diameter 5/16 inch, commonly 3/8 inch

Eyebrow piercings lack any known historical precedent. They were once the province of rebels and punk rockers, but now elegant jewelry can elevate this piercing to a stylish, sophisticated adornment. It draws attention to the windows of the soul in a whole different way.

Though essentially a surface piercing, when appropriate jewelry is properly placed in pliable tissue, rejection is rare. Complications often occur if the brow is not sufficiently padded, which causes excessive pressure of the jewelry against the bone. Wearing a piece that is too heavy for the delicate tissue, or a straight bar instead of a curved one, can also be problematic. If your skin does not seem ample or pinch up well in the area you would like to be pierced, you should consider a different placement, especially if you are concerned about visible scarring.

EYEBROW PIERCING: PLACEMENT

There are many options for placing eyebrow piercings. The standard spot is toward the outer third or quarter of the brow. While referred to as "vertical," it is usually most aesthetically pleasing when situated more perpendicular to the eyebrow with a slant mirroring the angle from the outer corner of the eye to the outside edge of the brow. When placed *too* vertically, the jewelry can look awkward; and, if a ring is worn, it will stick straight out. Many eyebrows are narrower than the channel, in which case, the piercing looks balanced when situated equidistant from the brow hairs.

In a more central location or vertical orientation, curved bars are preferable. A horizontal alternative may be situated slightly above, below, or among the hairs and should be angled to suit the anatomy. (The two basic forms are still referred to as "vertical" and "horizontal," even though a slant is usual for either.) Jewelry can be worn anywhere along the eyebrow, *if* the tissue is plentiful and pliable.

Piercings at the inner edge of the brow, vertical or angled, are less prevalent. One challenge is that this tissue is often tighter and more challenging to pinch, and therefore harder to pierce and to heal. Multiple piercings are possible, and the variations are limited only by your anatomy, imagination, and your piercer's skill.

EYEBROW PIERCING: PROCEDURE

Eyebrow piercings can be performed freehand, with forceps, or using a receiving tube. The key to a comfortable experience is to prepare the area with tissue manipulation first, especially if your skin is at all taut.

If clamps are applied correctly or not used at all, most piercees find the eyebrow to be a relatively painless piercing. Plenty of piercees have said that plucking or waxing the brows causes more severe or unpleasant sensations. When I had my horizontal eyebrow piercing done, I described it as a "warm fuzzy" feeling (for a piercing).

EYEBROW PIERCING: HEALING AND TROUBLESHOOTING

Eyebrow piercings are apt to bruise, bleed, or swell afterward, which may persist for several days. Immediately following the procedure, a small percentage of eyebrow piercings swell considerably.

You may be concerned about sweat getting into your eyebrow piercing, but this is not problematic with proper hygiene and aftercare. If you need to mop your brow, pat the pierced area gently with clean paper towels or tissues. It is essential to avoid getting skin care products such as moisturizers, facial cleansers, and cosmetics on the piercing during healing. It is safest to keep them an area about the size of a quarter away from the jewelry. Make sure tweezers are clean before plucking eyebrows.

EYEBROW PIERCING: CHANGING JEWELRY

Once your eyebrow piercing is healed, you may be able to change the jewelry yourself, but it can be tricky: your hands obscure your view, you must manipulate something right above your eye, and your image is reversed in the mirror.

The eyebrow piercing can be challenging to conceal, but a snug barbell with tiny 3/32-inch (2.5 mm) balls will minimize visibility, and anodized titanium can blend with certain skin tones.

EYEBROW PIERCING: STRETCHING

This piercing is not suited to stretching. Only the meatiest of brows can support jewelry as large as 12 gauge. On some, 14 gauge proves too heavy. This is *not* a spot where bigger is better. I've seen piercees attempt to enlarge eyebrow piercings and regret it when the piercings rebelled and, in some cases, rejected.

EYEBROW PIERCING: RETIRING

A healed eyebrow piercing is likely to leave some visible evidence of a scar if you remove the jewelry. However, if the holes were within or close to the hairs, the marks might be partially obscured. Unsightly scarring is rare unless you experienced healing complications or stretched thicker than average.

OTHER FACIAL PIERCINGS: TEARDROP/ANTI-EYEBROW, BRIDGE, VERTICAL BRIDGE, AND SIDEBURN

Several less-common piercings are done in the facial tissue. They aren't considered traditional placements, and they are not as easy to heal as the more popular ones. Fewer people are anatomically suited to them; many have tissue that is too taut for success. If the idea of a visible mark on your face is unappealing, you should not attempt any of these variations because they are more prone to rejection and scarring. They are all essentially surface piercings, but as above-the-neck placements, they are addressed here briefly. In any delicate facial tissue, small, flat barbell ends are preferred.

TEARDROP/ANTI-EYEBROW PIERCING
- **Description:** Placed in the tissue atop the highest crest of the cheekbone toward the outer edge of the eye. It is like a traditional eyebrow piercing but flipped down below the eye instead of above. The angle may be diagonal, horizontal, or any orientation in which the tissue can be pinched and, therefore, pierced.
- **Differences:** In this area, it might be preferable to have a slightly narrower piercing channel than is generally used for the bridge variations described next.
- **Healing time:** 3 to 4 months or longer
- **Initial jewelry style:** Mini curved bar or surface bar
- **Initial jewelry gauge:** 16 or 14 gauge
- **Initial jewelry size:** Minimum ⅜ inch

THE BRIDGE OR MID-BROW PIERCING
- **Description:** The bridge is a horizontal piercing through the *glabella* (tissue between the brows) or the *nasion* (between the eyes). It ranges from as high as the top of the eyebrows to the bridge of the nose. Multiples are rare but sometimes possible. Most piercers surveyed (89 percent) perform bridge piercings.
- **Differences:** Jewelry that is a little thicker than some of the other facial areas may be preferable, and healing time may be longer.
- **Healing time:** 4 to 6 months or longer
- **Initial jewelry style:** Straight barbell
- **Initial jewelry gauge:** 14 or 12 gauge
- **Initial jewelry size:** Minimum ½ inch to ¾ inch or even ⅞ inch
- **Warning:** Even if the jewelry is in your field of vision, it won't make you go cross-eyed. But there are other dangers, including a relatively high rate of rejection and scarring. Far more critical, however, is having insufficient padding between your jewelry and the structures beneath. Direct pressure can cause diminished blood supply to the bone. This may lead to bone density loss and, in a worst-case scenario, bone *necrosis* (death).[2] If you don't have plenty of pliable tissue, a bridge piercing is not advisable. Visible pitted scars are likely if you abandon this piercing.

VERTICAL BRIDGE OR THIRD EYE
- **Description:** A vertical surface piercing placed between the eyebrows or somewhat above them. If the tissue is pliable enough, it may be placed slightly higher, on the lower portion of the forehead.

- o **Healing time:** 4 to 6 months
- o **Initial jewelry style:** Surface bar
- o **Initial jewelry gauge:** 16 or 14 gauge
- o **Initial jewelry size:** From ⅜ inch to ½ inch
- o **Warning:** The same hazards of horizontal piercing in this region also apply (see the warning for the bridge piercing, above)

SIDEBURN PIERCING

- o **Description:** A vertical piercing on the facial surface in front of the tragus.
- o **Healing time:** 4 to 6 months
- o **Initial jewelry style:** Surface bar (a regular curved bar is not usually suited to this placement)
- o **Initial jewelry gauge:** 16 or 14 gauge
- o **Initial jewelry size:** Minimum 7⁄16 inch
- o **Warning:** These are apt to bleed more than many other areas and may scar significantly. Your piercer should observe while you open and close your mouth and make facial expressions because migration and other issues are likely when these are placed in an area with much movement.

THE POINT

Earlobe piercings are among the fastest and easiest to heal. The nearby cartilage of the ear presents plenty of options and also more challenges. Even so, many piercees find these piercings to be well worth having. You may want to go for the total package and have a customized, curated ear with multiple piercings.

Facial anatomy is relatively welcoming to piercings when principles for appropriate placement and jewelry are followed; but give careful consideration because they can leave visible scarring if abandoned later (except for the nasal septum). An above-the-neck piercing can enhance your appearance and effectively customize the way you face the world.

12

KISS OF THE NEEDLE: TONGUE AND ORAL PIERCINGS

Before attempting to clean or care for any oral piercing, carefully review and follow the instructions in "Aftercare for Oral Piercings," page 243.

ORAL PIERCING RISKS

You should be aware of the dangers before you decide to get an oral piercing. Once you know what they are, you can take precautions to minimize them, but these piercings are not risk-free. If you have a history of bad teeth or problem gums, a tongue or lip piercing is probably inadvisable. Studies show that piercees are not being advised about the risks, and their piercers are to blame for not educating them appropriately beforehand, so they can make informed decisions.[1]

Contrary to what people might think, infection rates for oral piercings are low, despite the large number of bacteria present in the mouth.[2] The oral cavity is not prone to infection because the lymphatic system, mucous membranes, and saliva provide formidable defenses. The most significant hazard is damage to teeth, gums, and underlying oral structures from jewelry. The delicate tooth enamel will get cracked or chipped if you play with your jewelry. Biting or clicking jewelry often or hard—for fun or by accident—results in *wrecking ball fractures* (small cracks in the teeth).[3] Continuous pressure from hard metal can diminish the density of the underlying bone over time.[4] Gum recession is caused by jewelry that is too big or improperly placed, or from the excessive rubbing of hard metal against the delicate soft tissue of the palate or gums.[5] Enamel, bone, and gum tissue *do not* regenerate. Damage to these oral structures is irreversible and can be critical.

You dramatically reduce the likelihood of complications when you adhere to accepted practices, wear properly sized jewelry that does not rub inside your mouth, and avoid playing with it. For more information, see the APP's brochure, "Oral Piercing Risks and Safety Measures" (www.safepiercing.org).

THE TONGUE PIERCING

- **Healing time:** 4 to 8 weeks
- **Initial jewelry style:** Straight barbell
- **Initial jewelry gauge:** Most commonly 14 and 12 gauge; sometimes 10 gauge
- **Initial jewelry size:** Bar length is anatomically dependent and must be long enough to allow for swelling. Initial jewelry for centrally placed piercings ranges from 9/16 inch for slim tongues to 7/8 inch for thick ones; a 3/4-inch length is common. An 11/16-inch post is a good fit for many builds, and others need 13/16 inch, though not all piercers stock these in-between sizes.

The tongue is a unique body part because it is situated inside the mouth—the tool with which we express ourselves, a center for sensuality, and the way we ingest our sustenance. A tongue piercing can be private or public, and it can be fun alone or with a friend.

If asked whether tongue piercing is erotic, some piercees would say, "Yes, absolutely!" but an equal number would earnestly respond, "Certainly not." None of these people would be insincere; they simply differ in their perspectives. A tongue piercing is what you make of it. For some, it is merely an ornament; for others, it is a useful sensual device. The wearing of tongue jewelry will not magically transform you into an oral virtuoso, but it will provide you with an additional tool, should you desire to use it.

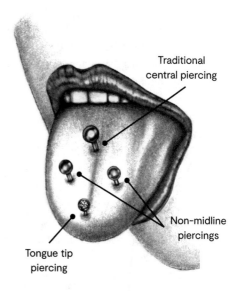

Traditional central piercing

Non-midline piercings

Tongue tip piercing

A DIFFERENT FUNCTION

Nowadays, everyone knows about tongue piercings, but they were unheard of in the 1980s. I'd tell people that my tongue jewelry was an acupuncture stud for weight control. I explained that the metal stud diminished my appetite, satisfied my palate, and prevented me from eating too quickly. Everyone believed me, and nobody *ever* asked, "Didn't that hurt?" Instead, they would inquire with interest, "Does it work?"

I'd share my secret with people who seemed open-minded: I actually did it for fun!

TONGUE PIERCING: PLACEMENT

The piercing can be positioned nearly anywhere along the tongue, from the tip to the back. Before marking, your piercer should carefully evaluate your anatomy. Bring up any considerations regarding concealment, and whether you have thoughts about placement, or plans to stretch or add more piercings later. Multiple piercings are not possible for all tongues.

A central position is popular because it minimizes visibility and keeps the jewelry well away from the teeth but still allows for fun and function. Piercing along the midline is safest. The tongue's major veins are visible underneath, distant from the center, alongside the nerves and arteries. Vessels are seldom located on the midline, but if one is detected, it must be avoided.

On standard anatomy, the piercing can rest right in the center, generally just in front of the attachment of the *lingual frenulum* (the thin band of tissue that attaches the tongue to the floor of the mouth). If your web is exceptionally thick or connects farther forward than usual, the underside of the piercing can be placed just a little off to one side. However, if you physically cannot stick your tongue out, then a piercing will be difficult or impossible to perform. When the lingual frenulum is tight and restricts tongue movement, this condition is called *tongue-tied* (or *ankyloglossia*, from the Greek for "crooked tongue"). A simple medical procedure can often correct it, but this is outside of the scope of services piercers are permitted to perform.

For safety and comfort, the piercing is commonly placed a bit farther forward underneath. This will cause the top of the barbell to slant back slightly toward the upper palate's highest point, where you have the most space for it in your oral cavity. This tilt also prevents the jewelry from standing straight up in your mouth, which could jam the bottom ball against your lower palate. It should not have too steep an angle, or that ball will rub behind your lower front teeth.

If concealment is a crucial factor, discuss your concerns and goals with a competent piercer. Allow them to help you select the best placement and jewelry to minimize visibility for your anatomy and circumstances. Often the right jewelry choice will be the most effective way to disguise the piercing. Using a certain shade of anodized titanium disc, M&M end, or setting on a pink coral cabochon can blend in nicely. Concealment jewelry can be changed, but placing the piercing farther back than usual in an attempt to obscure it would be permanent.

HELPFUL HINT

You may find your gag reflex kicks in when you stick your tongue out with your mouth open. If you can push it out of your mouth far enough for marking and piercing while keeping your lips closed, this usually solves the problem.

TONGUE PIERCING: ANATOMY AND CHOICE OF JEWELRY

The initial barbell should be just long enough to accommodate anticipated swelling. An excessively long bar can cause severe damage to delicate intraoral structures, so wearing the correct size is vital. Your piercer must weigh several elements to figure the length that will be ideal for initial healing. The farther back the piercing is placed, the greater the expected swelling. Piercings close to the tip are not inclined to expand as much, so 1/16 inch extra may be sufficient. Thick tongues are apt to swell more than slim ones. Share any history of swelling from previous piercings or injuries to help pinpoint the measurement. Steer clear of any piercer who puts a "standard-length" barbell in every tongue piercing. Anatomy is variable and must be evaluated on an individual basis for a safe fit.

When you stick out your tongue, it might look thin, and your new jewelry might seem long. But the piercing heals with your tongue inside your mouth, where the anatomy becomes thicker and more wedge shaped. It may also appear that a proposed placement is close to the tip, but when your tongue rests inside, you will find that the location is much farther back than it seemed.

Wearing balls made of an approved polymer (see "Jewelry Materials for Initial Piercings," page 91) inside the mouth could reduce the risk of damage to teeth. This is prudent if you have veneers or caps or wear dentures, bridges, or other oral appliances. Inert polymers are also a better choice if you are concerned about oral health or have a tendency to play with your jewelry, because they are softer than metal. Acrylic is not considered safe; therefore, it is not recommended, especially in oral piercings.

A small (3/16-inch) ball is a safe size for underneath, where space is limited. Some piercees prefer a disc on the bottom or an M&M end. This shape distributes pressure more evenly and may be safer and more comfortable for the soft palate's delicate tissues. A matching size or slightly larger (7/32- or 1/4-inch) ball or gem can be worn on the top, where there is more room for jewelry.

ALTERNATIVE TONGUE PIERCING PLACEMENT: TONGUE TIP

A piercing within the first 1/2 inch of the tongue is considered a *tongue tip* piercing. It can be worn as close as 5/16 inch from the end of the tongue. Due to the distribution of nerve endings, this spot is more sensitive than a traditional placement. You can try out a ring after healing, but a barbell is preferred initially.

Speaking clearly with jewelry at the tip of your tongue is possible, but getting accustomed to it is more challenging than with a central placement. A ring or bar is more apt to get caught between your teeth when the piercing is so close to them. You must be extremely careful to avoid biting the jewelry when you eat, especially at first. These piercings are rare, and they're riskier than those placed farther back.

ALTERNATIVE TONGUE PIERCING PLACEMENT: MULTIPLE PIERCINGS

Piercees with a personal desire, suitable anatomy, and an accomplished piercer can get multiple tongue piercings. Planning is needed to make the best use of the limited space, even on those with very long tongues. More than three along the midline is possible for the few who are lingually endowed. Two tongue piercings can be done in the same session if there is enough space between them, and the first one does not swell significantly. Getting more than two at a time is not advisable due to the likelihood of excessive swelling and discomfort.

The surface area is greater on top of the tongue, so multiple piercings in a straight row there might rest in a cluster underneath. Depending on anatomy, arrangements for multiple piercings include one (or more) along the midline plus a pair of piercings off to the sides. Some dedicated individuals wear piercings configured in triangle, diamond, and other shapes.

ALTERNATIVE TONGUE PIERCING (NON-MIDLINE) PLACEMENT: SNAKE BITES, VENOMS, VIPERS, OR VIPER BITES

These terms may be used for a pair of tongue (or lip) piercings placed off to either side of the midline. Before deciding to get such an arrangement, take a close look at the underside of your tongue with a bright light to familiarize yourself with any visible vessels. Note that they are present even if you can't see them. Your piercer must be extremely precise, or you risk a punctured vein, nerve, or artery. Non-midline tongue piercings are significantly riskier than centrally positioned ones. After the procedure, side-placement piercings are apt to bleed more, even when a major vessel is not nicked.

Off-center tongue piercings can take longer to heal and become accustomed to than a midline piercing. Depending on where you want them to be on the top, they may need to angle somewhat inward or outward underneath to avoid the vital structures. However, if the slant is too steep, complications can occur. Excess scar tissue may develop, or the jewelry can get caught between your teeth if it rests too close to them.

TONGUE PIERCING: PROCEDURE

First, your mouth should be prepped with mouthwash, and/or your tongue scrubbed with gauze, which may be saturated with an oral rinse. Alternatively, you could be asked to swish with plain water or saline solution. Next, your piercer will mark the placement on the top and bottom of your tongue, commonly using a single-use surgical pen.

A seated position is safest for the procedure. Tipping your head back isn't helpful because it draws your tongue into your mouth; but tilting your head forward slightly and moving your chin toward your chest helps to extend your tongue. If you are reclining, your tongue must fight gravity; worse, jewelry (or, heaven forbid, the needle!) could be dropped into your throat. A CSR drape can be used to protect the area if you are lying supine, which will help to avoid this risk.

Your tongue should be dried with sterile gauze, making it easier to grasp. Forceps or a freehand procedure are both common techniques for this area. The piercing can be performed successfully from either direction.

When you bite your tongue, you experience a painful crush injury, so some piercees are understandably concerned about the intensity of putting a needle through this part of the body. But a traditional tongue piercing is placed where the nerves primarily transmit signals for taste and temperature. It is more painful to get pierced at the tip or edges of the tongue than in the center.

QUICK TRICK

When internally threaded jewelry is used, a small *transfer pin* can be placed into the lumens of both barbell and needle, creating a single unit. The jewelry is inserted as the piercing is made. The needle and connector easily disassemble, and the second end gets screwed into place; the piercing is complete. This ensures the briefest procedure possible.

I've had more than one observer remark, "Wow! That was *fast*. I was watching, but I missed it." Some piercers work sequentially, piercing first, and then getting the barbell and transferring it in, which takes slightly longer.

TONGUE PIERCING: HEALING AND TROUBLESHOOTING

Sipping cold water from a clean cup immediately after receiving an oral piercing can help minimize initial swelling, and it feels soothing, too.

During the first week, significant swelling, light bleeding, bruising, and tenderness are normal. After that, the swelling should diminish, but some often remains for several weeks. There's no need to panic if you see a whitish discharge coming from your tongue. All healing piercings secrete fluids; however, inside the wet environment of the mouth, the substance doesn't dry to form the crust you often see in other areas.

Don't worry; you *can* eat with a new tongue piercing, but it isn't easy at first. You have the initial swelling to contend with, plus there's unfamiliar jewelry right in the middle of your mouth. Fasting or a liquid diet is not required, though some piercees prefer to eat only soft or blended foods for the first couple of days. Piercings heal better if your body is well nourished, so eat whatever feels comfortable, and in a week or so you should feel back to normal. Follow the instructions in "Healthy Habits for Rapid Healing" (page 229) and these tips for a safe, smooth course:

- Eat *slowly* and take small bites.
- Focus on keeping your tongue level. The jewelry can get between your teeth when it turns.
- Avoid sticky foods like mashed potatoes or oatmeal; they may be soft, but they can be challenging to eat because they adhere to your mouth and jewelry.
- Smoothies, shakes, energy drinks, ice cream, soups, and the like are good menu mainstays.
- Use clean fingers or utensils to place small bites of solid food between your molars. The tongue moves food to the back of the mouth, so food that is already there requires less manipulation.
- Cold and frozen foods are soothing and help to minimize swelling.
- Chewing gum or sucking on candy may be injurious during healing.
- Salty, spicy, acidic, or hot foods and beverages may irritate. (No specific foods need to be avoided, despite various urban myths.)
- A certain amount of speaking is unavoidable, but when your piercing is fresh, try to let your tongue rest as much as possible.
- Sleep with your head elevated to minimize overnight swelling.
- Do not play with your tongue or jewelry!

Plaque can form on oral jewelry just like it does on teeth. Generally, it adheres under the tongue at the juncture of the ball and the post, and on the ball itself. You can use dental floss around the bottom of the post to help keep this area clean. See "Regular Maintenance: Oral Piercings," page 269, for additional cleaning measures you can take once the piercing has healed.

TONGUE PIERCING: CONCEALMENT

Many professionals have successfully worn tongue jewelry in work environments where body modification is not acceptable. Polymer concealment balls, discs, or domes on the shortest post that fits could minimize jewelry visibility. Your tongue piercing is apt to go unnoticed if you avoid opening your mouth wide when you speak.

TONGUE PIERCING: SPEECH PROBLEMS

Your speech will probably be affected during a brief period of accommodation when your piercing is new. After the swelling has gone down (as quickly as three to five days) and you have had a little time to adjust, there is usually no impediment. With a properly placed piercing, speech is seldom altered after a fitted post is inserted.

TONGUE PIERCING: SCAR TISSUE

Scar tissue can appear as a pinkish or whitish raised ring of hardened skin that partially or entirely surrounds one or both openings of your piercing. It is usually temporary if it develops during healing. Most commonly, it is the result of using a harsh care product or too much talking, playing with the jewelry, or other activity. The oral cells regenerate exceptionally quickly, and they tend to go into overdrive if a tongue piercing is traumatized while healing. Limiting tongue activity is very important, so even if your piercing feels fine, take it easy for the first month. Sometimes the issue is caused by unknowingly manipulating the jewelry in your sleep, and this can be problematic to resolve.

TONGUE PIERCING: DOWNSIZING AND CHANGING JEWELRY

It is *absolutely vital* for your oral health that you wear the shortest post that fits once you are healed. In addition to harming teeth, persistent wear of an overly long barbell causes loss of jawbone density and gum recession.[6] These two structures play crucial roles in holding your teeth in your mouth. Your initial post, which has extra length to allow for swelling, must be changed to a shorter one. It doesn't matter if you like the way the long bar feels or looks, or if everything seems okay in your mouth—downsize!

A professional piercer can put a shorter bar in as early as a week after piercing if swelling is down. If you cannot visit a studio for help and do not have experience switching your own jewelry, wait until after the four-week minimum healing time to avoid damaging the tissue with an inept swap. If externally threaded jewelry was used initially, wait the full month before passing the post through the channel. If your piercer has a taper to avoid exposing your delicate new cells to the threaded post, they can change it for you once your swelling is gone.

Experimentation may be needed to find the most comfortable jewelry size and shape for you. Once your piercing has healed, feel free to try some of the many different options. Large or heavy ornaments are seldom safe here for extended periods. Think twice about vibrating tongue barbells or any jewelry that requires you to place a battery (which could leak) inside your mouth.

TONGUE PIERCING: DOWNSIZE POLICY

Anyone who pierces your tongue without educating you about the need to downsize the jewelry is remiss in their duties to safeguard your dental health. Does your piercer encourage downsizing by offering clear, detailed information and perhaps a discount on a shorter post? They will if they are knowledgeable and caring.

TONGUE PIERCING: STRETCHING

The tongue piercing is generally easy to enlarge by a gauge or two. But stretching tends to become more difficult as you expand to larger sizes. A disadvantage of creating an oversized hole is that the jewelry becomes heavier and bigger, too, increasing your risk of oral damage. In general, jumbo jewelry is dangerous to wear in tongue piercings. Discs are preferable to balls for large-gauge pieces in this area.

TONGUE PIERCING: RETIRING

When you remove your jewelry, the hole may shrink or close right up, even if you have had it pierced for years. On the other hand, it is not uncommon for an established tongue piercing to remain viable without jewelry. If it seems to stay open, apply the principles described in "Resting," on page 281, to determine how long you can comfortably leave it out.

If you want to abandon your piercing, simply remove your jewelry. Unless you stretched it to an unusually large size, the piercing will shrink, so there is little likelihood of food working its way inside the hole. An abandoned large-gauge tongue piercing that remains open could benefit from a periodic spray through the channel with a Waterpik or similar water jet device.

GOOD DENTIST, GOOD PATIENT

I know most dentists aren't nearly as enthusiastic about my five tongue piercings as I am, but I was fortunate to find one with an open mind who treats me with all of my metal in place. I have had panoramic X-rays, regular teeth cleanings, and even a root canal, all without removing a single bar. My hygienist spruces them up with a bit of polish on each ball. I visit the dentist every six months, floss and brush daily, use a tongue scraper regularly, and avoid clacking jewelry against my teeth or chomping on the posts. My dentist reports that my oral health is "perfect," which demonstrates that it is possible to wear multiple oral piercings without causing damage.

THE LABRET PIERCING

- **Healing time:** 6 to 8 weeks or longer
- **Initial jewelry style:** Flatback labret stud or ring-style
- **Initial jewelry gauge:** 16 through 12 gauge, depending on placement and jewelry style. The smaller sizes are most common.
- **Initial jewelry size:** Labret posts from 5/16 to 7/16 inch; ring diameters from 3/8 to 1/2 inch. To allow for swelling, rings should be one diameter larger than the size that will be worn in the healed piercing.

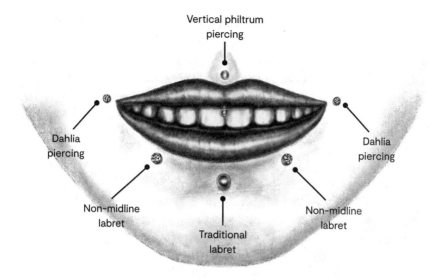

After the ear and nose, the lip is one of the most popular piercings in indigenous cultures around the world. Throughout the ages, people have worn ornaments of horn, bone, gold, and other natural materials in piercings of the lips.

LABRET PIERCING: PLACEMENT

Labret derives from the Latin word *labrum*, meaning "lip." Any piercing surrounding the mouth is a labret, though some use the term to denote only the placement centered beneath the bottom lip. There is a maximum distance from the orifice that can reasonably be pierced because the tissue connects to the gums. Within the limitations imposed by anatomy and aesthetic preferences, there are many options for piercings around the mouth.

The traditional labret is centered under the lower lip, below the *vermillion border* (where the pigmented area meets the face). It is best to avoid piercing through that juncture, as migration into the softer lip tissue is possible. Labrets may be worn higher or lower, in pairs or multiples, centrally, or off to the sides. Situating the piercing so that the jewelry rests at a neutral angle is critical for comfort and safety. All labrets (including the variations described below) must be placed with this principle in mind. Excess pressure against teeth or gums—even from the slightest slant—can result in discomfort and damage. The thin tissue inside the lip allows many of the blood vessels to be easily seen and avoided.

If you wish to switch back and forth between ring- and stud-style jewelry after healing, discuss this with your piercer, because the angle of the piercing and the distance from the edge of your lip must be considered.

LABRET PIERCING JEWELRY: THE LABRET STUD

A *labret stud* is a short barbell with a slim disc that is worn inside the mouth. A ball, gem, spike, or other adornment shows on the facial surface. Some piercees prefer the slightly more domed backing design of an M&M end.

One type of labret stud is composed of three separate pieces, which include a post and two removable threaded ends: a disc for the inside, and an ornament worn on the front. Others have just two parts: a disc with an attached post, plus the front end. An advantage of the two-piece style is that you can't possibly lose the disc. A disadvantage is that you will need to replace this whole portion to downsize your jewelry after the initial swelling is gone. Two advantages to the three-piece style are that you can replace just the post once it is time to downsize, and it allows you to change both ends. The usual starting disc is 5 millimeters, but you may wish to try a 3 millimeter or other size after healing. The disadvantage is that you have a slightly increased possibility of jewelry loss because both ends unscrew. Many piercers use threadless posts, and only the front is removable. The threaded style is preferred if a large ornamental end is worn, to avoid bending or breaking the connector pin.

The length of the post is anatomy-dependent, and a good fit is imperative. The lip tissue is so soft and quick to regenerate that there is a risk of the jewelry rapidly becoming embedded if it is too short. However, an overly long bar is apt to cause trauma and irritation. Once your piercing has fully healed and you have a fitted post inserted, you may see the disc *nesting* (sinking a millimeter or two into the inside surface of your lip). If you have no discomfort, this indentation is acceptable, and it may help to protect your teeth and gums by keeping the disc from directly pressing against them.

LABRET PIERCING JEWELRY: THE RING

Rings work best on lip piercings placed close to the vermillion border. If you have a full lip or your piercing is located far from its edge, a hoop would need to be overly large.

A tight fit has to wait until after healing if you want to wear a ring that hugs your lip. You must have a slightly larger diameter at first to accommodate initial swelling. When a hoop fights gravity (as with a lower lip piercing), it will rest over to one side. The ring will not sit straight up unless it is snug. Drinking from a cup or glass can be a tad tricky when you first wear a lip ring. Clean dishware and a little patience and practice are required.

LABRET PIERCING: PROCEDURE

The piercing may be done freehand or using forceps, and from the outside, or the inside. Those with facial hair need not trim or shave, even if the piercing will be placed within the whiskers. It will be more challenging for your piercer, but an adept technician will be able to do the job, even through a heavy beard.

LABRET PIERCING: HEALING AND TROUBLESHOOTING

It is typical for jewelry to nest somewhat into your lip; however, if you suspect tissue is actually growing over it (inside or out), visit your piercer immediately, or medical intervention may be needed to remove an embedded ornament.

The facial surface of labret piercings may discolor, usually pinkish or reddish, and crust up throughout the healing period. Wearing lipstick or lip balm is fine, but keep the container clean and don't share it. Applying it from a tube is safer than using your finger. Don't open your mouth too wide when you wear a labret stud because the disc on the inside might catch on your teeth.

Plaque can accumulate on the jewelry inside your mouth, especially at the juncture of the disc and the post. This area is difficult to access and scrub with a toothbrush, but dental floss can help to keep it clean. Most of the tips in the "Tongue Piercing: Healing and Troubleshooting" section on page 137 apply to lip piercings.

You may shave as normally as possible, given the obstacle of the jewelry. Avoid getting aftershave, especially alcohol-based products, into a healing piercing. See more shaving tips on page 169.

A new ornament in your lip is hard to ignore, and you may be inclined to fiddle with the jewelry, but you must leave it alone. Once your labret is well healed, playing with the jewelry shouldn't irritate your piercing, but if the activity involves your teeth or gums, it will damage them.

If you experience sore gums as you adjust to the jewelry, you can apply dental wax to minimize the impact. It is inexpensive and available at drugstores. Problems are generally resolved by wearing smaller or shorter jewelry once healing is complete. If pressure on your teeth or gum irritation persists regardless of jewelry size and style, the piercing will have to be abandoned.

LABRET PIERCING: CHANGING JEWELRY

Depending on your healing process and how long your initial bar is, you might need to downsize the post more than once. Safety must come first, so wait until healing is over before inserting tight-fitting jewelry.

The slippery nature of saliva makes changing your own jewelry in oral piercings tricky. Keep clean paper towels handy, because you are probably going to need them. Separate disc-back labret ends can be challenging to screw on because of their flat shape and small size. It may be easier to insert a labret post from the inside and screw on the front or wear a threadless version. Small, smooth-jaw hemostats are helpful to hold the jewelry during this process. Or pay a visit to your piercer, as many piercees do.

LABRET PIERCING: CONCEALMENT

Unless you have a thick beard, total concealment of a healing labret is not possible, even with the most discreet jewelry. Additionally, the extra post length required to accommodate initial swelling makes it more apparent when new. After healing, camouflaging options improve and include clear and "flesh tone" glass or silicone retainers, but this area is still challenging to hide. If you have facial hair, a concealment end in a color that blends with your whiskers may be less visible than the skin-tone options. See the sections on retainers, page 305.

To avoid the possibility of embedding, initial healing should be over before you wear ends as small as a ⅛ inch (3 millimeters) unless you have 1/16 inch of extra post length.

LABRET PIERCING: STRETCHING

Historically, lip piercings are among those most commonly stretched, and some modern piercees wear impressive sizes. Do not stretch lip piercings beyond 10 gauge without due consideration. The tissue is relatively elastic, but the risks increase with larger sizes. Bigger and heavier adornments against teeth and gums compound oral health hazards. Depending on how much you enlarge, your hole might not shrink enough to prevent saliva from leaking if you abandon the piercing later. Some individuals with large-gauge lip piercings experience saliva leakage while eating, even with jewelry in place. Permanent damage to the lower front teeth or adjacent gums is to be expected with extreme lip enlargement.

LABRET PIERCING: RETIRING

Should you take out your jewelry, a small divot or spot that looks like an enlarged pore usually remains if healing was uneventful, and the piercing was not stretched. If it was positioned under the curl of your lip, the natural crease might obscure the mark.

If your tissue was expanded to a large gauge or stretched too quickly, a permanent void will likely remain, and it can be unsightly; surgery may be the only way to restore a semblance of your previous appearance.

LIP PIERCING: VARIATIONS

The healing time and jewelry information are the same as for the labret piercing.

LOWER LIP SIDE PLACEMENT

The self-explanatory *side lip piercing with ring* is ordinarily placed at or just below the vermillion border. There is generally space for the hoop to rest at the corner juncture of the upper and lower lip, though some piercees prefer to have the jewelry lean toward the center.

The tissue inside the lip is very soft, so the piercing tends to rise a millimeter or two from its original position on the interior when you wear a ring. In anticipation of this, experienced piercers will cheat the initial placement down just a little on the inside. Then, the hole will heal in the desired position (usually equidistant from the edge of the lip, inside and out). Wearing a snug ring (after healing, of course) is less likely to cause gum damage, though there is still some risk of injuring your teeth by biting the jewelry.

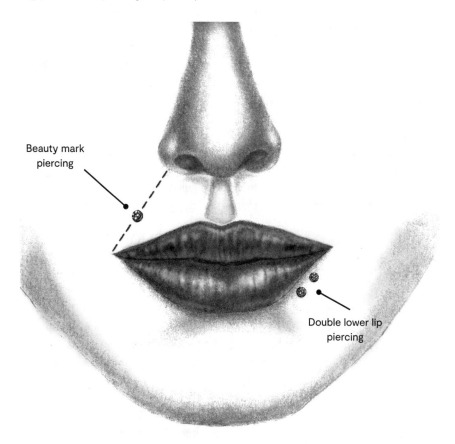

Beauty mark piercing

Double lower lip piercing

UPPER LIP SIDE PLACEMENT: BEAUTY MARK, MONROE, OR MADONNA

This glamorous piercing is a beauty mark of metal worn off to one side above the upper lip. It is often embellished with a sparkling jewel. The names derive from the legendary ladies known for an unpierced version near their own mouths.

Other than a longer healing time of two to three months or more, this piercing shares many characteristics with all of the lip area placements. Initial jewelry is usually a labret stud in 16 or 14 gauge.

UPPER LIP PLACEMENT

This style is placed toward the corner of the mouth, normally 5/16 to ½ inch above the vermillion border. This ornament is intended as a lip enhancement, but some practitioners place them closer to the nose. While piercings often work best in the natural creases of the body, an upper lip piercing that sits in the *nasolabial fold* (smile line) is much more difficult to heal.

Your piercer should take great care to see that the angle is neutral when your face is at rest and consider how the area changes with different facial movements. On some anatomy, the gums join the lip relatively low; a spot that seems reasonable on the outside sometimes sits above your gumline inside. If your piercer is not meticulous and skillful, your jewelry could end up at an awkward angle that is difficult or impossible to heal, and potentially damaging to your teeth and gums.

UPPER LIP PIERCING: HEALING AND TROUBLESHOOTING

Some individuals heal this piercing rapidly, yet others find it takes commitment and patience over many months before it settles.

Regardless of proper placement, these piercings can catch when you open your mouth wide. Be careful when eating burgers, big sandwiches, and the like.

UPPER LIP PIERCING: CHANGING JEWELRY

Jewelry changes at home can be tricky, especially once the short post is in place or if you wear a tiny ornament. Many piercees return to a professional for help.

UPPER LIP PIERCING: RETIRING

The permanent mark left after jewelry removal may be more evident than one from a central lower labret. It is apt to look like an extremely enlarged pore, so this is not a piercing to get as a temporary ornament; it may well leave a noticeable scar.

UPPER LIP CENTER PLACEMENT: PHILTRUM

This style may appeal to you if you favor midline placements. Some alternative names for the anatomical term *philtrum* include *Medusa*, *divot*, and *upret*.

The philtrum piercing also takes an average of two to three months to heal and commonly uses a 16- or 14-gauge labret stud.

The piercing is situated in the natural divot (also called the *infranasal depression*) between the mouth and the nose. Depending on personal preferences and available space, it may be seated closer to the lip, nearer the nose, or right at the midpoint.

During this procedure, you may feel as if you're getting a strong bop on the nose rather than an oral piercing. Your eyes may water, too.

PHILTRUM PIERCING: RETIRING

Like all labrets other than the lower central placement, this is likely to leave a visible mark if abandoned.

VERMILLION PIERCINGS—LIP SURFACES: UPPER OR LOWER, VERTICAL OR TRANSVERSE, AND VARIATIONS

These piercings pass through the pigmented portion of the lip. This tissue is thinner and more delicate than other skin, so the risk of migration or rejection and scarring is higher. However, when well-placed on suitable anatomy, they tend to heal without issues. If the ornament sits directly on the line where the lips meet, there may be more trauma and complications.

The *Ashley* piercing rests in the center of the lower lip. Depending on your anatomy, it may be done as a *reverse (or inverse) vertical labret*, which exits inside the mouth and uses a curved barbell and flat disc on the interior. Alternatively, it may be like a high labret, through the lip instead of below it, with the same type of jewelry and angle.

Vertical lip surface piercings do best on full builds. They can be placed entirely within the pigmented zone or may exit at the vermillion border or slightly lower, on the facial surface. Another variation that goes through both types of tissue is the vertical philtrum or *jestrum* piercing. It extends from the philtrum to the upper lip surface, close to or where the lips meet.

Transverse (horizontal) lip surface piercings are located entirely within the vermillion region and are at higher risk for migration or rejection and scarring.

DAHLIA OR JOKER PIERCINGS

Also called *Dahlia bites* or *Joker bites*, this is a set of piercings on either side of the mouth, near the juncture of the upper and lower lips. The same considerations for other oral piercings apply. Dahlia piercings are a safer option than cheek piercings. See more on those below. Depending on anatomy and jewelry fit, there can be a high likelihood of damage to the teeth—especially at first, when longer jewelry must be worn to accommodate swelling, which can be considerable in this region.

QUESTIONABLE ORAL PIERCINGS

Some oral piercings have a higher potential for complications than others. This isn't to suggest they never heal, but they do not have the same likelihood of success as more traditionally placed labrets, and they have greater risks. Before deciding on any of the following spots, weigh the dangers.

THE LINGUAL FRENULUM PIERCING

This is a piercing of the web under the tongue. It is not a viable option for people who do not possess sufficiently pronounced anatomy and superb tongue control for the procedure. Those who are well enough endowed usually wear a small 16-gauge ring or curved bar (5/16 or 3/8 inch). The piercing should be through the base of the web, but it must not be placed deep into the *sublingual* (under the tongue) tissues. Vital structures and vessels are there, including the sublingual veins and a pair of sublingual salivary glands. You must be able to cooperate by lifting your tongue and holding it still for the procedure. When placed correctly in suitable anatomy, this piercing usually heals quickly and easily.

SMILEY/SCRUMPER AND FROWNY

Smiley and *scrumper* are both names for a piercing of the upper frenulum that attaches the center of the lip to the gums. Most people have only a tiny web of flesh there that is insufficient to support a sturdy piercing. Migration and rejection are obvious risks. The proximity of jewelry to the teeth and gums can lead to irritation and erosion. For the same reasons, the *frowny* (piercing of the lower lip frenulum) is also questionable.

NONRECOMMENDED ORAL PIERCINGS

There are several placements in the tongue and oral cavity that are not advisable, and it would be sensible to avoid them, though plenty of piercers will perform these piercings despite their dangers.

CHEEK PIERCING/DIMPLE

Dimples are often considered attractive facial characteristics, and some people wish to enhance natural indentations or create dimples via piercing. Unfortunately, that region of the face contains a host of significant structures, including blood vessels, nerves, and the *parotid duct* (a conduit for a component in saliva). Piercing into any of these can be disastrous. If abandoned, this piercing can cause permanent scars and excessive dimpling of the skin. See "The Worst Piercing Story," page 150. Due to the elevated risks, only 37 percent of the piercers surveyed perform cheek piercings.

MANDIBLE OR SPRUNG PIERCING

The mandible is a bone, but this vertical piercing passes under the tongue, through the floor of the mouth, to the underside of the jaw. It traverses a lot of tissue and could puncture vital anatomy. Due to the force of gravity and the presence of saliva, this could become a spit drain and funnel liquid out the bottom.

TRANSVERSE TONGUE PIERCING

There are nerves, veins, and arteries inside the tongue that make piercing it from side to side *extremely* dangerous. Another problem with a horizontal tongue piercing is that you are almost certain to bite the jewelry. Piercees risk uncontrolled bleeding and critical, permanent damage from this piercing. Shallow or surface transverse ("scoop") piercings are apt to reject and scar.

TRANSVERSE TONGUE TIP PIERCING ("SNAKE EYES")

This is essentially a horizontal scoop piercing across the tip of the tongue. It is subject to the same problems and risks as the transverse tongue piercing, but is more likely to damage the teeth and gums by being at the front of the mouth. Its position right where certain speech sounds are made means it may cause an impediment. Fortunately, this should resolve once the jewelry is removed, if no damage has been done to vital structures.

LOWBRET AND VERTICAL LOWBRET

These are both placed as low as possible inside the lip and pierce through to the surface of the face. The *lowbret* is perpendicular to the tissue like a regular labret, and the vertical placement exits closer to or at the jawline. Gum and bone erosion are likely consequences due to the limited space for jewelry at this location inside the mouth.

PERIL PERSPECTIVES

Millions of people engage in hobbies and activities like skiing, motorcycling, scuba diving, and rock climbing. Though some of these are of interest to me, they seem unacceptably perilous, so I don't do them. I find my oral piercings to be rewarding and enjoyable; to me, they are worth the risks.

THE POINT

Because oral piercings have significant hazards, they deserve due consideration. However, if your anatomy is suitable, your piercer is qualified, and you adhere to all safety guidelines, the dangers are minimized. Each person must weigh the factors and decide for themselves if it is worth the risks.

THE WORST PIERCING STORY

In my entire career, this was the worst disaster to befall someone I pierced—and it happened to me.

In 1998, I pierced my own cheeks to mark a significant personal milestone. I placed the piercings in the natural indentations that appeared when I smiled. I had long fantasized about wearing dainty, sparkling diamonds in my dimples.

I carefully inspected each side, didn't detect any anatomical structures, and performed the piercings without any issues.

During the following week, the only discomfort I experienced was the distinctive sensation of smiling too much. I had an uneventful healing course of about seven months. On a daily basis, people admired my unique adornments and made complimentary remarks. I loved the way my fancy dimples looked, and I felt at least 33.3 percent cuter with them.

About a year and a half post-piercing, the right side started to leak. Periodically, a drop of clear liquid came from the piercing, wetting my cheek. It was lighter than water and not viscous like saliva. I tried everything I could think of to resolve this unusual problem, including changing my soap and detergent, trying larger discs, and swapping jewelry materials. Still, the leaking worsened, and my cheek became sore and chapped from the liquid and the friction of wiping it away. I consulted my dentist and an orofacial surgeon. Although my parotid gland and duct were fine, a portion of the tube that delivers saliva to the mouth had opened into my piercing channel. The doctors' advice: "Take those things out."

No. Way. I was resolved to keep my beloved piercings, no matter what.

But the leaking got progressively worse, and when the liquid dripped onto someone I was about to pierce, I knew I'd lost the battle. With extreme reluctance, I abandoned the piercings. I was devastated but figured out a way to glue small rhinestones where my jewelry used to shine.

My right cheek continued to leak. In desperation, I used a medical device called a cautery pen to burn the hole shut (not a service offered at piercing studios!). It took three attempts, but finally, the tool generated enough scar tissue to seal the channel. I sure wish I'd known the risks of piercing cheeks farther back than the first molars. Now that you do, you can avoid repeating the nightmare I experienced.

13

TORSO PIERCINGS: NIPPLE AND NAVEL PIERCINGS

The torso is a substantial region of the body, yet its surfaces provide anatomy suitable for only a few standard piercing placements: the navel and nipples. These piercings differ in many ways, but both areas can be somewhat tricky and take a long time to heal. Therefore, all aspects must be handled properly.

THE NAVEL PIERCING
- **Healing time:** 6 to 9 months or longer
- **Initial jewelry style:** Curved bar; rarely, a J-curve or ring
- **Initial jewelry gauge:** Minimum 14 gauge; sometimes 12 gauge and rarely, 10 gauge
- **Initial jewelry size:** Lengths ⅜ to 9/16 inch, with 7/16 inch the most common.

Like the ear, the navel is simply another spot for adornment. Unlike the earlobe, however, navel piercings are not quick and easy to heal. In fact, this piercing is among those with the longest average healing time.

One issue is that the abdomen is *avascular* (lacks blood supply), which causes slow healing.[1] The region is also subject to stress from normal movement of the body and friction from clothing. Because navel piercings can be troublesome, they take some patience and dedication to proper care during the extended healing time. Teenage girls were the original recipients when navel piercings gained popularity, but adults of all ages and gender identities can—and do—get them. Nearly all piercers surveyed perform navel piercings (98.7 percent).

NAVEL PIERCING: PLACEMENT AND CHOICE OF JEWELRY
This piercing frames the tissue surrounding the *umbilicus* (navel) at the epicenter of the body. Local anatomy differs substantially from one individual to the next, but piercers may fail to take these variations into account. A superior professional

will carefully assess you and suggest placement and jewelry that fit your unique build. Suitability for this piercing depends on the configuration of your navel itself—not your weight or fitness level.

A traditional vertical piercing is placed in the center through a fold of tissue on top of the navel. If your skin is inflexible, the procedure can be harder to perform, and the piercing will be more at risk for migration and rejection. If your navel area is flat, there is no lip, and the skin is not supple, pierce a different site.

Your navel's size and configuration should be evaluated while you are sitting, standing, and reclining. The shape and dimensions of the area can transform dramatically with the changes in position, and this has to be factored in when determining placement and selecting jewelry size. If your navel flattens and closes when you're seated, this must also be taken into consideration. For success, the piercing must be situated so that your body will accommodate the jewelry in all usual positions and postures.

PAINFUL MISTAKE

Before your navel is pierced, your piercer should check the marks while you are reclining *and* standing. An unfortunate man whose piercer skipped this crucial step once came to me for help. He was nearly doubled over by jewelry that constricted his abdomen. The width of his piercing required jewelry that was twice the diameter of the ring that his piercer had inserted!

NAVEL PIERCING: BARS VS. RINGS

Ring-style jewelry gained early favor as the navel ornament of choice because it was the most readily available design. The 1990s belly piercing craze preceded the availability of curved bars—and even the mass production of body jewelry. But a ring is far more obtrusive than a bar, especially if your navel is not deep. Curved bars have been the preferred navel jewelry for quite some time. An extra post length of ¹⁄₁₆ to ⅛ inch is generally sufficient to accommodate the expansion of tissue when you recline.

A hoop may be safe if your navel has a distinct lip and substantial depth. When a ring is the initial jewelry for a vertical navel piercing, the underside must be pierced well away from the edge to keep the hoop from protruding excessively. But if you

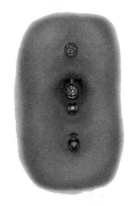

A navel with a jeweled navel curve in the traditional central placement and a curved bar on the bottom

change to a curved bar later, its bottom end will be hidden inside your navel, which may or may not be desirable.

If you are among the minority of people who have a flap only on the bottom of your navel, you might be a candidate for a piercing there. A bar is the preferred jewelry style for lower-navel placement.

NAVEL PIERCING: JEWELED NAVEL BARS AND J-CURVES

Curved barbells set with sparkly synthetic stones or genuine gems are among the most popular jewelry designs worn in vertical navel piercings. There are several standard varieties (curved bar, jeweled navel curve, and J-curve) and innumerable variations. See chapter 10, "Jeweled Navel Curve" and "J-Curve" (page 89) for photos and more information.

The jut of the J-curve projects the bottom adornment forward to make it more visible and prevents it from resting inside your navel. This can minimize irritation and allow for better circulation and comfort. The J-curve is useful if your navel piercing is deep on the underside.

NAVEL PIERCING: WEIGHT AND WEIGHT LOSS

Regardless of your weight, if your navel folds in and disappears when you sit down, traditional piercing placement and jewelry would cause mechanical stresses that all but guarantee healing complications. If you have a horizontal crease across the area, even when you are standing, the same concerns apply. Some heavy abdomens are still able to support standard navel piercings because body size isn't as key a factor as your configuration in the area of the piercing. However, the diminished blood supply caused by excess abdominal fat makes healing even more difficult. If you have diabetes and carry excess weight in this area, navel piercings are inadvisable because complications are likely and can be more serious.

If you are planning to lose weight, your navel area's overall shape is still the primary consideration. Usually, the abdomen gets smaller with weight loss but maintains the same basic contour unless the reduction is extreme.

Rapid weight gain or loss during healing could cause irritation only if the region changes shape quickly enough to prevent the piercing from settling. It is unlikely that a weight fluctuation could impact a healed navel piercing unless it is substantial enough to alter your navel's shape or location.

NAVEL PIERCING: FLOATING NAVEL PLACEMENT

This newer alternative works for some navels that are unsuited to traditional placement. It may be an option if your abdomen creases at the navel when you sit or bend, or if your anatomy is too small or closed to accommodate the usual size ball or gem on the bottom. A defined lip is still required, and the piercing is generally positioned deeper on the underside than usual. A flat disc, M&M-shaped

bead, or small ball is typically used on the bottom. This takes up less space underneath and gives the appearance of the upper ornament floating on the navel since the bottom of the jewelry isn't easily seen. The bar lengths are typically longer for these than for a traditional navel piercing.

NAVEL PIERCING: "OUTIE" ANATOMY

A protruding *outie* navel is fundamentally unsuited to piercing. I have never perforated one, but some piercers do, and this is referred to as a *true navel piercing*. A hardened outie that is scar-like may be a remnant of your umbilical cord, and it could be connected to the interior of your abdomen. Infection of an outie piercing could travel rapidly to your *peritoneum* (the membrane lining the abdominal cavity) or internal organs, presenting severe health risks.[2]

An outie that is softer and pushes in easily is probably an umbilical hernia. Some of your intestines can poke through this breach, which is a weakness or hole in the abdominal lining near your navel.[3] If this tissue is pierced, there is a possibility of puncturing your small intestine, which is a life-threatening scenario. Most navels are recessed, but if your anatomy protrudes, consider carefully whether the hazards of piercing are acceptable to you. A flap of skin surrounding the bulge might be pierceable if it is distant enough. An experienced piercer can determine if the nearby tissue presents any safe options for piercing.

NAVEL PIERCING: ALTERED ANATOMY

The *abdominoplasty* (tummy tuck) is a popular procedure to remove excess skin and fat from the area. Unfortunately, post-surgical anatomy often can't or shouldn't be pierced. Incisions cause scar tissue, which is not a welcoming place for piercings. During a full abdominoplasty, the navel is cut free from its original position and sutured into a new location.[4] The skin is often pulled so taut that it cannot be pinched up, making piercing difficult or impossible. Even if the tissue is pliable or has been formed into a lip-shaped fold, it is less vascular and much harder to heal. If you wish to show off an ornamented and surgically flattened midriff and find a piercer willing to attempt it, jewelry made of a flexible polymer may be preferable to metal. Unfortunately, post-abdominoplasty piercings are often not successful.

The navel is a frequent site for *laparoscopy*, a common medical procedure involving small incisions to insert instruments for exploratory and microsurgical purposes. Most often, the cut is on the bottom of the navel, so it does not interfere with a traditionally placed piercing. If you have had an incision in the region you wish to have pierced, the scar will need to be evaluated by a piercer. When there is a minimum of scar tissue, piercing is usually possible. Occasionally a surgical scar does not heal correctly and continues to secrete fluid. Navels with weeping, active scars are potential passageways for bacteria to travel into the abdominal cavity; they should not be pierced.

Stretch marks are a form of scarring caused by stretching and tearing of the skin. They are frequently present in the navel region, and they are weaker than other skin, so it is best to avoid them. Piercing near a stretch mark is preferable to going right through it because of the increased risk of migration or rejection.

NAVEL PIERCING: PROCEDURE

Though you must expose the area to get a navel piercing, you should not have to remove all clothing and bare your entire torso unless you've worn a bodysuit. Navel piercings are usually performed while you are in a supine or semi-reclining position. If your skin is especially taut, tissue manipulation can gently improve its suppleness. Also, if you are slightly propped up (rather than stretched out flat), it may be easier to grasp the tissue for the procedure. These can be done with forceps, freehand, or a receiving tube.

Some people have sensitive navels, but many piercees experience nothing more intense than discomfort from the piercing. "It just felt like pressure" and "It was a pinch" are common descriptions of the sensation. A few piercees report that cleaning is the worst part of the process because it tickles.

When compared to most other piercings, navels are less likely to bleed, but the ones that do might heal more rapidly. A superior blood supply makes it easier for your body to bring nutrients and oxygen to the region and process a wound.[5]

NAVEL PIERCING: HEALING AND TROUBLESHOOTING

The navel is no more prone to infection than other piercings; however, it is more likely than many others to become irritated. It also has an extended healing period, and therefore, a longer window of time for potential infection.

Piercees and medical professionals alike frequently see an ordinary, healing navel that has become irritated and pronounce it infected. Some discoloration (pinkish, brownish, or purplish), secretion of clear or cloudy fluids, and *induration* (hardening of tissue) can all be present in a typical healing navel piercing. A misdiagnosis of infection is highly unproductive if a doctor prescribes antibiotics: they won't resolve your irritation or address the actual cause of the problem.

Wear low-rise pants or loose, breathable garments to prevent clothing from pressing or rubbing against the piercing and to allow for good air circulation. Sometimes a change as simple as switching to the fetal position for sleeping will help diminish irritation. Effective solutions aren't always complicated.

NAVEL PIERCING: MIGRATION AND REJECTION

If your navel tissue is very taut, you are more likely to suffer from these complications. See your piercer to check the fit of your jewelry and consider trying a flexible polymer substitute. Sometimes nothing will help, and you can only contemplate your navel with disappointment.

NAVEL PIERCING: BUMPS

Complications arise if you sleep on your stomach, wear tight clothing over the piercing, or have an abdomen that creases and folds near the jewelry. Keeping this area dry is challenging, but moisture contributes to healing problems. Friction, pressure, and trauma can cause a bump, tenderness, swelling, redness, and delayed healing. Try to determine whether your irritation is from inferior quality jewelry, an improperly sized or shaped piece, or other external forces; you must resolve the issue if you are to have a chance of healing.

An unattractive, scary-looking growth can form at one or both openings of your piercing due to moisture or irritation. If it is dark red and resembles raw hamburger, you probably have *hypergranulation* (excessive growth of granulation tissue–small particles that grow to cover healing wounds). It may not be as sore as it looks, but it might bleed easily or drain clear fluid. Navels are more prone to develop excess granulation tissue than many other areas. Hypergranulation is not always indicative of a need to give up on your piercing (though a doctor is apt to tell you otherwise); some piercings heal successfully following a bout or two with such growths. Keeping the piercing as dry as possible may provide the best chance for resolution. See chapter 16, "Trouble and Troubleshooting," for more details on excess granulation tissue and other healing problems.

NAVEL PIERCING: UPS AND DOWNS

Throughout the healing process, many piercings tend to go through cycles of getting better and then regressing. These phases are particularly characteristic of navel piercings and one of the reasons patience is vital for success. Even if you experience some trouble-free periods during healing, continue with the aftercare protocols for at least six months.

NAVEL PIERCING: EXERCISE AND ACTIVITY

Of all the piercings, navels are most vulnerable to stresses caused by physical activity. Because the navel area is so affected by the torso's movement, this piercing is often a challenge for active individuals. During your entire healing period, you should be cautious with actions that affect your torso. When working your abdominal muscles, especially during initial healing, avoid full sit-ups. Perform only controlled crunches that don't crease your abdomen, or do exercises that simply contract the muscles. You must prevent physical impact to the site for the piercing to heal. Avoid injury to your piercing during exercise or sports by wearing a plastic eye patch over the jewelry (see "Protective Patch," page 231).

Sexual activity can be perilous to your navel piercing due to friction on the wound and the potential for contamination from your partner's bodily fluids. Wearing waterproof bandages during sexual encounters helps to prevent problems.

NAVEL PIERCING: CHANGING JEWELRY

You should not change your own navel jewelry for about the first six months, though if you are wearing a bar, the removable ends can be switched carefully at any time. Should your initial jewelry cause problems, visit your piercer to replace it as soon as possible. In as little as four months, a professional piercer might change the jewelry to another piece that is still suited for the healing phase, *if* the piercing appears to be doing well. You must avoid wearing elaborate body jewelry until your piercing is completely settled. Healing navels are touchy enough without the added weight, motion, and potential for catching that come with a large or dangling ornament.

NAVEL PIERCING: STRETCHING

Once a navel piercing is seasoned (at least a year), you can stretch it up a gauge. After you wear the larger size for nine months or longer, if you have a substantial amount of tissue between the entry and exit holes, you may be able to stretch again. Enlarging beyond 14 gauge is not advisable if your piercing is close to the surface.

Navels are rarely sites for jumbo jewelry, but with an adequate amount of pierced tissue and a slow stretching timetable, they can safely be enlarged.

NAVEL PIERCING: RETIRING

If you wish to abandon an unhealed navel piercing, it is best to do so when it is not irritated, infected, or needing to drain. Navel piercings frequently leave a visible scar, which tends to be more evident if you experienced healing difficulties. The residual mark may benefit from a scar-reduction product (see page 257). Refer to "Navel Piercings and Pregnancy," page 309, for information about having a baby when your belly is pierced.

If you abandon your piercing after healing is over, it might not seal up. The holes will tend to shrink, but full closure is not always dependent upon how long you had the piercing. Some navel piercings that are quite old will shut after jewelry removal, and others that were in for less than a year will remain permanently viable. Navel piercings that are very shallow but fully healed tend to stay open. There is no health risk or medical necessity to wear jewelry in the channel, even if it doesn't seal shut; the matter is aesthetic.

THE POINT

Despite the lengthy healing period, navel piercings can be very rewarding. They make an alluring accent to an appealing abdomen, and some piercees enjoy showing them off, to the delight of other fans of the art. Ironically, when they became exceptionally popular, some people decided against getting one because of their prevalence. Piercing is a personal decision, so if you want one (and have suitable anatomy), you should get it!

THE NIPPLE PIERCING

While the piercings discussed so far are the same for any gender, some considerations for nipple piercing will differ depending on your specific anatomy and biology. These factors are described in the following discussion of nipple piercings.

- o Healing times:
  - Small nipples (less than 3/8 inch in width), 3 to 4 months or longer
  - Large nipples (wider than 3/8 inch), 6 to 9 months or longer
- o Initial jewelry style: Straight barbells, rarely rings (harder to heal)
- o Initial jewelry gauge: 14 gauge minimum, 12 gauge for rougher play or larger builds, and 10 gauge only on well-developed anatomy
- o Initial jewelry size: Anatomy-dependent. For barbells, 1/16 to 1/8 inch longer than the relaxed nipple
  - For small nipples, minimum ring diameter is usually 9/16 inch, but 1/2 inch may be suitable for small nipples that protrude
  - For large nipples, minimum ring diameter will be double the diameter of the nipple itself; often 3/4 inch or larger may be necessary. Rings are not recommended as initial jewelry for wide nipples

The contrast of metal jewelry through the flesh of a nipple is exotic and striking. This piercing defines the region, frames the tissue, and makes the nipple stand at attention (though it doesn't necessarily cause it to remain erect at all times). Prior to the early 1990s, when navel piercings became popular, nipples were the most prevalent location for body piercings, and they remain in widespread demand today.

Some piercing enthusiasts—particularly in the gay and SM subcultures—explored the erotic potential of their bodies and started what has become the current style of nipple piercing. These days, people from all walks of life are experiencing their delights. For some, it is an aesthetic preference or fashion statement; for others, it reigns as a favorite in the realm of sexual and sensual pleasures. Virtually all piercers surveyed offer nipple piercings (99.1 percent).

HISTORICAL NIPPLE PIERCING

The Karankawa, a now-extinct Native American tribe who lived along the Gulf Coast of Texas, widely practiced nipple piercing. There are rumors that it was historically practiced among other groups, including the Kabyle of northern Algeria, and women in rural Poland, but concrete evidence of prior nipple piercing activity is lacking until the Victorian era.[6]

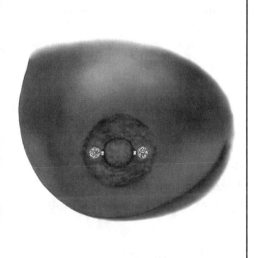

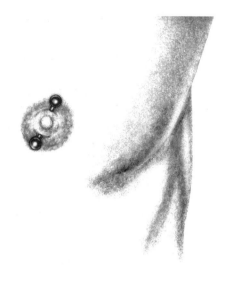

A well-developed nipple with a
barbell in a horizontal piercing

A small nipple with a barbell
in an angled piercing

NIPPLE PIERCING: PLACEMENT
AND CHOICE OF JEWELRY

Virtually all adult nipples—even tiny flat ones—are pierceable if they are pliable. Whether you prefer the position to be horizontal, vertical, or somewhere in between, nipple piercing works best when placed in your tissue's natural creases. Depending on the angle and shape of your breasts or pectoral muscles, the "horizontal" placement may be more visually appealing if the outer edge is just a bit higher than the inner side. This tilts the jewelry up at a slight slant that often frames the area nicely. A geometrically horizontal placement can look a little droopy at the outer side on certain chests.

If you have well-developed anatomy, the piercing should be placed in the grooves at the base, where the nipple rises from the areola. If your nipple is defined with substantial height, the piercing can safely go in as little as 5/16 inch of tissue. If you have flat nipples, the piercing should generally encompass a minimum of 3/8 inch between entry and exit when the area is relaxed. However, some practitioners will pierce the nipple through much less skin, which raises concerns over safety and long-term durability. If your nipples are featureless, without an elevated tip, the tissue in the nipple's visual center might be pierced so that the jewelry rests evenly within your areola. (While this type of piercing routinely extends into the areola, especially on very small anatomy, it is still considered a nipple piercing.) If you want a pair of piercings and have large, protruding nipples that are uneven in size, it is often best to position the jewelry at the natural base of each nipple, and not make one side shallower (or deeper) in an attempt to make them match.

You may like the accent of a single nipple piercing or prefer the symmetrical appearance of adorning both sides. If you wish to have a pair of nipple piercings, you may wonder if it is preferable to pierce one, let it heal, and later add the second; or to get both during the same session. An advantage of having them done at once is that your piercings are complete after a single studio visit and healing period. Also, it may be easier to get more symmetrical results if you have them both marked and performed at the same time, because alterations in the tissue as a result of piercing can be substantial. Then again, a benefit to sequential piercings is that you will still have one nipple to play with while the other is mending.

If you find that your nipples are more sensitive just before or while menstruating, consider this when scheduling your piercing.

NIPPLE PIERCING JEWELRY: RINGS OR BARS?

Rings were the standard initial jewelry style for nipple piercings for many years, but healing is easier with barbells, so they are recommended. Threadless bars are an excellent option if you wish to change the ornamentation on your jewelry, but threaded barbells are superior for rougher play (after healing, of course).

Rings have more potential for catching accidents, and if a bra or chest binder is worn, it can put excessive pressure against the jewelry and cause healing complications. Over time, rings acquired a reputation as being bad for healing, in part because piercers often inserted jewelry that was too small in diameter. If you wish to start with a ring, the portion of the hoop that passes through your piercing must be relatively straight. Too snug a ring will pinch your tissue at the entry and exit and cause irritation, discomfort, and other healing problems. A good rule of thumb is to multiply the width of your nipple by two for the appropriate diameter. Piercees are frequently surprised that a safe diameter for a nipple ring is considerably larger than they had imagined. When properly sized, both bars and rings can be worn in traditionally placed nipple piercings. But the barbell is the only practical style for steeply angled variations.

Your jewelry, whether ring or bar, must have sufficient room for the tissue to relax to its widest natural state, and some extra space to allow for swelling or tissue *development* (see "Nipple Piercing: Post-Piercing Nipple Development," page 162). To safely accommodate a piercing that measures just ⅜ inch across, a ½-inch diameter ring will be too small if there is normal swelling or development.

MULTIPLE NIPPLE PIERCINGS

A nipple can be pierced only once in a session; however, after healing, depending on its configuration and dimensions, it may be pierceable a second time. Few nipples are substantial enough to accommodate more than two piercings. Typical arrangements include two horizontal piercings (ordinarily moving closer toward the body for the subsequent hole), a cross (usually with a horizontal placement in front and a vertical behind it), or an *X* shape formed by two diagonal barbells. Exceptional skills may be required to place additional holes accurately in an already-pierced nipple.

PIERCING INVERTED NIPPLES

When performed on suitable candidates, piercings can be a remarkable resolution for inverted nipples. If the tip can be coaxed out sufficiently, then the nipple can probably be pierced, and jewelry will block it from retracting. However, the tissue can fight against the jewelry, so 12 gauge is a preferable minimum if the anatomy is sufficient to accommodate it. If this pressure is too forceful, migration is likely. Flexible polymer jewelry may be needed for healing if mechanical stress is too extreme. The full alteration may not be seen until metal jewelry is inserted later. Inverted nipples frequently swell more than usual following piercing, so the initial jewelry should be sized accordingly.

NIPPLE PIERCING: PROCEDURE

All undergarments and clothing above the waist need to be removed for nipple piercings to make sure the tissue rests naturally. Marking should be done while you're standing; you may then be positioned anywhere from seated to reclining flat, depending on your piercer's preference and the furniture in the room. I generally use forceps to perform nipple piercings. For your comfort and to make the procedure smoother, I do tissue manipulation before applying the clamps, especially for tight skin or underdeveloped nipples. If the forceps don't go on readily, I use a freehand method, as many piercers do. Others prefer a receiving tube technique.

Some studios offer *tandem piercings*, in which both nipples are pierced simultaneously by two synchronized piercers. This is an excellent option if you are planning to pierce both sides, and you are concerned about being able to tolerate the process. One of the piercers may mark the placement for both nipples to assure symmetry. Nipple sensitivity is dramatically different from person to person. If you have tender nipples, it is all the more important to seek an accomplished technician; it will have a significant impact on your comfort.

> **"My new nipple piercings are healing up well, and I am thrilled with them! For the first time in my life I am happy with how my breasts look, and I didn't even have plastic surgery!"—P.**

NIPPLE PIERCING: HEALING AND TROUBLESHOOTING

Tenderness may come and go due to clothing fit, sleep habits, physical activities, and other factors. Since this area is affected by hormonal fluctuations, many piercees find that they experience a *flare-up* (secretion, swelling, or discomfort) just before and during menstruation, even long after the healing period.

Nipple piercings can take an extended time to heal completely. They may regress for no apparent reason after months of stability. Should your piercing take an excessively long time to settle, try different jewelry or change care regimens until you figure out what works best. Experimentation can require patience, but adjust at least one aspect before giving up. If you endured the procedure and some of the healing period, it is worth preserving the piercing.

You will probably find that a snug undershirt or smooth-cup bra is helpful for protection and

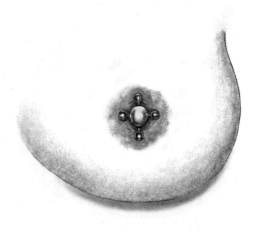

A double-pierced nipple with barbells forming an iron cross

comfort, including while you sleep. A minute or so after settling into a tight garment, the piercing usually feels less tender. Those who are not partial to sleeping in a shirt or bra can wrap a length of clean elastic bandage across the chest and around the body. This type of compression dressing protects the area while still allowing it to breathe, and avoids adhesives that could irritate skin or pull hair upon removal. A disposable nursing pad or cut-to-fit piece of panty liner worn inside a bra will absorb any blood or sweat and also help to conceal your jewelry. Nipple tissue is often rigid and unyielding, so your jewelry might not move easily unless wet or lubricated, even after healing. See "Tightness Is Normal," page 226.

NIPPLE PIERCING: POST-PIERCING NIPPLE DEVELOPMENT

Certain piercings are subject to swelling after the procedure. Nipples, however, are prone to *development* (a semipermanent or lasting change in the shape, dimensions, and texture of the localized nipple and areola tissue). This is often mistaken for swelling, though it is quite different. This effect is most common in *underdeveloped* (small) anatomy, and the change can be relatively dramatic. Still, it is not a universal response to nipple piercing. In essence, the nipple grows from the stimulus of the jewelry and the piercing. When the piercing is placed in the natural creases of the body, this development is usually attractive and well formed. If the piercing is not made in the proper spot, however, the tissue can develop a blobby, awkward appearance. These changes may not dissipate even if the jewelry is removed; think about whether this is acceptable before getting a nipple piercing.

NIPPLE PIERCING: CONCEALMENT

Nipple piercings may be discernible under light-weight or white clothing, but adding an undershirt, bra, or any extra layer should help to diminish the visibility of average-sized jewelry through clothing.

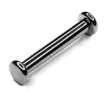

Snug-fitting barbells capped by small balls or discs are effective for concealment under clothing in most situations. Using a cylinder-shaped bead instead of a round one in a captive ring can eliminate the appearance of a second nipple protruding below your own.

A post with small disc ends helps to diminish the visibility of nipple piercings

NIPPLE PIERCING: BREAST HEALTH

There is no medical evidence that piercings increase the risk of cancer.[7] Nipple piercings won't interfere with breast exams or self-examinations; they may even remind you to pay attention to your breasts. Piercings might also encourage or inspire a partner to assist you with regular breast checks.

Health care personnel routinely require you to remove all metal from the area before a mammogram or other medical procedure. See your piercer for a suitable nonmetallic jewelry alternative to keep your piercing open, such as a polymer retainer. In the time it takes for a mammogram appointment, even a well-healed nipple piercing can shrink so much you won't be able to get your jewelry back in without the aid of an insertion taper—or a piercer.

NIPPLE PIERCING: SURGICAL CONSIDERATIONS

Many people experience substantial increases in sensation from nipple piercing after suffering diminished feeling from breast surgery. However, before piercing, it is essential to wait until you heal thoroughly after any operation in the region. Whether you have a breast reduction, augmentation, or other procedure, it is prudent to delay *at least* a year—even if your doctor says sooner is acceptable. If you have implants, use sound judgment when selecting a piercer and strictly comply with all post-piercing guidelines. The risks are real: an infection from the piercing can spread to your implant, which could require surgical intervention and might cause the loss of your augmentation.

You may not be a candidate if you have undergone radical breast surgery and reconstruction with nipple replacement using non-areolar tissue. Piercing might be possible if the donor tissue is a type that heals readily, such as labial skin. You should consult both an expert piercer and your surgeon.

Should you plan to undergo surgery in which your nipples will be entirely or partially removed and repositioned, it is advisable to leave in nonmetallic retainers so your doctor can reattach the tissue with the piercings at the same angle. More than one piercee has awakened from an operation to find a horizontal piercing had become diagonal or vertical. If necessary, have your surgeon discuss the matter with a trusted piercer.

NIPPLE PIERCING: BREASTFEEDING
Healed nipple piercings do not ordinarily prevent breastfeeding. For detailed information, see "Nipple Piercing and Breastfeeding," page 309.

NIPPLE PIERCING: IRRITATION, INFLAMMATION, AND BUMPS
In response to even slight trauma, nipple piercings can become tender and inflamed, and may secrete clear or cloudy fluid. It is relatively common for bumps to appear on one or both sides of a piercing. They may be inflamed tissue, excess scar formation, or what I term a "localized piercing pimple." See page 254 for information. Each type of bump requires a different approach, so check the relevant sections in "Trouble and Troubleshooting," chapter 16. Provide aftercare for your nipple piercings consistently throughout the entire minimum healing period. Treat them gently and do your best to avoid trauma, including excessive friction or pressure from clothing, and impact during sleep.

NIPPLE PIERCING: MIGRATION AND REJECTION
When most piercings migrate, they usually move directly outward from the body, but nipple piercings sometimes rise or twist instead. Consult your piercer at the first sign that your piercing is closer to the surface, there is less tissue between the entry and exit, or if it has moved from its original position. It is best if you make an effort to stop the progression right away. Options include changing to a different jewelry style, size, or material. Wearing nursing pads for protection or altering your sleeping position to minimize irritation are other possibilities. You will have to retire the piercing if you can see the jewelry right through the skin or there's just a small amount of fine tissue left between the entry and the exit.

NIPPLE PIERCING: CHANGING JEWELRY
Some piercees are comfortable changing their own nipple jewelry once the piercing has healed. This is not particularly challenging for the dexterous, though the tightness of the skin can make moving your existing jewelry difficult. Take a shower or apply a warm compress first to loosen the tissue. Use sterile lubricating jelly to ease out the old piece and facilitate the transfer of the new one.

Don't dally in the middle of a jewelry change; nipple piercings are notorious for being among the quickest to shrink and the most difficult to reinsert once left empty, even momentarily. An insertion taper can help you get the channel open and reinsert jewelry if you run into trouble. Unless you feel confident about what you're doing, it is best to visit your piercer for help.

NIPPLE PIERCING: STRETCHING

Most nipple piercings are not easy to stretch, and the tissue responds irritably if you attempt to expand too quickly. Wait a minimum of nine months to a year from the initial piercing, and don't force it, or you are likely to end up with a rejected piercing, not a larger-gauge hole. An enlarging schedule of one gauge per year is a steady pace. A double stretch (from 14 to 10 gauge, for example) is seldom possible, even with an old piercing of many years. Unless the next size slides right in without pushing and the thicker one does not need to be forced, keep to the one-size-at-a-time plan. With time and patience, however, some nipple piercings can be stretched to impressive sizes.

NIPPLE PIERCING: RETIRING

Expect some permanent modification from piercing your nipple. If you have had tissue development, much or all of it may remain, even if you abandon the piercing. A divot at the entry and exit might be the only lasting marks if you did not experience much change.

Do not impulsively remove nipple jewelry. Many a piercee has returned in regret to redo a closed nipple piercing they wished they'd left in place. It is significantly easier to keep in an existing nipple piercing than to get a reinsertion or repiercing later.

THE POINT

Nipple piercing is a favorite among many well-adorned body art fans and plenty who don't have any other piercings. Healing this placement sometimes requires patience, but you will likely find it well worth the effort. A piercing in your nipple can highlight the area in an enticing way and may add a whole new dimension of sensation and enjoyment. The subject of physical pleasure leads us right into the next chapter.

14

BELOW THE BELT: GENITAL PIERCINGS

Disclaimer: This chapter openly discusses adult matters, including genital anatomy and sexual function. Intimate piercings are not available to minors; these sections are not intended for individuals under eighteen years of age.

The first section in this chapter contains general introductory information about genital piercings. The next portion covers piercings of the *vulva* (external genitalia surrounding the vagina), followed by those of the penis and adjacent anatomy. For more information about living with these piercings, see chapter 20, "Sex!" Also refer to "Safer Sex," page 312, for essential facts about maintaining hygiene while healing a genital piercing.

Our Western culture does not foster genital pride, so many people feel disconnected from their nether regions. Intimate piercings encourage self-awareness and often educate piercees about their own bodies. Countless clients have said to me, "I want my clit pierced." When I show them a photo of a clitoris piercing, they shout, "Oh, no! Not *there*." They really wanted a *clitoral hood* (tissue above the clitoris) piercing but were not sufficiently acquainted with the territory or terminology to know the difference.

Below-the-waist piercings aren't for everyone, but many people get them to enhance their sex lives, and some seek them to feel adventurous or naughty. Others get genital piercings to reclaim or connect to their bodies, or for their extraordinary liberating and empowering effect. If they are of interest to you, there is much to know.

SELECTING THE RIGHT PIERCER

Genital piercing is unique because it has the potential to affect your sexual pleasure. A poorly placed piercing can result in a missed opportunity for enhancement or a temporary or permanent loss of sensation. Because of variations in genital anatomy and personal preferences for sexual stimulation, each piercee must be evaluated (even counseled) on an individual basis before deciding on a genital piercing.

Locate an experienced authority who has had specific training in placing and performing genital piercings. Some studios now offer services above the waist (or even above the neck) only, and many piercers have never done any genital work. The right practitioner will communicate with you openly and have a professional manner that helps you feel comfortable and safe.

Your piercer must be able to undertake their role with sensitivity, and you should be prepared to describe what you want from your piercing with honesty and candor. Many piercers simply do not have enough knowledge to guide you. They cannot determine, for instance, whether a particular placement would be stimulating or simply ornamental on your anatomy. A good piercer will have an in-depth conversation with you to be sure that you have all the education you need to make an informed decision about your piercing. Don't settle for a piercer who does not impress you with their vast knowledge and outstanding qualifications.

To properly place piercings, your piercer must scrutinize your genitals and may need to do some stretching, tugging, and pinching of your tissue to take a close look for veins or other vital structures. For accurate placement, the area must be marked, and then the skin may need to be moved. If you have a foreskin, it may need to be retracted, and the tissue pulled taut (as it is when you are erect). If you are a novice piercee, you might misconstrue these activities as being sexual in nature, but these procedures are invaluable for accurate placement. Nonetheless, always listen to your intuition. It is appropriate to call off your piercing if you believe your piercer is behaving inappropriately.

In my capacity performing professional online (photo) consultations for piercing problems, I see a never-ending parade of improperly placed genital piercings. Some are dangerous and excruciatingly painful, including accidental punctures of the clitoris. Please believe me when I say that it is crucial to vet your piercer carefully!

HOW MUCH DOES IT HURT?

Merely the thought of genital piercing is enough to cause many people to slam their knees together protectively. But intimate piercings are not particularly painful, contrary to what the uninitiated usually think. You should anticipate feeling well; however, you probably won't want to ride a bicycle or wriggle into your tightest jeans that day.

Many clients have compared the intensity of genital piercings favorably over other areas. Exceptions include ampallangs, apadravyas, dydoes, and the serious (though rare) clitoris piercing. These are sensitive spots, but getting them pierced can also be very rewarding.

BLEEDING

Just like any other piercing or break in the skin, a new genital piercing might bleed off and on for a few minutes to a few days. Specific placements in this vascular region tend to bleed. I address these in the sections covering each piercing.

Following any genital piercing, you should either be bandaged (see "Penis Region Piercings: Bleeding," page 193) or wear a panty liner or sanitary pad to protect your clothing, home furnishings—and your piercing. You may not bleed immediately, but once you stand and move, it often begins. Piercees of any gender can use panty liners or sanitary pads while healing. Initially, these absorb blood and help cushion the piercing; later, they also help keep it clean and dry. They come in a wide variety of thicknesses, sizes, and designs. To maintain hygiene, keep your fingers from the surface that will rest against your body; handle the pad or liner only from the back or the edges. First, pull your underwear to your knees and then stick the pad or liner into place to avoid contaminating it with your feet or shoes.

If you experience heavy bleeding, you may benefit from a potentially embarrassing purchase: disposable adult diapers. These are extremely absorbent and can help prevent messy accidents, especially overnight, as they are able to handle a much larger volume of blood than any pad. Clotted blood is normal and healthy; it is nothing to be concerned about when you maintain regular hygiene.

UNDERWEAR AND HYGIENE

"Going commando" might sound appealing, but snug undergarments help to hold your jewelry in place and reduce discomfort and tissue trauma. The extra layer of fabric helps maintain cleanliness, and, of course, it is hard to wear sanitary protection without some underwear to which you can attach it. Cotton fabric is more absorbent and permits better air circulation than synthetics. Make sure your underwear has no holes or loose threads to snag your jewelry. Yanking your skivvies down when they are caught on your ring or bar can damage—or even tear out—a genital piercing.

If you accidentally step on the crotch of your underwear and then pull them up against your piercing, that's as filthy as putting your open wound on the floor! When you don your undies, make plenty of room for your feet.

During healing, always put on underwear or clothing, or set down a clean towel before sitting on upholstery or another questionable surface.

URINATING

Bodily fluids are apt to get on certain genital piercings, which is not a problem—*if* they are your own. Urine will not harm your healing piercing if you are healthy, and it may even facilitate healing.[1]

The regular passage of fluid over the jewelry helps minimize crusting, too. Highly acidic urine can sting during the first few days, so drink lots of water to lower the acidity and decrease discomfort. Eat a diet rich in vegetables and fruits (including citrus), and low in animal foods to produce alkaline urine. Additionally, you can pour a clean cup of water—warm or cool, as you prefer—over the area as you urinate. This rinses off the urine so it doesn't linger uncomfortably, and the water feels soothing.

SHAVING AND WAXING

Depilating (removing hair via shaving, waxing, depilatory creams, etc.) your pubic region before visiting a studio for genital piercing is helpful. Depending on placement, trimming might work, but often leaves too much hair in the way. Clearing the area will make it easy for your piercer to see what they are doing. It could also make the experience easier for you, since having your hair accidentally pulled during a procedure might be more uncomfortable than getting pierced.

Shaving with a new genital piercing in place can prove a little tricky at first. Let the piercing heal for several weeks before grooming close to it. Once the piercing is healed, some jewelry (such as outer labia or scrotum rings) can be used as handles to hold the tissue taut while you shave. See "Depilating," page 307, for more tips.

TRANSGENDER CONSIDERATIONS

Anyone on hormone replacement therapy (HRT) for gender transition should take it for at least two years before seeking genital piercing to allow the expected local tissue changes to occur. Following genital gender confirmation surgery (GCS), delay piercing for at least one year (preferably two), for scar tissue to mature and the region to settle—as is recommended following any operation. Also, be frank with your piercer about your history to be sure they feel competent to work with surgically modified anatomy. Not all piercers have experience or familiarity with GCS, and any post-surgical area can present challenges.

VULVA PIERCINGS

Below you'll find general information about vulva piercings, followed by a detailed discussion of each of the most common placements.

VULVA PIERCING: ANATOMY

Genitals have tremendous—though sometimes subtle—variations. Very few piercees are candidates for all of the placement options. In fact, some with petite anatomy are suited only to outer labia piercings, and nothing in the hood region. Most vulvas are not configured for a triangle piercing, and many are not built for a horizontal hood piercing either. Everyone is different; heed the advice of an expert, and don't take it personally if the piercing you want doesn't anatomically suit you.

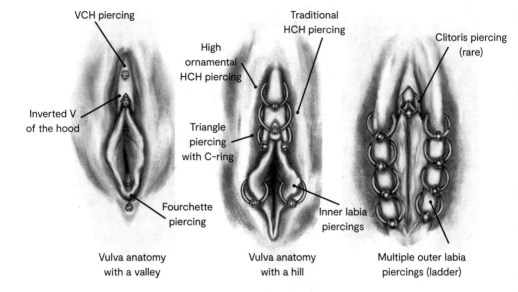

VCH piercing

Inverted V
of the hood

High
ornamental
HCH piercing

Traditional
HCH piercing

Clitoris piercing
(rare)

Triangle
piercing
with C-ring

Fourchette
piercing

Inner labia
piercings

Vulva anatomy
with a valley

Vulva anatomy
with a hill

Multiple outer labia
piercings (ladder)

VULVA PIERCING: HILLS AND VALLEYS

The following terminology helps us to identify and discuss two basic shapes of vulva anatomy. You might hear the terms *innie* and *outie* used to describe these shapes, but I'll reserve those words for navels.

If you have a *valley*, your outer labia are higher than your hood, which is flat or concave. You are very vertically shaped and are poorly suited to horizontal placements; the tissue is not the right shape to accommodate jewelry between your legs.

If you have a *hill*, you have a substantial hood that is higher than your outer labia. You may be a better candidate for triangle and/or HCH piercings, depending on other aspects of your anatomy. People with hills are better suited to horizontal piercings than those with valleys, but some still wear vertical placements, or both. A third configuration is a combination: a hill situated within a valley. Horizontal piercings may be possible, but they are more challenging on this type of shape.

VULVA PIERCING: THE STARTLE OF THE STICK

Even if your piercer guides you through deep breathing and you know a piercing is about to happen, the stick may startle you, causing you to jump or move. An experienced piercer will anticipate this, but it is also good for *you* to prepare yourself by being aware that this is a predictable response. Try to keep your knees apart and your hands away so your piercer can put in your jewelry and finish the job.

VULVA PIERCING: HYPERSENSITIVITY

This is not a frequent problem, but should you ultimately feel your genital piercing is too intense, you can try a different size or style of jewelry. If you still have discomfort, the piercing can be abandoned with no permanent changes to your sensation (if it was placed correctly). See "Overstimulation, Sensation, and Desensitization," page 314, for related information.

VULVA PIERCING: MENSTRUATION

Since menstrual fluid is your own bodily secretion, it is not harmful to a healing piercing. Nor is it problematic to get pierced while you are menstruating.[2] Exceptions include the Princess Albertina, due to its internal placement—and perhaps the fourchette. Individual piercers may prefer not to pierce you during your cycle, but there are no safety concerns. If your body is more sensitive at that time, this would be a reason to postpone piercing.

VULVA PIERCING: YEAST INFECTIONS

A yeast infection isn't an invasion of foreign pathogens, but an overgrowth of candida, a fungal flora that is routinely present in the body.[3] Therefore, it doesn't represent the same risk to your piercing that a bacterial infection could. Candida can cause the tissue to become irritated or sore, and a genital piercing could be affected the same way. Yeast infections are easily treatable, and it is unlikely that such an episode will cause lasting issues with your piercing. Note that the same symptoms (discharge, soreness, itching, painful intercourse) can be caused by other types of vaginal infections, which could affect a healing piercing. You should see a doctor for an accurate diagnosis and appropriate treatment.

THE VERTICAL CLITORAL HOOD (VCH) PIERCING

- o **Healing time:** 4 to 8 weeks
- o **Initial jewelry style:** Curved or straight barbell, or ring-style jewelry
- o **Initial jewelry gauge:** Commonly 14 or 12 gauge; maximum 10 gauge
- o **Initial jewelry size:** On average, ⅜ to 9⁄16 inch, sometimes longer

Many adults like the idea of making their genitals more functional and attractive at the same time. Having an extra spot to wear a diamond or ruby is pretty fabulous, too. These are some of the driving forces behind the expanding popularity of the vertical clitoral hood piercing. All types of people, from sorority sisters to empty-nest retirees, are getting VCH piercings. Numerous piercees who have no other body art wear the VCH. It is suited to anyone with a vulva who wants to explore new avenues of erotic sensation—if they're anatomically built for it. This piercing is liberating and stimulating, appealing, and inspiring. The momentary pinch and quick, easy healing period are a small price to pay for the pleasure you can derive. This is the genital placement performed by more practitioners than any other: 80 percent of the piercers surveyed offer VCH piercings.

Dr. Vaughn Millner and associates at the University of South Alabama conducted a research study on VCH piercings as they relate to sexual satisfaction. The results led to the following statement: "In this exploratory study, we identify a positive relationship between vertical clitoral hood piercing and desire, frequency of intercourse and arousal." These encouraging findings were published in the prestigious (and conservative) *American Journal of Obstetrics and Gynecology.*[4]

> "My VCH healed beautifully, and our first 'test drive' with some safe, gentle sex yielded not just one but MANY orgasms with just penetration alone. No additional clitoral stimulation needed, which was always needed for me in the past to reach orgasm. My mind is BLOWN. This piercing has changed my life. I wish every woman could experience this. My time on earth will be forever better."—A.

VCH PIERCING: PLACEMENT AND CHOICE OF JEWELRY

The VCH is, by far, the most popular vulva piercing for several reasons. The piercing and anatomy are oriented in the same direction, so jewelry nestles comfortably in the area. Approximately 80–90 percent of vulvas have a deep enough *prepuce* (the protective fold of hood tissue above the clitoris), in which jewelry can be placed for a safe and stimulating piercing.

This hood is typically configured like a tiny one-ended tunnel, and the VCH pierces just the (usually thin) skin above your clitoris, not through the glans itself. Most of the jewelry rests under the hood, so your clitoris receives direct action from contact with the jewelry during sexual activities. Many piercees enjoy this a great deal, but if you would describe your clitoris as hypersensitive, you will probably not want to wear jewelry in this location.

Whether your hood is formed like a hill or a valley, its depth is the primary consideration for suitability. To determine if your hood is deep enough for the piercing, try the "Q-tip test." Remove some of the fluff from the tip of a cotton swab, lubricate the end well, and attempt to slide it underneath your hood. If most of the cottony portion fits beneath the tunnel, you have sufficient depth for a VCH. (You must also lack a visible vein along the midline to be pierceable). If you are shallow and cannot accommodate most of the swab underneath, you are probably not a candidate. On some petite builds, the piercing can be cheated a little further from the edge of the hood for safety and durability. Still, a *minimum* of 5/16-inch natural depth is needed, along with pliable tissue.

Traditional placement for the VCH is at the *apex* (the deepest part) underneath the hood, along the midline. The piercing is commonly situated 3/8 to 9/16 of an inch up from the edge of the hood, depending on its depth. The VCH should be essentially equidistant from the edge on the top and underneath. Because of the tunnel shape, only a small amount of skin is pierced; I can often see right through it!

I use curved barbells in fresh VCH piercings, though some piercers favor straight ones. The curve conforms well to the area, enables the jewelry to rest a little closer to the clitoris, and provides a small amount of extra room without added length. In snug hoods, straight bars can cause pressure against the tissue. I would start with a ring only if you have an especially deep valley, so the jewelry doesn't protrude. If you are configured with a hill, a bar is the only suitable style, and even so, the piercing may be subject to a bit more trauma and irritation than those whose hoods rest more protected within their labia.

If you have a deeply recessed and hidden hood, you may still be suited to a VCH piercing if it has adequate depth, and your piercer can access the area to perform the procedure. If necessary, you or a studio employee, wearing clean gloves, can help to expose your hood. Even if your jewelry will be entirely tucked in and obscured by surrounding tissue, the VCH generally heals well. One concern is that irritation or embedding can result if the pubic mound puts excessive pressure against the top of the jewelry. A 7-millimeter silicone disc worn on the bar post beneath the top ornament will prevent these issues.

Inexpert piercers frequently place the VCH too low and close to the edge of the hood. Shallow piercings provide less sensation because the jewelry rests farther from the clitoris. Also, if too little tissue is pierced, you have a higher risk of tearing, migration, and rejection. Worse, many untrained "pros" perform inappropriate hood surface piercings, which don't contact the clitoris at all, and have a high risk of excessive scarring and other complications.

When you wear a bar for healing, the bottom end should show below the inverted V that forms the hood's peak. It should not be hidden entirely underneath. However, this is an option once healing is concluded and might be more pleasurable if your hood covers your glans. A ring worn as initial jewelry must be large enough to avoid constricting the tissue.

VCH PIERCING: PROCEDURE

Before you sign up, ask the piercer how they perform the piercing. If the reply is, "With forceps," turn around and leave! Clamping the tissue for a VCH can endanger your clitoris and cause the jewelry to rest too far from it. Or you might get one of the misplaced surface piercings that is just through a pinch of superficial skin on top of the hood. Unfortunately, these placement blunders are widespread.

A more suitable procedure is to use a needle receiving tube under the hood. I pierce through the dot that I marked for placement, and into the tube protecting your clitoris underneath. Alternatively, your piercer may carefully insert the needle under your hood and pierce upward using a freehand technique. The pierced tissue is often much thinner than that of an earlobe. A small percentage of piercees have thicker skin here, which is usually a little more sensitive during the procedure and may take longer to heal.

When performed capably, the sensation of the piercing itself is very brief, and afterward, there is seldom lingering discomfort. By the time you get dressed, you're likely to find that your VCH piercing feels good already, or simply that you notice something is there. It is also possible to feel nothing different at all. *Even if a VCH feels healed sooner, you must still follow all aftercare protocols for the minimum four-week initial healing period.*

> "When I got my VCH piercing, there was maybe just a half second of a dull ache. That was it. Then immediately no pain. I swear my piercing has already healed and it's only ten days old. No pain. No throbbing. My ears and cartilage hurt more than my VCH."—S.

VCH PIERCING: HEALING AND TROUBLESHOOTING

Occasionally, a bump will form at the top of the piercing, beneath the ornament. It is critical to avoid friction and tight, constrictive garments. Wearing cotton underwear or unscented panty liners and keeping the area dry might be helpful.

If you have a hill with an exposed hood, you may find healing more challenging, and the first week or so it might be a little more sensitive. Wearing the smallest jewelry that is safe will help to minimize irritation. If your initial jewelry is still uncomfortable or troublesome after the early accommodation period, its size or style will need to be changed by a professional as soon as possible.

A properly positioned VCH does not pierce through any significant nerves, so there is no basis for a loss of sensation.

VCH PIERCING: PHYSICAL ACTIVITY

Engaging in physical activities after getting a VCH piercing is fine; just listen to your body. Take a break from bicycling or horseback riding for a few weeks. With the exception of these activities, you will probably find that your new piercing doesn't cause discomfort while exercising; in fact, you may not even notice it. Then again, it may inspire you to work out. More than a few piercees have discovered that the stair-stepper or other gym equipment holds new interest for them after getting a genital piercing!

VCH PIERCING: CHANGING JEWELRY

The VCH piercing can feel quite different when you change the style or dimensions of your jewelry. Consider experimenting with other sizes of bars and threaded ends after you have healed. You might delight in the sensations from a short post with a ball resting under your hood, or you might enjoy a longer bar. Then again, you could prefer the feeling of a ring, and how it can be looped onto your partner's tongue barbell during oral sex. For maximum stimulation, especially if you have a recessed clitoris, a J-curve is a good option. Personal preferences vary, but the research can be fun.

VCH PIERCING: STRETCHING

The VCH is usually easy to stretch at least a size or two, and most wearers have sufficient anatomy to support gauges thicker than the initial size. Heavier jewelry may produce different sensations. After three months or so, the piercing should be ready to enlarge one gauge. Extensive stretching and heavy jewelry could disfigure this fine tissue.

VCH PIERCING: RETIRING

The VCH tends to shrink and close quickly; few piercees find they can easily take their jewelry in and out after healing. Since the clitoral hood is not a public area, any residual mark is apt to go unnoticed. If initial healing was uneventful, only someone looking for the spot would be likely to tell you had ever been pierced.

> "How funny it sounds to say that a piercing has changed my life, but it has. Not only did I find a lifelong friendship with someone special (Elayne Angel), I got a VCH piercing that has freed me. In the past, I'd had a few multiple orgasms, but the norm was one, and I was done. Well, now I have multiples often, and very strong, too. I never knew it could be this good.
>
> I had been molested as a child, so my genital area was something I looked at in shame. . . . This piercing has freed me from the bonds of the molestation. I can look at my genitals with pride and joy . . . I look at my piercing every day, and love it more and more. I didn't think a piercing could have this effect on me, but surprisingly, it has. No amount of therapy could have healed me the way this piercing has—by taking ownership of my body and choosing to have the VCH—by a piercer who is loving, kind, and very knowledgeable."—J.

THE PRINCESS DIANA/DUKE PIERCING

- Healing time: 4 to 8 weeks
- Initial jewelry style: Straight or curved barbell
- Initial jewelry gauge: Commonly 14 or 12 gauge; maximum 10 gauge
- Initial jewelry size: On average, ⅜ to ½ inch, sometimes longer

Princess Diana (or simply Diana) piercings are identical to the VCH, except that they are off to the side(s) of the hood instead of in the center. Some piercees, especially trans or gender nonbinary individuals, refer to these by their alternative name: *Duke piercings*. Ordinarily, they are worn in pairs; however, if you have more tissue on one side of your hood than the other, a single piercing could be a great way to celebrate your asymmetry. These are angled as high as eleven and one o'clock, or as wide as nine and three o'clock. Dianas are not nearly as popular as the VCH, since many builds are not full enough or are too asymmetrical for a matched pair. Some ample anatomy boasts all three: a VCH and two Princess Dianas/Dukes.

I named this piercing after the first woman I performed them on, and Princess Diana was in the news at the time, too. I thought female royalty should get some industry exposure since the popular Prince Albert piercing (see page 194) has had so much of it.

THE HORIZONTAL CLITORAL HOOD (HCH) PIERCING

- o **Healing time:** 6 to 8 weeks
- o **Initial jewelry style:** Customized circular barbell (C-ring or U-ring), fit to the anatomy; ring style
- o **Initial jewelry gauge:** Minimum 14 gauge; maximum 10 gauge
- o **Initial jewelry size:** Ring diameter ⅜ to ½ inch

The HCH piercing traverses a pinch of hood tissue above the clitoris, which many find aesthetically appealing. Unfortunately, because of the way most vulvas are configured, the HCH won't be able to deliver the added sensation the majority of piercees desire. If you're among those seeking genital piercing to enhance your erotic pleasure physically, a different placement may be more worthwhile. Of course, a vulva piercing can be visually delightful and boost self-image, even if not placed for extra stimulation. Most of the piercers surveyed (62 percent) perform the HCH.

HCH PIERCING: PLACEMENT AND CHOICE OF JEWELRY

Ample tissue in the configuration of a hill is needed for an HCH piercing. If you have a valley with a flat, concave, or deeply recessed hood, you are not a candidate. If your build is not symmetrical, which is common, the jewelry tends to twist or lean to one side, causing discomfort, migration, or other healing difficulties. Most vulvas are formed with a hood that nearly—or completely—covers the clitoral glans, preventing jewelry from touching it. For an HCH piercing to be stimulating, your clitoris must be exposed, the piercing perfectly placed, and the jewelry accurately sized. Then the bead on a ring can touch your clitoris to add sensation; otherwise, the HCH will be . . . just a hood ornament.

The piercing should go in the natural creases at the base of the hood tissue where it forms from your body. Your piercer should carefully check for blood vessels because they are sometimes located in this area. If a vein cannot be avoided, then the piercing should not be attempted. Your piercer must also be sure that your hood tissue is pliable enough to pinch up and lift away from your clitoral shaft below, so they don't unintentionally pierce it.

The best level for an HCH depends on your anatomy and your goal. You may prefer to have it positioned toward the top of your hood for visibility if you want the piercing solely for adornment rather than sexual enhancement. For sensation, the placement works in conjunction with the ring diameter so that the ball rests on the desired spot. The correct diameter ring will encompass the tissue without pinching. A bar is seldom comfortable or safe. If it is short enough to avoid twisting, it may embed or pinch. If it is long enough to accommodate your hood, it will be prone to shifting and causing problems when you close your legs. A modified circular barbell is superior for safety and comfort during healing, especially if your build is tall, with a lot of height from the base to the edge of your hood. See "Customized Circular Barbell (C-Ring or U-Ring)," page 87, for details.

HCH PIERCING: MULTIPLE PIERCINGS

If you have a long enough hood, multiple horizontal piercings (among other options) may be possible. Two or three are not unheard of, but more than that is rare. Rings are usually positioned so that they overlap somewhat. But there has to be enough space between them so that the jewelry does not pinch your sensitive tissue. You need highly symmetrical, well-developed anatomy and a skilled piercer for multiple hood piercings. It is best to get them one at a time unless they are relatively far apart. More than two hood piercings per session could be excessively traumatic to the area.

HCH PIERCING: PROCEDURE

I find forceps well suited to the HCH piercing. They not only secure the skin, but they also help to assure that only the hood is clamped and pierced, and not the nerve bundle just underneath. Tissue manipulation can help to separate the hood from the clitoral shaft. I am careful to pinch up the skin from the midline in anticipation of its tendency to fold in on itself. Otherwise, you can end up with a channel that is too shallow in the middle and wears through over time, or an unsafe double piercing that misses the center completely and just passes through an unstable sliver of skin on each side of your hood. If the tissue cannot be lifted and kept elevated in the center for the procedure, do not attempt this piercing. Some piercers use a freehand technique or receiving tube.

HCH PIERCING: HEALING AND TROUBLESHOOTING

It can be challenging to accommodate horizontal jewelry in a vertical space, so this is not a practical piercing for many builds. The most common complaint during healing is that the jewelry twists. Prevention is key: if your anatomy is not well suited, don't get an HCH piercing. If your build is not too asymmetrical, twisting should be minimized by wearing a *C-ring* or *U-ring* (widened circular barbell). Visit your piercer if you experience trouble, as you may need a jewelry adjustment or change—even during healing. Early intervention can prevent more severe issues.

HCH PIERCING: CHANGING JEWELRY

Sometimes a smaller ring can be worn after you are healed, which may improve your comfort by reducing the tendency for the jewelry to twist. Changing the ring's diameter might alter the way the piercing feels, however, since the bead will rest in a different spot. A ring with an oval or inverted teardrop shape may be more comfortable and also functional. Bar-style jewelry cannot add sensation since it will not touch the clitoris.

HCH PIERCING: STRETCHING

If you have a substantial amount of tissue in the piercing, you can safely enlarge it to rather hefty sizes over time. You may find the HCH more stimulating when you wear heavier jewelry. After six months or so, it should be ready to expand one gauge.

HCH PIERCING: RETIRING

If you remove your jewelry, the piercing can shrink or close quickly. Because the HCH should be placed in the natural creases at the base of your hood, if you abandon it, even your gynecologist may not notice any residual traces. There is no physiological basis for a lasting change in sensation from getting this piercing and later retiring it.

THE TRIANGLE PIERCING

- o **Healing time:** 3 to 4 months
- o **Initial jewelry style:** Customized circular barbell (C-ring or U-ring), fit to the anatomy
- o **Initial jewelry gauge:** Commonly 12 gauge, rarely 14 or 10 gauge
- o **Initial jewelry size:** Circular barbell 3/8- to 9/16-inch diameter before widening

The *triangle* is a modern innovation. According to *PFIQ magazine*, Gauntlet piercer Lou Duff performed the first one in the early 1990s (see "The Inventor," page 179). The triangle is a horizontal piercing of the hood tissue, but unlike the HCH, it passes just beneath the clitoral shaft. Sensations from the triangle are quite unlike the stimulation from genital piercings that contact the clitoral glans.

The triangle is a very advanced piercing because it is placed primarily by feel in an area where unfortunate and unacceptable damage could be done if a mishap occurs. Scrutinize the qualifications of any piercer who is under consideration to perform your triangle. Find out exactly where and how they learned to do this piercing and how many they have done. If you aren't thoroughly impressed with their training and experience, keep looking. Only 34 percent of piercers surveyed offer them. I can report from vast experience doing online consultations that many piercers are unaware of the suitable anatomy, proper location, or ideal jewelry for the triangle, but perform them anyway.

THE INVENTOR

I didn't conceive of the triangle piercing myself, but I performed one on Lou Duff, the San Francisco piercer who did invent it. She originally called it the "Triangle of Submission," after the basic shape of the area through which the jewelry runs (a triangle formed by the pubic bone, the clitoral shaft, and the edge of the clitoral hood), and for the *bottom* (the submissive partner in a BDSM relationship) on whom she first performed it. Since Lou felt such a name wouldn't be popular with the general public, she shortened it to "the triangle" when she brought it to Gauntlet, and thereby the world.

TRIANGLE PIERCING: PLACEMENT AND CHOICE OF JEWELRY

Optimal anatomy is symmetrical, with a substantial protruding hill formation. Your piercer must be able to locate your clitoral shaft and pinch behind it, at the base of your hood. Any veins in the area must be avoidable. If your anatomy is very narrow, petite, flat, or concave, you are not a candidate. Unfortunately, most vulvas are not configured for a triangle piercing.

This piercing should support and stimulate the clitoral shaft, *not* the glans. Because the skin of this region is exceptionally soft and pliable, positioning jewelry behind the clitoris does not add sensation. Regrettably, this is a widespread placement error. The triangle belongs at the natural juncture where the base of the hood joins the body, at the highest point just beneath (not through!) the clitoral shaft.

A triangle and an HCH both pierce through the same type—and often a similar amount—of hood tissue. However, for most piercees, a triangle is the far more pleasurable option. Many people ask whether a VCH or a triangle is more stimulating, but they are entirely different. Lots of piercees get one of each. Wearing both the VCH and triangle creates a tantalizing clitoris sandwich because jewelry surrounds it, front and back.

Due to the recessed location of the piercing and the vertical orientation of the vulva, the safest and most comfortable jewelry for a healing triangle piercing is a custom-fit circular barbell. Your piercer should adjust the size and shape to suit your build. The gap between the circular barbell's ends must be wide enough to accommodate your hood so that the jewelry tucks down to cradle your inner labia. The surrounding structures hold the jewelry securely in place. The part of the ring that passes through your tissue fits in the limited space without twisting like a hoop or shifting like bar-style jewelry. For more on this jewelry, see "Customized Circular Barbell (C-Ring or U-Ring)," page 87.

FAILED GEOMETRY

Unfortunately, many of the so-called "triangle" piercings I see are not correctly placed because they are not located behind the clitoral shaft. Fortunately, most of these failed piercings have not resulted in damage or dysfunction, but they can cause grave disappointments and lost opportunities for enjoyment. These misplaced piercings often cause unnecessary pain and must frequently be abandoned. I have also seen incorrectly placed piercings that accidentally passed through the clitoral glans or shaft (all performed by piercers who claimed to be trained and experienced in triangles).

TRIANGLE PIERCING: PROCEDURE

I use small Pennington forceps to perform triangle piercings, though some piercers prefer septum clamps, and others use a receiving tube or freehand technique. First, I perform tissue manipulation to lift and isolate the clitoral shaft and assure correct placement. This also makes it safer and easier to apply the forceps. The piercer *must* keep your clitoral shaft elevated throughout the procedure. If they let go, the cordlike structure will drop down, and the piercing will not be in the correct position. Your clitoral shaft itself might get pierced, or you will end up with a low or deep hood piercing, but not a triangle. If your piercer does not seem concerned with keeping your clitoral shaft lifted, they probably do not know where a triangle should be placed.

I've had piercees comment that the triangle was less tender than a nipple or VCH piercing, but others find the experience more intense and draining. Still, when skillfully executed, the process should be brief.

> "The triangle piercing is my absolute favorite and the one I love and cherish the most. It really has transformed my life both personally (a confidence thing) and sexually. Sex with the triangle and VCH together is a total game changer in the bedroom, with a partner . . . or without!! Prior to the triangle piercing I just couldn't reach orgasm, period!" —B.

TRIANGLE PIERCING: HEALING AND TROUBLESHOOTING

The triangle is the vulva piercing most likely to bleed heavily, so don't be surprised if you spot, or even flow, for several days afterward.

If your jewelry doesn't rest evenly between your legs, migration is to be expected. It may move just a little and then stop, or you may need to abandon the piercing. Some settling or movement is common even when the placement and jewelry are ideal. If your C- or U-ring does not comfortably tuck down or upward close to your body, the ring, threaded ends, or gap size may need to be adjusted. If your piercing is not healing well and you are not wearing a custom-fitted circular barbell, you should have one inserted.

TRIANGLE PIERCING: CHANGING JEWELRY
After healing, you can try wearing a captive or bead ring, teardrop, curved or straight barbell, or another jewelry style. Because the anatomy is manipulated (the clitoral shaft lifted) to do the piercing, removing the jewelry can result in a total loss of your triangle, instantaneously. The hole can be very difficult or impossible to locate immediately following jewelry removal. Always use insertion tapers for jewelry changes to keep something in the channel at all times.

TRIANGLE PIERCING: STRETCHING
The triangle is a sturdy piercing, although it is not always easy to stretch. But it can be expanded to large sizes with time and patience. Some piercees enjoy the way heavier or thicker jewelry looks and feels after enlarging a healed triangle to a bigger gauge.

TRIANGLE PIERCING: RETIRING
Consider carefully a decision to remove triangle jewelry; reinserting it later is often impossible. When the piercing is positioned correctly against the body at the natural folds, evidence of an abandoned triangle is seldom very visible if healing was uneventful.

SUCCESS!
I have had multiple clients confide that they had never experienced an orgasm until after I performed their triangle piercings. Their partners and sexual activities were the same as before, so the piercings were responsible for the desired effect. (That validates my life's work right there!)

OUTER LABIA (LABIA MAJORA) PIERCINGS

- o **Healing time:** 3 to 4 months or longer
- o **Initial jewelry style:** Ring or curved bar
- o **Initial jewelry gauge:** Most commonly 14 or 12 gauge; 10 gauge for generous anatomy
- o **Initial jewelry size:** ½- to ⅝-inch diameter ring-style jewelry; ⁷⁄₁₆- to ⅝-inch length curved bar

These piercings are worn on the sides of the vulva in the thick, fleshy folds of tissue where hair grows. *Labia* mean "lips" in Latin; the awkward singular form of the word is *labium*.[5] Outer labia piercings are often done in pairs, with one on each side, or in multiples, to form a *ladder*. In general, you are unlikely to experience erotic sensations like those often derived from a VCH or triangle; piercing here is apt to be primarily visually pleasing. Seventy percent of piercers surveyed perform this placement.

PUTTING THE *FUN* BACK IN *FUN*CTION

Labia piercings have *some* potential for function. At least one inventive piercee I know has used multiple outer labia rings to hold up her stockings on occasion.

OUTER LABIA PIERCINGS: PLACEMENT AND CHOICE OF JEWELRY

The piercings can be situated nearly anywhere along the pliable rim of the outer lips. They pass through denser tissue and take longer to heal than hood and inner labia piercings. On some builds, they can be positioned adjacent to the clitoris, where the jewelry might provide stimulation from the sides. You can wear them higher up on the lips, to make them more visible, or lower, next to the vaginal opening, where a partner might feel them during intercourse.

To determine the most comfortable spot for your piercing(s), consider the size and shape of your anatomy when your legs are together and apart. A curved bar is generally a better choice if you have large thighs and the space between your legs is crowded. The jewelry diameter is dependent on the size and shape of the area. If your labia are more defined and convex, then a smaller diameter can be used because it will encompass sufficient tissue. When the area is flatter, a wider diameter is needed to include the optimal width between entry and exit. If you have undefined lips or large thighs, you might find outer labia piercings hard to heal.

The piercings can be placed to frame the most exposed portion of your lip (the surface that faces the floor when you are standing), or they can be tucked inward, to frame the edge of the labia—half on the smooth, hairless part, and half on the surface where hair grows.

You can make a statement with multiple labia piercings—inner and outer—depending on your build. Six or eight is not unheard of, and some piercees have even more. If you plan to wear a single piece of jewelry to join both sides together after healing, let your piercer know so the placement can be aligned accordingly. Matched piercings can be directly opposite one another. The tissue is malleable, so pairs need not be offset.

OUTER LABIA PIERCINGS: PROCEDURE

I use a forceps technique to perform outer labia piercings, though some prefer freehand. Even when a pair is done directly across from one another, they are pierced one at a time. Many would describe the feeling of getting outer labia piercings as "biting and pinchy." Once the procedure is over, you may experience some tenderness or bleeding afterward. When you receive a pair of outer labia piercings, it is normal if one side bleeds, and the other doesn't.

OUTER LABIA PIERCINGS: HEALING AND TROUBLESHOOTING

Your bleeding could continue for a week or so, and swelling may remain for longer. Snug underwear helps to support the jewelry, but tight pants will cause discomfort and irritation, so wear loose or stretchy clothing at first.

You might experience thickened or hardened tissue, excess scarring, or other problems around the openings during healing; don't panic. This is generally caused by the unavoidable trauma of walking and sitting. It tends to come and go throughout healing. Try one or more of the troubleshooting techniques suggested in chapter 16. If your problem is persistent, a change in the size or style of your jewelry is warranted. These complications frequently resolve over time, and the piercings heal without ill effects—except for a drain on your patience.

OUTER LABIA PIERCINGS: CHANGING JEWELRY

Unless you are very flexible or your piercings are located closer to the front, you may require assistance to change your jewelry. After healing, adding weights, bells, or charms on your piercings could be pleasurable. Some piercees also enjoy the feel of tugging on these sturdy labia piercings during sexual activity.

OUTER LABIA PIERCINGS: STRETCHING

Wait nine months or more before stretching. If you had troubled healing, wait a year or longer. This is a durable piercing; if the channel is reasonably wide, you can safely wear jumbo jewelry. If you have especially pliable tissue or wear weights (or attach your stockings to your jewelry), you might be able to skip a gauge.

OUTER LABIA PIERCINGS: RETIRING

Outer labia piercings may not close upon removal, but they do shrink. Because the area is not in public view and may be masked by pubic hair, these piercings will not leave much of a mark. If you depilate and/or had healing problems, more noticeable signs of your piercings may be visible to a doctor or lover.

LABIA MINORA (INNER LABIA) PIERCINGS

- o **Healing time:** 4 to 8 weeks
- o **Initial jewelry style:** Ring-style
- o **Initial jewelry gauge:** Most commonly 14 and 12 gauge
- o **Initial jewelry size:** Diameters from ⅜ inch to ½ inch

Inner labia are the delicate, hairless folds of flesh situated between the outer labia. This tissue is nearly identical to that of the clitoral hood; it is quick and easy to heal. Some labia are not large enough to pierce or have only one side that is suited. A single ring on either side is popular, or they can be pierced in pairs or multiples. Few piercees report experiencing erotic sensations from this placement, but a partner might feel them during intercourse. Most of the piercers surveyed (68 percent) offer labia minora piercings.

INNER LABIA PIERCINGS: PLACEMENT AND CHOICE OF JEWELRY

This area is frequently shaped much like an earlobe, and traditional placement for a single piercing is at the lobe's visual center. However, any spot along the labia is acceptable if the piercing is least ⅜ inch from the edge of your lip. Your piercing should be equidistant from the edge on both sides to frame the area aesthetically and comfortably. Unlike most other piercings, this skin is usually so slim that a ring without any added diameter won't constrict the tissue. If you wear jewelry that is too thin, it can cut your skin or stretch it unintentionally. Even short (¼-inch) barbells are generally too long for labia minora piercings because the tissue is so slender. When a post is long, the bar doesn't sit evenly, and one ball rests too heavily against the fresh piercing. Rings are best for initial jewelry; bars are acceptable later.

INNER LABIA PIERCINGS: PROCEDURE

I use forceps to secure the tissue for piercing, though other techniques can be used, including a receiving tube or freehand. Few describe inner labia piercing as intense; most would say it is a brief pinch or sting. Afterward, you can expect minimal discomfort, though there may be some bleeding.

INNER LABIA PIERCINGS: HEALING AND TROUBLESHOOTING

Inner labia piercings are generally trouble-free to heal, thanks to a good blood supply and fine tissue. The main concern is to avoid excessive trauma during healing from sexual or physical activity. On fuller anatomy, they may be subject to additional irritation, and therefore, be more tender. Supportive underwear may minimize this issue. Labia minora is one of the piercings in the pathway of urine, which could sting at first. To increase your comfort, follow the suggestions on page 168, "Urinating."

INNER LABIA PIERCINGS: CHANGING JEWELRY AND STRETCHING

The subjects of changing jewelry and stretching are usually discussed separately in this book, but inner labia piercings stretch so readily that the two must be covered together.

You may enjoy the sensation of tugging on healed labia minora piercings or wearing weights, bells, or charms; however, these activities usually result in stretching because the tissue is very fine. Twelve-gauge jewelry is a safe minimum if you want to wear some extra weight or play with your piercing in this way.

Labia minora are the vulva piercings most frequently expanded to oversized gauges: some determined wearers stretch to ¾ inch or larger! This thin tissue is also sturdy and resilient. Large holes are normally stable if set sufficiently distant from the edge. Although rare, it is not unheard of for inner labia to have tissue development, just like a nipple. Some asymmetrical piercees will even receive an inner labia piercing on their less-developed side, seeking to make things match up. While not a guaranteed result, it could be worth a try.

INNER LABIA PIERCINGS: RETIRING

If you abandon inner labia piercings, they will leave small marks that are not highly visible—unless you have stretched them or hold an unconventional job. The holes may shrink, but even when they are left empty for an extended period, this is one of the few areas of the body that routinely remains open once fully healed.

THE FOURCHETTE PIERCING

- ○ **Healing time:** 6 to 8 weeks
- ○ **Initial jewelry style:** Curved bar
- ○ **Initial jewelry gauge:** 12 or 10 gauge
- ○ **Initial jewelry size:** ⅜ inch or longer

The melodious anatomical term for the site of this piercing is the *frenulum labiorum pudenda*, also known as the *fourchette* (French for "little fork"). This piercing is located in the perineum, like the guiche piercing. But it is more practical and comfortable because, like the vulva, it is oriented vertically. It could be challenging to find an experienced professional, however, as only 37 percent of piercers surveyed perform the fourchette.

FOURCHETTE PIERCING: PLACEMENT AND CHOICE OF JEWELRY

The fourchette piercing frames the rear border at the bottom of the vaginal opening. The lower portion of the piercing rests between the vagina and the anus, and it should be no closer than ½ inch from the rear orifice. If you have had a midline tear or *episiotomy* (incision to facilitate childbirth), you are not a candidate due to localized scarring. Because this tissue is so fine, the jewelry must be thick enough to prevent tearing. A 12 gauge is a safe minimum size. If you don't have a substantial, defined natural fold or ridge of tissue in this location, you should skip the fourchette piercing.

THE RIGORS OF RESEARCH: THE FOURCHETTE

The fourchette piercing is an innovation of the 1990s. I got the first three of them on different occasions, each in a slightly different spot. I tried diligently to identify perfect placement. While enjoyable, my investigation revealed that the required anatomy for a fourchette has a defined lip of tissue in the region. Unfortunately, I do not. The research was worthwhile, though, because many of the piercees who wear them find that the fourchette produces unique and enjoyable sensations. Mine did, too, while they lasted. Sitting on a powerful speaker at a live concert was an unforgettable experience!

FOURCHETTE PIERCING: PROCEDURE

The procedure can be a little tricky for your piercer because of the fourchette's almost-internal placement. I generally use forceps, but have also performed it using a receiving tube. Others may prefer a freehand technique. Most do not find this to be a particularly intense piercing, though the procedure can be a little awkward. These don't tend to flow, but some bleeding is always possible.

FOURCHETTE PIERCING: HEALING AND TROUBLESHOOTING

You must be careful not to sit on unclean surfaces unless you are wearing underwear or clothing. To increase comfort throughout healing, sanitary napkins or panty liners can provide extra padding and wick away moisture. Maintain excellent hygiene due to the proximity of the piercing to the anus: shower regularly and be careful to wipe away from the jewelry after visiting the toilet.

FOURCHETTE PIERCING: CHANGING JEWELRY AND STRETCHING

This spot is nearly impossible to access yourself, so expect to require assistance for jewelry changes. Similar to the inner labia, this fine, elastic tissue easily accommodates larger sizes, but it does not withstand heavy jewelry because of a propensity to stretch more than desired. You may find it expands so much with normal wear that an ordinary barbell end (³⁄₁₆ inch, or 5 millimeters) can pass right through the piercing! To prevent jewelry loss, if the channel appears to be widening on its own, avoid wearing ends that are too small. If your fourchette piercing continues to stretch, you may need to switch to a ring—unless you wear ends that are significantly bigger than average. The catch-22 is that large balls or gems may cause unintentional stretching, yet a ring might be problematic for penetration. Most wearers find a curved bar is the preferred jewelry style.

FOURCHETTE PIERCING: RETIRING

The area is not subject to public view, and the piercing is placed within natural creases, so it will not leave a visible mark. A divot or slight pit may be observable on the outside surface, but the inner portion will be invisible. Once the piercing is well established, it is fairly likely to remain open without jewelry in place.

THE CHRISTINA PIERCING

- o **Healing time:** 6 to 9 months or longer
- o **Initial jewelry style:** Surface bar, curved bar, or L-bar
- o **Initial jewelry gauge:** 14 to 10 gauge
- o **Initial jewelry size:** ½ inch or longer

The *Christina* (or *Venus*) piercing is a vertical surface piercing at the top of the *cleft of Venus* (top of the *vulva*) that extends up the *pubic mound* (soft rise of flesh just above the genitals).

The jewelry does not contact the clitoris, so this placement is ornamental. Though the Christina will not add erotic sensation and takes a long time to heal, if you are a motivated piercee, these aspects may not prove to be barriers. Half of the piercers surveyed perform this placement, but I am not one of them. (Though I specialize in genital piercings, I eschew this one because it is a surface piercing, which is not my area of expertise.)

CHRISTINA PIERCING: PLACEMENT AND CHOICE OF JEWELRY

You are suited to a Christina piercing if you have plenty of pliable tissue on your pubic mound and also a defined valley or divot at the very top of your hood (where the vulva separates into two sides). This is where the bottom end will rest. However, if your mound is so pronounced that the jewelry would lean forward on the top or face the floor, this is not a good piercing for you. An L-bar is sometimes used to conform to the area. It has a right-angle bend for the top of the piercing and is straight on the bottom. A disc, flat gem, or another low-profile threaded end is likely to be safer and more comfortable than a ball on the top.

CHRISTINA PIERCING: PROCEDURE

It is best to depilate before visiting the studio for a Christina piercing. If you fail to do so, your piercer will usually have to trim your hair closely. Tissue manipulation can help to prepare the area before applying forceps or supporting the tissue for a freehand procedure.

CHRISTINA PIERCING: HEALING AND TROUBLESHOOTING

For a Christina piercing to be successful, you must avoid trauma, but this region is subject to considerable stress from ordinary clothing. Don't wear lace or mesh underwear, which can snag your jewelry. A somewhat frequent complication is the enlargement of the top hole. This is more likely if you're wearing a curved bar (rather than a surface bar), or a ball-shaped end instead of a flatter one. If the jewelry starts sinking in or embedding, visit your piercer immediately. As with all surface piercings, migration and rejection are not uncommon.

Sanitary pads can help to shield and cushion the Christina throughout healing. Place it farther forward than usual to protect the piercing. Frontal sexual contact is inadvisable during the entire lengthy healing course. Consider your lovemaking preferences before deciding to get a Christina piercing, because even after healing, this type of friction may prove uncomfortable and irritating.

CHRISTINA PIERCING: CHANGING JEWELRY/STRETCHING

This area is a little more accessible for home jewelry changes. It is safest to use a taper to minimize trauma and facilitate the swap. Large gauges are not usually desirable because the Christina is a surface piercing. If you do want to stretch, wait for a year or more following the piercing.

CHRISTINA PIERCING: RETIRING

Abandoning this piercing will leave a mark on your pubic mound. Should you plan to be depilated on a long-term basis and are not fond of scars, the Christina is not a wise choice for you. However, if you grow your pubic hair, residual scarring may not be visible.

THE CLITORIS (CLITORAL GLANS) PIERCING

- o **Healing time:** 4 to 8 weeks
- o **Initial jewelry style:** Ring- or bar-style for horizontal placement, bar-style for vertical
- o **Initial jewelry gauge:** Usually 16 gauge, rarely 14 gauge
- o **Initial jewelry size:** ⅜-inch minimum diameter, up to ½ inch for the well-endowed

If you are familiar with human anatomy, you surely comprehend that the clitoris is a profoundly sensitive part of the body. This small but significant structure contains approximately eight thousand nerve endings,[6] twice the number found in the glans of the average penis.[7]

Piercing of the *clitoral glans* (visible beneath the hood) is rare, and it is serious business. A piercing mishap can result in the loss of your clitoral sensation and the termination of your erotic pleasure from that zone. Only a highly experienced master should perform this piercing, and only on candidates who are ideally suited to it. Exercise extreme caution before embarking upon a clitoris piercing; this is not an area with which to take risks.

Out of the limited number of people who genuinely desire a clitoris piercing, only about 5 percent are suitably configured. Those who are sufficiently endowed and properly pierced usually do experience increased sensitivity. However, you could lose sensation if the piercer is not masterful enough to carry out the job perfectly, you are anatomically unsuited, or you experience healing complications. The diminished feeling *might* return upon removal of the jewelry.

CLITORIS PIERCING: PLACEMENT AND CHOICE OF JEWELRY

Chances are, your clitoris is too small to withstand a piercing; the average one is less than 5 millimeters in width (no bigger than a pencil eraser).[8] Therefore, 16 gauge is the most common initial jewelry size. This is the only below-the-neck piercing that I will start with jewelry so thin. To preserve the sensitivity of your diminutive but precious organ, jewelry must not comprise too great a proportion of the anatomy.

Even when your clitoris is large enough to pierce, if the hood tissue fits too tightly or heavily over it, this would interfere with the jewelry. For safety, your clitoris must be relatively large (*at least* a full ¼ inch wide) and be easily exposed beneath a short or loose hood. Most builds are simply not made this way.

The proper placement is always in the groove at the base of the clitoral glans. For a horizontal placement, when the head is oval, the piercing is made at the midpoint. If the glans is teardrop-shaped, it goes a small distance below that, at the widest point. Some hoods cannot be comfortably retracted enough to expose the upper part of the clitoris for a vertical piercing. Most lack space to accommodate the end of a barbell there.

A perfect jewelry fit is critical. If a ring or bar is even slightly too large, it can interfere with the way your hood naturally rests. Pressure against the jewelry will be painful and can lead to scarring, migration, and healing problems.

CLITORIS PIERCING: PROCEDURE

If your clitoris can't be clamped because your anatomy is too small, your hood is in the way, or the process is too intense for you, then you aren't a suitable candidate for the piercing. Even if forceps aren't used, these remain reasonable criteria for would-be piercees. Slow, deep breathing is especially important to help keep you as relaxed as possible. Moving during the procedure can be ruinous. Most of the brave, determined individuals who do receive a clitoral glans piercing find that it is a very intense (though ultimately rewarding) experience.

Give yourself some extra time to recover before arising. You may want to take a day or two off from work and physical activities. Always wear a pad or liner following the procedure. Due to the vascular nature of this area, bleeding is normal. It can be relatively heavy and may last for several days. The trade-off is the same as other spots with a good blood supply: this piercing usually heals quickly.

CLITORIS PIERCING: HEALING AND TROUBLESHOOTING

You can expect intense discomfort or actual pain for several days after piercing this exquisitely sensitive area. Excessive distress beyond the first week or two may indicate that your jewelry isn't resting properly and that you have too much pressure against it from your hood or labia. See your piercer for an evaluation and possible jewelry change. If you cannot find a size or style that situates comfortably, your piercing will need to be abandoned. Do not persist in trying to heal, because scarring from this problem is to be expected. It can be extensive, permanent, and may cause diminished feeling or hypersensitivity.

CLITORIS PIERCING: CHANGING JEWELRY

You will probably want some help with jewelry changes. Altering the style and size can impact the mechanics of your sexual activities and satisfaction, so consider experimenting with different options to find your favorite, once you are fully healed.

CLITORIS PIERCING: STRETCHING

You can stretch a clitoris piercing if your anatomy is substantial enough to support thicker jewelry. Increasing one or two sizes is usually possible if you allow plenty of time between stretches. After that, the tissue may be more challenging to enlarge. A few hardy piercees have expanded their clitoral piercings to 6 gauge and even larger.

If you have your mind set on a sizable clitoral glans piercing, once healed, put in the heaviest jewelry you can wear comfortably. Try adding light charms or bells as tolerated to help it stretch over time. Never endure discomfort for the stretching process; if your piercing does not enlarge easily, do not force it. Even after healing, this can cause migration.

> "I had my clitoris pierced (not the hood) and I have never regretted getting it done. Over the years it stretched to a 4 gauge. The pleasure never stops, the feeling is still intense, and my sex life has never been this good. I'm seventy-five now but still going strong in that department. What a rewarding experience!"—G.

CLITORIS PIERCING: RETIRING

When you leave jewelry out of a well-healed clitoral glans piercing, it may stay open. However, if the channel shrinks much, this spot could be too tender to stretch for jewelry reinsertion. The piercing is recessed at the base of natural folds, so there will not be any visible mark left if you abandon the piercing, unless there was scarring. A clitoris piercing often causes some enlargement of the area, and this can be permanent, but other evidence of piercing will be difficult or impossible to see.

THE PRINCESS ALBERTINA PIERCING

- o **Healing time:** 4 to 6 weeks or longer
- o **Initial jewelry style:** Captive ring
- o **Initial jewelry gauge:** 10 gauge, though some piercers will use 8 gauge
- o **Initial jewelry size:** ⅜ inch

The Princess Albertina is a rare piercing of the female urethra. Its name derives from the Prince Albert, which pierces the equivalent anatomy on the far-more-accessible penis. If you haven't experimented with urethral stimulation, it is advisable to try it out before deciding on this piercing. The jewelry will produce a lot of sensations, and you may not find them enjoyable if they aren't familiar.

PRINCESS ALBERTINA PIERCING: PLACEMENT AND CHOICE OF JEWELRY

The piercing enters the *urinary meatus* (urethral opening) and exits through the bottom with a ring resting at or in the vaginal opening. Variations in placement result from different anatomy: a higher urethra can cause the piercing to be more prominent and forward; a lower opening can make the jewelry rest more hidden and tucked into the vaginal canal. The Princess Albertina should not be prohibitive to penetration—and it is intended to enhance it. James Weber of Infinite Body Piercing is the piercer responsible for popularizing this version of the PA. He advocates 10 or 8 gauge for initial jewelry, though I use the smaller 10 gauge as a maximum for any piercing. The ring should be thick enough to withstand the pressure and tugging of sexual activities.

PRINCESS ALBERTINA PIERCING: PROCEDURE

This piercing is tricky to perform due to its recessed location, and its rarity makes it challenging to find a professional with experience. Having an assistant to spread the labia and expose the area is extremely helpful during the procedure. I insert forceps into the urethra and pierce from inside it, though some practitioners use a receiving tube. A curved needle may be helpful in the limited space here.

PRINCESS ALBERTINA PIERCING: HEALING AND TROUBLESHOOTING

Bleeding afterward is to be expected. Though quick and easy to heal, the Princess Albertina piercing is not very forgiving if you mistreat it. As a rule, you *must* wait at least two weeks after getting pierced before penetrative sex, which is a departure from my usual post-piercing guidelines. (See "Safer Sex" on page 312.) Migration and rejection are likely if you abuse the piercing too early (or possibly at all).

Since the vulva has a significantly shorter urethra than the penis, there may be an increased risk of urinary tract infections when this piercing is healing. Drinking lots of water is essential, and cranberry juice may be helpful.[9] Jewelry is unlikely to affect the flow of urine, though some spraying is possible. Urination may sting initially, so follow the advice on page 168, "Urinating," to reduce discomfort. You should not use soap on this piercing, but saline is fine, and your own urine flushes out the wound.

PRINCESS ALBERTINA PIERCING: CHANGING JEWELRY

You will require assistance with jewelry changes due to the recessed location of the piercing within the vaginal opening.

PRINCESS ALBERTINA PIERCING: STRETCHING

The Princess Albertina stretches readily, much like its princely counterpart. However, heavy jewelry is not suggested, since the piercing is made relatively close to the urethra's edge.

PRINCESS ALBERTINA PIERCING: RETIRING

The Princess Albertina won't leave a visible mark or any noticeable residuals since the site is internal. Like the Prince Albert, the channel tends to stay open if the jewelry is removed. You would need to leave this piercing empty for childbirth.

PENIS REGION PIERCINGS

All of the genital piercings described in the prior section fit neatly into the single word "vulva." Unfortunately, the English language lacks an equally concise way to refer to the genital piercings discussed next, which include those of the penis, scrotum, perineum, and pubic area.

Introductory information common to all genital piercings is at the beginning of this chapter. A few additional points are covered below, followed by detailed explorations of each of the standard placement options for this anatomy.

PENIS REGION PIERCINGS: URINATING

Urine will run directly over certain piercings, including the Prince Albert and foreskin (when not retracted). To soothe stinging, follow the suggestions under "Urinating," page 168. Alternatively, put some water in a big, clean cup or other vessel, submerge the piercing, and urinate underwater.

Putting unwashed hands anywhere near your piercing or jewelry poses some risk of infection, even if you don't touch it when you use the bathroom. To avoid contamination from dirty fingers, wash your hands before you urinate, use a tissue or paper towel to handle yourself, or sit down, but make sure your piercing never touches the toilet bowl.

PENIS REGION PIERCINGS: BLEEDING

I always apply the amusingly named "rubber chicken" wrapping for piercings on the head or shaft to help you avoid an embarrassing mess. This dressing consists of sterile gauze around the piercing, covered by a medical glove. (The drooping fingers look like a chicken comb.) I secure it with a rubber band that is snug enough to keep the bandage in place, but not so tight as to diminish your circulation. Prince Albert, ampallang, and apadravya piercings regularly bleed enough to fill a glove, multiple times. Keep the rubber chicken on until it is full and needs to be changed or until you must urinate. Reapply a leak-proof wrapping if there is any sign of bleeding, and for a day or two longer. If your penis retracts into your body, this type of bandage won't stay on. Should you receive a piercing that bleeds much, heavy-duty sanitary pads or adult diapers may be needed.

PENIS REGION PIERCINGS: SENSATION

You need not be concerned about feeling distracted and continuously aroused by your new genital piercing. Unless a piercing is being handled or moved, it will produce almost no physical sensations. This is true even for a fresh piercing once the procedure is over and your nerve endings settle down. It is possible, however, that the idea or the appearance of your new ornament will result in an excited state. The penis and scrotum have a wide distribution of nerve endings, so desensitization and hypersensitivity are seldom issues with genital piercings.

PENIS REGION PIERCINGS: COCK RINGS AND CHASTITY DEVICES

If you wish to wear a cock ring with a genital piercing, discuss this openly with your piercer if it might conflict with the jewelry. This can be of concern for pubic, guiche, and high scrotum piercings. You may need to put on your favorite model so your piercer can see if there is room for both. Even if you have space for a cock ring, you'll probably need to forgo wearing it for a while to avoid excessive pressure on your new piercing.

If you are hoping to use piercing(s) in conjunction with a chastity device, be sure to bring this up with your piercer beforehand, as this is a critical factor for determining the best placement. Also see "Infibulation," page 316.

PENIS REGION PIERCINGS: ERECTIONS

It is natural to get an erection during the cleaning or marking phase of a genital piercing, and this will not surprise an experienced piercer. An erection can assist in obtaining an accurate jewelry measurement, which is advantageous for certain piercings. If you are still rigid when the time comes for your piercing, the procedure will be more difficult or impossible for your piercer, and you will surely bleed more. Try to think about baseball or dinner at Grandma's house for a few minutes to alleviate your condition. Getting an erection from seeing your new piercing with the jewelry in place is also a frequent occurrence. Again, bleeding is a common consequence.

The jewelry you wear in genital piercings must accommodate your largest engorgement. If your jewelry is too tight when you are erect, return to your piercer for a new piece right away. Jewelry that is too small can cause discomfort, migration, and healing problems.

When your piercing is new and tender, you may want to keep a glass of ice water by the bedside to douse any nighttime or morning erections. If there is dried matter on your jewelry, getting an erection can be painful as the crust gets pulled into your piercing. This rough material can also be detrimental to the delicate healing tissue.

THE PRINCE ALBERT (PA) PIERCING

- Healing time: 4 to 8 weeks or longer
- Initial jewelry style: Ring, customized circular barbell (C-ring or U-ring) preferred, or a curved bar
- Initial jewelry gauge: 12 gauge minimum, far more commonly 10 gauge; some piercers do larger
- Initial jewelry size: Minimum ⅝ inch, but anatomically dependent

In the world of modern piercing, the *Prince Albert* is a historic piercing, but not because Queen Victoria's consort wore one—he didn't. Claiming he did was a

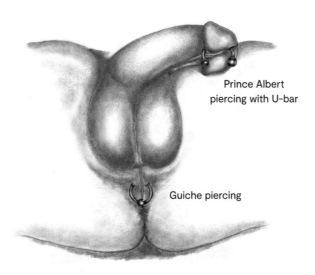

Prince Albert
piercing with U-bar

Guiche piercing

fanciful fabrication (see sidebar below). It is notable because, during the early years of Western body piercing, this was the most popular genital placement. Many among the heavily pierced describe the Prince Albert as their favorite.

The PA looks like a severe puncture of the penis. However, the piercing traverses the thinnest pierceable tissue on the body, encompassing much less skin than the average earlobe piercing. I often hear unfounded concerns that the Prince Albert is more dangerous, harder to heal, or more susceptible to infections because it pierces the urethra. If you are healthy, your own urine is not harmful to the piercing. Two-thirds of piercers surveyed offer PA piercings, though only 45 percent perform them on *intact* (uncircumcised) penises.

A TITILLATING TALE BY DOUG MALLOY

"The *Prince Albert*, called a 'dressing ring' by Victorian haberdashers, was originally used to firmly secure the male genitals in either the left or right leg during that era's craze for extremely tight, crotch-binding trousers, thus minimizing a man's natural endowment. Legend has it that Prince Albert wore such a ring to retract his foreskin and thus keep his member sweet-smelling so as not to offend the Queen. Today its function is strictly erotic, providing the ultimate in sexual pleasure to men of both persuasions. Piercing is through the urethra at the base of the penis head. The procedure is quick; the pain, minimal; the healing, rapid; and the pleasure, lifelong."

—Excerpt from a pamphlet circulated by Gauntlet in the 1970s and '80s called *Body Piercing in Brief,* which provided almost entirely fictitious "histories" of a dozen piercings (courtesy of Jim Ward, from his book, *Running the Gauntlet)*

PRINCE ALBERT PIERCING: PLACEMENT AND CHOICE OF JEWELRY

The piercing is made on the underside of the penis at the juncture of the head and shaft. The jewelry rests within the urethra and is worn out the tip of the *urinary meatus*. Many piercees greatly enjoy the sensation of an object inside the urethra, though it may take a short time to become accustomed to its presence. The urethra is not in the center of the penis—it runs along the bottom—so the piercing passes through just a membrane of skin.

The 10 gauge is a reasonable maximum starting thickness, and the most common I use. Let your piercer know if you have plans to stretch to jumbo sizes because this should be factored in when deciding on the placement. If you don't have a large penis or a high urethra (allowing for an ample distance between the natural juncture and the lower edge of the urethral opening), you can be pierced a little further down the shaft to make the piercing more substantial. Even if the piercing is distant from the tip of the penis, the skin isn't any thicker. You should have no less than ½ inch of tissue between the piercing and the edge of your urethra when your penis is flaccid. If you want to stretch larger than 8 gauge, the piercing should encompass at least ⅝ inch when you're flaccid.

I suggest the customized circular barbell jewelry style for healing. It conforms better to the area than a curved bar and doesn't protrude from the body as far as a hoop would. This lower-profile design is more conducive to wearing condoms, which are required for sexual activities during healing. Other advantages include a more precise, adjustable fit, greater comfort, and less trauma. When you wear a bar (of any shape), the ball at the tip of your penis should be large enough to prevent it from slipping into your urethra. The jewelry must be sized to fit when you are erect, though you need not achieve that state during the procedure. Your piercer can get a measurement by pulling the skin between the spot for the piercing and the tip of your penis.

Instead of a flat, pierceable surface, a cordlike web often rests in the center of the area where the Prince Albert is worn. In these cases, the piercing must be set a little further down the shaft, or, more commonly, slightly off to one side. The web must be avoided because penetrating it makes an unstable, uncomfortable PA and tends to result in little flaps of cut tissue. If the skin is not webbed, then the piercing can safely go right in the center (if no visible blood vessels are identified).

Several factors can help you and your piercer decide whether the piercing should be placed to the left or right of the web if it can't go in the center. Your piercer should look for visible veins and select the other side. If both are clear, they can put it on the one that aligns better with your urethra so that the jewelry sits straighter.

If your penis is intact, you may still be built for a PA piercing. You must be able to comfortably retract your foreskin far enough for the piercing to be placed in the appropriate location. The piercer should check your tissue with your foreskin in both positions to be certain the jewelry will fit properly, and you must not wear a piece so large that it prevents your foreskin from resting in its natural position.

PRINCE ALBERT PIERCING: ANATOMY/HYPOSPADIAS
Approximately one in every two hundred fifty male children is born with a form of *hypospadias*, a congenital anomaly in which the urethral opening is not located at the tip of the penis.[10] The Prince Albert piercing is impossible or inadvisable in severe cases. In milder forms, the urinary meatus is still on the glans (sometimes in the spot where a PA is traditionally placed). If the urethra is large enough, a piercing might be possible by situating it further down the shaft. You must consult an expert piercer if you have hypospadias.

PRINCE ALBERT PIERCING: PROCEDURE
This procedure may be challenging for you mentally, but it is not particularly intense physically. Some have compared it favorably to an earlobe piercing.

I perform the Prince Albert using a needle receiving tube. I lubricate it before inserting it a short distance into your urethra. The NRT is not overly large, but some piercees still find its presence to be the most unpleasant part of the procedure, so I leave it in as briefly as possible. My technique is to overshoot the dot slightly when I insert the tube, so when I draw it back into position underneath the mark, I am confident the tissue inside the urethra is taut and flat. In most cases, I can see right through the skin to the tool inside. I make the piercing from the outside, through the mark, into the protective tube, safely guiding the sharp tip of the needle out your urethra. I transfer in the jewelry following the same direction.

PRINCE ALBERT PIERCING: HEALING AND TROUBLESHOOTING
The amount of post-PA bleeding that frequently occurs can be alarming even if you think you are prepared for it. It is cruel and unprofessional for a piercer to perform your Prince Albert without educating you about what to expect during the aftermath. Rest assured, intermittent blood flow for several days is absolutely normal. After that, it can continue to bleed off and on for a few more days. Keep bandaged up for a while longer than you think you need to (in the "rubber chicken" or adult diapers), even if it seems your bleeding has stopped.

Healing of Prince Albert piercings is usually quick and trouble-free unless you are overzealous with sexual activity too soon.

PRINCE ALBERT PIERCING: URINATION
Many piercees are apprehensive about being able to urinate standing up after getting a PA. A few easy maneuvers can help you to normalize the act once you have

healed. When a ring sits in the middle of your urethra, it can split the flow and cause a splashy mess. Also, many Prince Albert piercings stretch on their own, leaving extra room around the jewelry, which results in leakage from the piercing hole. A simple solution is to plug the hole on the bottom manually when you urinate. Place a finger on the underside of your penis just at the front of the jewelry. If you wear a ring, put your fingertip within the hoop. This draws the jewelry to the lower edge of your urethra, so it doesn't interrupt the flow. Or, rotate your penis so that the ring faces the ceiling. This helps to merge urine leaking from the piercing hole back into the stream.

PRINCE ALBERT PIERCING: CHANGING JEWELRY AND STRETCHING

It is usually easy to change your own Prince Albert jewelry, especially if you insert it from the outside, rather than feed it into your urethra. Sometimes the PA stretches so readily that you may be able to skip sizes. However, once expanded, the tissue may not shrink back much if you remove your jewelry later. This is the most popular body piercing for jumbo expansion; jewelry of 0 or 00 gauge (8 or 9 millimeters) is not unusual. Many piercees and their partners enjoy the sensations of a Prince Albert sporting big, heavy jewelry. Sizable rings do not prohibit urination because when thicker pieces are added, the urethra stretches, too. Caution: hefty rings or bars can be dangerous to your partner's teeth during oral sex.

PRINCE ALBERT PIERCING: RETIRING

Unlike most piercings, once a Prince Albert is healed, it is usually there to stay. Even if you abandon it, you can probably reinsert jewelry later. Depending on how large the hole was stretched, it could remain open enough to leak once empty. Covering the hole with your finger during urination is an acceptable resolution for most piercees. If not, consult an understanding urologist or surgeon to learn about the pros and cons of a procedure to excise and stitch up your unwanted aperture.

PRINCE ALBERT PIERCING: ALTERNATE PLACEMENT— DEEP PRINCE ALBERT

When the piercing is made further down the shaft, this is called a *deep Prince Albert*. This is sometimes performed as a result of mild hypospadias; other times, it is just a personal preference, especially for those who want to wear jumbo jewelry. The tissue is still thin and pierceable, but the tube is inserted further into the urethra for the procedure. These tend to heal quickly, and other aspects are the same as a traditionally placed PA.

PRINCE ALBERT PIERCING: ALTERNATE PLACEMENT— DOLPHIN PIERCING

When a deep PA piercing is made (farther down the shaft), and jewelry is threaded between it and a traditionally placed PA, this is called a *dolphin piercing*. Unfortunately, this works much better in fantasy than in reality. Those who have a typical amount of size difference between flaccid and erect states do not often find any style of metal jewelry comfortable in a dolphin piercing. Flexible polymers may be more practical.

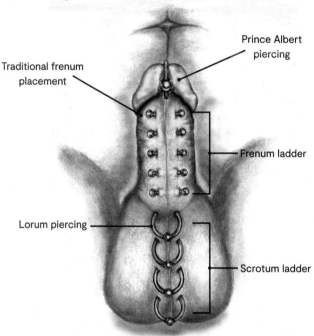

Prince Albert piercing

Traditional frenum placement

Frenum ladder

Lorum piercing

Scrotum ladder

THE FRENUM PIERCING

- o **Healing time:** 3 to 4 months or longer
- o **Initial jewelry style:** Straight barbell
- o **Initial jewelry gauge:** 12 or 10 gauge, some piercers do larger
- o **Initial jewelry size:** Anatomically dependent; commonly ⅝ inch, though sometimes 9/16 to ¾ inch or more

The *frenum* is a versatile genital piercing that is second in popularity only to the Prince Albert. The name comes from shortening the anatomical terms for the area: *frenulum* or *fraenum* (a fibrous cord of connecting tissue, in this case, on the underside of the penis). It joins the glans to the foreskin, and the bulk of it is commonly removed during circumcision.[11] Two-thirds of piercers surveyed (66 percent) perform frenum piercings.

FRENUM PIERCING PRECEDENT

A documented reference shows that a tribe in Southeast Asia practiced frenum piercing for sexual enjoyment long ago. According to an ethnological publication dated 1884, "Amongst the Timorese of Indonesia, the Frenulum beneath the glans penis is pierced with brass rings, the function of the ring is to enhance stimulation during sex."[12] Lacking other historical precedents, the frenum piercing appears to be primarily a modern innovation, intended for the pleasure of the wearer and possibly their partner.

FRENUM PLACEMENT

A traditional frenum piercing is placed on the underside of the circumcised penis about ½ inch down the shaft from the usual location of a Prince Albert. Poorly trained piercers frequently place the frenum too close to the glans, so there is not enough room for a PA. For intact anatomy, this high placement may be the only practical location for a frenum piercing near the usual spot. The classic frenum is on the bottom of the penis. It rests opposite the groove where the corona joins the shaft on the top. After healing, if you wear a large ring through the piercing and around the shaft, the hoop rests level. A ring wide enough for this is too cumbersome for healing.

The frenum piercing does not penetrate the shaft or the urethra; it simply goes through the fine, pliable tissue. If the skin can be pinched up, it can be pierced. "Frenum" initially referred only to the traditional spot on the underside; now, it is used to describe any piercing along the surface of the shaft, including the top and sides. Success rates vary for nontraditional spots. Some piercees can heal anywhere along the shaft, but many find alternative placements more apt to migrate or reject.

FRENUM LADDERS

Multiple frenums are common, and when placed in a row, they are referred to as a *frenum ladder*. You can wear a ladder on any surface of the shaft, but the bottom is most popular. The piercings, however, need to be an adequate distance apart to avoid pinching. Depending on how many you ultimately desire, one option is to put several evenly spaced piercings wide apart and add more between them over time. Each piercer has their own policy regarding how many they will perform in one session; my maximum is four. The more piercings you get at once, the longer they may all take to heal. When your body is taxed beyond its ability to repair, rejection is a frequent consequence, so patience and planning are required for ladders.

FRENUM PIERCING: PROCEDURE

I use the forceps method for frenum piercing, though some practitioners prefer freehand. Illumination is very useful for locating veins in the area. Anyone who has ever had a zipper accident will probably say it was considerably more intense than a frenum piercing.

FRENUM PIERCING: HEALING AND TROUBLESHOOTING

Because frenum piercings tend to experience a lot of friction during sexual activity, you must modify your behavior if you experience discomfort or irritation. Pleasure Plus condoms have extra room in the traditional frenum area.

Frenum piercings frequently migrate a small amount during healing, and those placed in nontraditional spots often lose even more tissue. A barbell that fits well at first can end up too long. Downsizing to a snug bar after healing makes your piercing more comfortable and less prone to issues. Frenum (and several other genital) piercings could result in thickening of the tissue, which becomes harder and denser around the jewelry. This does not indicate a complication, and the tissue changes can be permanent or may diminish over time.

FRENUM PIERCING: CHANGING JEWELRY

After a traditionally placed frenum piercing heals, you may want to replace your jewelry with a large ring or add a *frenum loop* (band of metal that encircles the shaft) by attaching it to your barbell. You might be able to add one onto your existing barbell. If the post is too snug, you will need a longer one to accommodate the attachment ends of the loop. A functional style variation has several balls around the outside of the piece for your partner's pleasure.

Determine the diameter you need for an around-the-shaft jewelry style while you are erect. Measure using a draftsman's circle template (available at office and art supply stores). The frenum loop or ring should be snug when you are erect. If you have a substantial size difference between flaccid and rigid states, this jewelry style will stay behind your glans only when you are erect.

A circular barbell is a good option because its two balls on the top of your penis may provide extra stimulation for your partner. You can also alter the diameter of a circular barbell to your exact size by spreading or narrowing the gap between the balls. If a pair of balls is good, a third might be even better; add an extra one to create a captive circular barbell. It could be tricky to find a bead that fits in a wide gap if you have spread the ring diameter.

FRENUM PIERCING: STRETCHING

If your frenum piercing is located in very loose excess skin, it will be a better candidate for stretching to a large size. A nontraditionally placed frenum or one that is through taut tissue will be less likely to respond well to attempts at expansion.

FRENUM PIERCING: RETIRING

Removing jewelry from a healed frenum piercing often results in complete closure of the channel. Some permanent changes in the appearance of the area may occur. Once hardened scar tissue forms, it generally remains fairly obvious because this skin is fine. Dimpling or pitting might also be evidence of an abandoned piercing.

THE LORUM PIERCING

- o **Healing time:** 3 to 4 months or longer
- o **Initial jewelry style:** Ring-style or curved bar
- o **Initial jewelry gauge:** 12 or 10 gauge (preferred)
- o **Initial jewelry size:** Minimum bar diameter ⅝ inch; minimum ring diameter ¾ inch

The *lorum* is a piercing at the natural fold that divides the penis shaft from the scrotal sac (see illustration, page 199). The name was coined in the 1980s while I was performing a genital piercing on the late Dan Kopka, my former coworker at Gauntlet, Los Angeles. He wanted a frenum, he said, only lower.

"Not a frenum, a lower-um," Dan declared, pinching the tissue at the desired spot.

"Oh, that would be a good spot. Yeah, a 'lorum,'" was my reply, and the name stuck: piercing in that particular location has been called a lorum ever since.

LORUM PIERCING: PLACEMENT AND CHOICE OF JEWELRY

The lorum is a horizontal piercing at the juncture of the penis and the scrotum. When positioned more toward the shaft, the jewelry can help to anchor a condom in place—though this would be uncomfortable and unsafe during healing. If you don't want it to rise onto the shaft when you're erect, request a lower placement.

This stretchy tissue changes substantially depending on temperature and arousal. Your piercer should carefully check the proposed marks before piercing you, because this skin can expand dramatically.

LORUM PIERCING: PROCEDURE

I perform the lorum with forceps, as I do other piercings in this area, though freehand is always an option. Your piercer may request that you don a glove to hold your penis out of the way. However, they may manage to access this spot without assistance.

If you have failed to trim or shave, the pulling of some hair could end up being the most uncomfortable part of your piercing experience; most piercees do not usually find the lorum intense. This area seldom bleeds much.

LORUM PIERCING: HEALING AND TROUBLESHOOTING

The piercing is protected by being sandwiched between the scrotum and the shaft of the penis; healing is often smooth and comfortable. Like other genital piercings, this one sometimes develops lumpy or hardened tissue around the openings as a routine part of healing.

You must apply a waterproof bandage to protect your piercing before sexual activities. Even if your lorum rests within the lip of a condom, that won't provide sufficient protection.

LORUM PIERCING: CHANGING JEWELRY

Once you are healed, it is not particularly difficult to change your jewelry. A minor challenge is that you must keep your penis out of the way to access the area.

LORUM PIERCING: STRETCHING

The lorum is a sturdy piercing that can be stretched to large gauges. It is not particularly challenging to expand, but you must have sufficient tissue in the initial piercing and wait long enough (nine months or more) between stretches.

LORUM PIERCING: RETIRING

Because the lorum rests beneath the penis, evidence of the piercing will not be obvious upon removal. Residual scarring will not be noticeable even on a nudist.

Lorum piercings tend to shrink and close quickly. Once you remove jewelry from a well-healed lorum, you cannot ordinarily reinsert it easily later.

THE SCROTUM PIERCING (HAFADA)

- Healing time: 3 to 4 months or longer
- Initial jewelry style: Ring-style or curved bar
- Initial jewelry gauge: 12 or 10 gauge (preferred)
- Initial jewelry size: Minimum diameter ⅝ inch; (for rings I favor ¾ inch for a sturdy piercing)

If you desire a genital piercing that is ornamental and not inserted during intercourse, a scrotum piercing may appeal to you (see illustrations, pages 199 and 217). The general location of a scrotum piercing is evident in its name, but the particulars are yours to determine. They can be placed pretty much anywhere the skin can be pinched. The piercing is called a *hafada* when placed on side(s) in the upper portion of the natural fold(s). Scrotum piercings can go along the midline from lorum to guiche, and in its most plentiful expression, multiples can form a chain mail pouch surrounding the entire sac. Over half of the piercers surveyed (56 percent) do scrotum piercings.

SCROTUM PIERCING: PLACEMENT AND CHOICE OF JEWELRY

The piercing traverses only the surface tissue and does not penetrate the interior of the scrotal sac. To help you decide on placement, imagine how jewelry will rest in your skin and how clothing and motion from your activities will affect the healing wound. The orientation of the piercing is not a limiting factor when you wear bar-style jewelry; vertical, diagonal, or otherwise, it will rest close to your body. A ring is suitable as initial jewelry only when the piercing is relatively horizontal.

Be patient with your piercer, because the scrotum can be tricky to mark. This tissue expands, contracts, and changes drastically and rapidly. Your piercer may require you to stand and sit several times to check the placement. A set of marks represents a baseline for the way the tissue rests at that particular time. Marks can appear level and then rise, fall, or spread to change position by as much as an inch. Asymmetry of the scrotum is standard, so matching up pairs can be challenging. If you are uncertain about the proposed placement, ask your piercer to let you wait for a few minutes to see if any tissue changes necessitate adjustments. If you plan to have a scrotum ladder, getting several piercings in one session can lead to more accurate spacing and alignment.

SCROTUM PIERCING: PROCEDURE

This procedure is essentially the same as the lorum piercing.

SCROTUM PIERCING: HEALING AND TROUBLESHOOTING

As far as sexual activity is concerned, it could be considered either a pro or a con that the piercing is not on your penis. It shouldn't be tender during penetration, but the healing wound still needs to be protected from your partner's bodily fluids. Since you can't cover this area with a condom, you must wear a waterproof wound-sealant bandage over the piercing during sex.

SCROTUM PIERCING: CHANGING JEWELRY

If you are comfortable changing your jewelry, you can swap out the frontal placements on your own. Toward the back of the scrotum, they may be more challenging to access without assistance. You might experience pleasurable sensations from adding weight to your scrotum piercing.

SCROTUM PIERCING: STRETCHING

These piercings can be expanded to relatively large sizes after healing. Wait at least nine months from the initial piercing before attempting your first stretch, and the same amount of time or longer between subsequent enlargements. Unless you wear weights, the one-gauge-at-a-time schedule is standard.

SCROTUM PIERCING: RETIRING

Once you take the jewelry out, the piercing could shrink or close; it might be diffi-cult or impossible to reinsert if you change your mind later. If you had substantial tissue changes during healing, some visible lumpiness or thickening could remain. These changes may not be as noticeable if the piercing is in the natural folds of the scrotum.

THE GUICHE PIERCING

- ○ **Healing time:** 3 to 4 months or longer
- ○ **Initial jewelry style:** Ring-style or curved bar
- ○ **Initial jewelry gauge:** 12 or 10 gauge (preferred)
- ○ **Initial jewelry size:** 9/16-inch minimum diameter

The *guiche* (pronounced "geesh") is a piercing in the *perineum* (between the scro-tum and anus). It straddles the *perineal raphe*, the faint vertical ridge of tissue that runs through the region (see illustration, page 195). This piercing is specifically for the pleasure of the wearer, and jewelry creates various possibilities for erotic stimulation. Ornamenting the perineum with a piercing calls attention to the region in addition to making it more sensitive. One of Doug Malloy's colorful fab-rications is a story about South Pacific Islanders who ostensibly pierced this area during puberty as a rite of passage into adulthood. He claimed they wore a shell hanging from a leather thong through the hole to help them to assess the tides as they squatted in the water. In reality, the guiche appears to be a modern innovation that originated in the gay leather community. Half of the piercers surveyed offer guiche piercings.

INSTANT GRATIFICATION

So many piercees find that the guiche piercing feels good as soon as the jewelry is in place that I became a little envious. Their immediate enjoyment—and my resulting guiche envy—was my inspiration for researching the fourchette piercing for those of us with vulvas.

GUICHE PIERCING: PLACEMENT AND CHOICE OF JEWELRY

The guiche is a horizontal piercing between the scrotum and the anus, near the location of your pants' inseam. The piercing should be placed at least 5/8 inch from your anus. You might have limited space, with only a single location where a guiche can be situated. If you are generously built in that region, you may have a range of options. Your piercer may point out (by gently pinching and prodding) the traditional central placement and then offer sites slightly north and south so you can select the one that feels best to you. Multiple guiches are possible if you have a long perineum, but more than one is not often performed in the same session. Vertical perineum piercings aren't common, but can be successful if the tissue is pliable, and there is sufficient space for the jewelry.

You are suited to the guiche if you have loose, pliable skin in this region. If your anatomy is flat, you will need to wear jewelry that is a little wider in diameter to encompass sufficient tissue. The size and shape of your thighs also affect the placement, and this should be considered during marking. A small amount of migration is normal while healing, so if your piercing starts with too little tissue, you can end up with a shallow guiche that might reject.

GIGANTIC GUICHE

The largest guiche piercing I've ever seen was at least 00 gauge (9 or 10 millimeters). It was the ever-present companion of a long-distance truck driver who attributed his patience for his job to the enjoyment he experienced while riding on his impressive guiche jewelry.

GUICHE PIERCING: PROCEDURE

It is appropriate to come in waxed or shaved for a guiche piercing. Some piercers position you on your back with your feet on the table or in stirrups. Others place you on your hands and knees. Your piercer may mark you in one position and double-check the placement and/or pierce you in the other. If you're on your back, your piercer might ask you to glove up and assist by lifting your scrotum out of the way.

As with all such piercings on pliable tissue, I use forceps. Tissue manipulation can be very beneficial on tighter skin. Some piercers prefer a freehand technique.

GUICHE PIERCING: HEALING AND TROUBLESHOOTING

You may want to wear sanitary napkins or liners throughout healing to help the area stay dry and provide protective padding. Keep the piercing as free from moisture as possible and maintain good air circulation.

Due to the wound's proximity to the anus, you must be careful to avoid contact with waste during healing and to shower once or twice a day. Following bowel movements, wipe away from the piercing to uphold good hygiene. If you use wet-wipe products after visiting the toilet, do not allow the towelettes to touch your piercing if they contain alcohol, detergents, fragrances, chemicals, or preservatives. These ingredients may be suitable for freshening up or post-potty cleaning, but they aren't meant for open wounds. Protect the piercing with a waterproof bandage before engaging in receptive anal sex during healing.

This region is subject to considerable friction from daily activities, which can cause the piercing to become irritated. A healing guiche doesn't prohibit exercise, though it is certainly best to avoid biking and horseback riding for the first few weeks. Lumpy, protruding scar tissue sometimes temporarily forms at the openings of the piercing during healing. You may need to change your jewelry style or size to resolve this problem.

GUICHE PIERCING: CHANGING JEWELRY

You will need to get a piercer or a capable friend to help because it is very tricky to access a guiche by yourself unless you are extraordinarily flexible. The added sensation of wearing weights on your guiche could be enjoyable.

GUICHE PIERCING: STRETCHING

Some piercees like the look and feel of large jewelry after healing. If you have sufficient tissue, your guiche can slowly be stretched to substantial sizes. A solid piercing in this sturdy and resilient area can support relatively heavy weight. You should be ready to stretch up one gauge approximately nine months after piercing.

GUICHE PIERCING: RETIRING

Guiche piercings tend to shrink quickly, though occasionally they will remain open without jewelry in place. The guiche generally leaves two divots that are not highly visible. An abandoned piercing is unlikely to be noticed if healing went smoothly.

THE PUBIC PIERCING

- o **Healing time:** 4 to 6 months or longer
- o **Initial jewelry style:** Curved bar is preferred, rarely ring-style
- o **Initial jewelry gauge:** 10 gauge
- o **Initial jewelry size:** ¾-inch minimum diameter

There is no apparent historical precedent for the pubic piercing, but it has made a showing in recent years. Rock star Lenny Kravitz has displayed his pubic piercing (which I performed) in a few of his more risqué photos. This is an attractive option if you desire a genital piercing that is noticeable when you are undressed, or one that is not on the penis. The pubic piercing is not involved in penetration, but it still has the potential to be sexually functional. A ring in your pubic piercing can stimulate your partner's clitoris when you are face-to-face during intercourse. Only 42 percent of the practitioners surveyed do pubic piercings.

PUBIC PIERCING: PLACEMENT AND CHOICE OF JEWELRY

A pubic piercing should be seated in the natural fold where the top of your penile shaft meets your torso (see illustration, page 217). If it is situated higher, on the flat portion of the pubic mound, it is a surface piercing, which is a different topic. Many piercers put them in too little tissue, or skin that is too taut, so this location developed an undeserved reputation for high rejection rates. For the pubic piercing to be successful, the initial placement needs to be wider than that of most body piercings: I encompass a minimum of almost ¾ inch of tissue. When the piercing is set wide enough in pliable skin at that juncture, healing is seldom eventful. I use standing as the baseline for marking and also check the placement while you are seated to see if the angle changes.

The curved bar is the safest, most comfortable style for initial jewelry; it is subject to significantly less friction and stress than a ring. If you do want a higher pubic mound surface piercing, you should wear a surface bar, and it will not have the capacity to add sensation for your partner. Some of the information below won't apply.

PUBIC PIERCING: PROCEDURE

Wax or shave before you go in for a pubic piercing. Following tissue manipulation to prepare the area, I use forceps to perform the pubic piercing. It may bleed, swell, or bruise afterward, but is not among the most vascular of the penis region piercings. Most wearers do not find the pubic piercing to be particularly sensitive or intense. Some piercers prefer to do these freehand.

PUBIC PIERCING: HEALING AND TROUBLESHOOTING

You might find it comfortable to wear a sanitary pad to protect the area with a layer of absorbent cushioning for the first few weeks or longer—or at least a panty liner.

Like the lorum, the pubic piercing may ultimately be able to help hold a condom in place. But a prophylactic won't cover this area, so you must wear a waterproof bandage to avoid sharing bodily fluids during sexual activity throughout healing.

PUBIC PIERCING: CHANGING JEWELRY

If you begin with a bar, you may want to change to a ring later, especially if the sexual pleasure of a partner with a vulva is among your motivations for getting this piercing. The captive circular barbell is one of the best options for that purpose, as the three balls provide the best chance of connecting with the right spot for your lover's enjoyment. Keeping your pubic hair trimmed will make home jewelry changes easier. Because the channel is wider than most, you should use an insertion taper during swaps.

PUBIC PIERCING: STRETCHING

It is not common practice to stretch pubic piercings to large sizes. A sturdy 8 or even 6 gauge is not unheard of, but jumbo jewelry is not usually worn here.

PUBIC PIERCING: RETIRING

If you depilate the region, residual marks will be noticeable. Pubic piercings are not likely to stay open well without jewelry in place because of the long channel and relative density of the tissue.

GETTING THE SHAFT: AMPALLANG AND APADRAVYA PIERCINGS

In the West, we have come to call the vertical placement an *apadravya* (pronounced "app uh drav ya"), although it is uncertain if this term was used the same way in ancient times. The name *ampallang* (pronounced "am puh lang"), used for the horizontal placement, is said to derive from the Dyaks in Borneo. Traditionally, when Dyak boys reached manhood, their rite of passage would be celebrated with the installation of the *palang* (crossbar) horizontally through the head of the penis; no reputable woman would marry a man without it.[13] Ampallangs are now more popular in modern culture than they are among tribal members; today, they are seldom worn in Borneo

A bar worn vertically through the glans may be capable of stimulating a partner's *G-spot* (a sexually sensitive area on the front wall of the vagina) and increasing sensation and pleasure for both partners. Sexual motivations remain an inspiration for most individuals who seek these. An *iron cross* or *magic cross* is when the same piercee wears both horizontal and vertical piercings. Approximately 45 percent of piercers surveyed perform these piercings.

THE AMPALLANG PIERCING

o **Healing time:** 6 to 9 months or longer
o **Initial jewelry style:** Straight barbell
o **Initial jewelry gauge:** Rarely 12, usually 10 gauge; some piercers will go larger
o **Initial jewelry size:** Anatomically dependent; bar length must fit your erect size

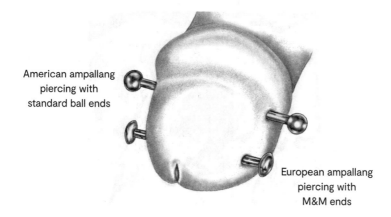

American ampallang piercing with standard ball ends

European ampallang piercing with M&M ends

The piercing procedure, healing course, and aftercare concerns are very similar for both glans piercings. Therefore, the ampallang will be described in detail first, followed by a section highlighting the differences and specific considerations of the apadravya piercing.

AMPALLANG: PLACEMENT AND CHOICE OF JEWELRY

The *American ampallang* goes horizontally through the head of the penis above the urethra toward the corona's ridge. The *European ampallang* is positioned considerably lower and more forward on the glans, and it passes through the urethra. The European version may heal faster because it pierces less tissue, being located where the anatomy is narrower. Also, because it traverses the urethra, urine may help promote healing. The jewelry will not interfere with urination unless the gauge is excessively large. Whether American or European placement is preferable is a matter of personal opinion.

The thinnest acceptable size is 12 gauge, but 10 is more common. Jewelry over an inch long (and sometimes 1.5 inches or more) is frequently used. The barbell must comfortably accommodate your maximum girth across the glans when you are fully erect, but extra length beyond that is not necessary or desirable.

It will be extremely helpful to measure yourself for the post length you'll need before coming to be pierced. However, the measurement must be taken at the spot where the piercing will be situated. If you have not premeasured and you do not get an erection during the cleaning and marking, your piercer may step out of the room to have you assess your maximum size. Having to achieve an erection and measure it in the studio right before a piercing may not be easy, but accuracy is crucial. Otherwise, you will have to estimate the appropriate barbell length. Strive for precision rather than to impress. If your bar is too short, it will pinch painfully when you are erect; if it is overly long, it will snag and cause trauma.

AMPALLANG PIERCING: PROCEDURE

The ampallang can seem rather daunting because of the lengthy piercing channel, though many of my clients have said that their nipple piercings were more sensitive. This piercing goes through the spongy tissue of the glans, where most nerve endings are capable of conveying the sensation of pressure. You will feel the greatest intensity as the needle exits, where the nerve endings inform you, "This *stings!*" Even so, piercees routinely say that it wasn't as bad as they thought it would be.

Because the area is large enough to support well with my fingers, I usually favor a freehand technique for the ampallang and apadravya. A skilled piercer can accomplish the procedure in just a few moments. The larger the initial gauge, the harder it can be to push through the dense tissue. Some ampallang piercings do not bleed at all, though many flow freely but intermittently for several days.

AMPALLANG PIERCING: HEALING AND TROUBLESHOOTING

If your initial jewelry is uncomfortable because it is shorter or longer than you need, have a professional piercer swap it out as soon as possible. It is generally more damaging to leave an ill-fitting barbell in place than to have it changed early.

You may find that the correct post length catches and causes soreness if you have a significant size differential between your flaccid and erect states. A telescoping bar that widens and shrinks with your changing anatomy would be ideal but does not yet exist. Loosely wrap the glans and jewelry in a figure-eight bandage with roll gauze to support and stabilize the exposed portion of the barbell and prevent excess movement.

AMPALLANG PIERCING: CHANGING JEWELRY

After the piercing heals, you might find it pleasurable to wear a barbell that is short enough to pinch slightly when you are erect. The fit between intimate partners is unique; some couples enjoy large balls, while others prefer minimal jewelry such as flat discs, M&M ends, or small balls. Because the channel is long, an insertion taper should always be used to facilitate jewelry changes for this piercing.

AMPALLANG PIERCING: STRETCHING

Patience is needed to stretch piercings with a long channel or dense tissue, and the ampallang has both. Making a full jump to the next gauge can be difficult. Jewelry in intermediate gauge sizes would be helpful, but it is not readily available.

Another challenge with piercings that have a long channel is that an average insertion taper is about 2.5 inches long. So, the entrance of the piercing may be stretched to the thicker gauge before the far side has even been expanded. To keep advancing the taper through, maintain constant pressure on it and closely support the skin around the exit side. You can have a piercer help you with a stretch in the studio, or you can purchase a taper and do it over a more prolonged session at home, perhaps after a warm bath to soften and loosen the tissue.

AMPALLANG PIERCING: RETIRING

Abandoning the piercing usually results in some pitting or scarring on the glans. If the piercing was no larger than 10 gauge, the marks could be minimal. Once your jewelry is removed for any length of time, it is rare to be able to reinsert it. The interior of the channel tends to shrink quickly, and it usually closes completely.

THE APADRAVYA PIERCING

The information below explains the placement of this piercing and highlights its few differences from the ampallang, described above.

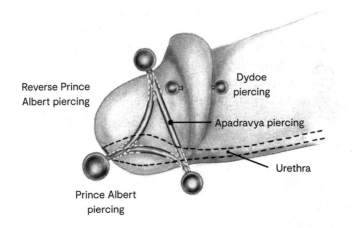

Reverse Prince Albert piercing

Dydoe piercing

Apadravya piercing

Urethra

Prince Albert piercing

APADRAVYA PIERCING: PLACEMENT AND CHOICE OF JEWELRY

The apadravya is pierced vertically through the glans. Traditional placement is where the *coronal ridge* (rim of tissue between the glans and shaft) begins to flare, but it could also be placed forward of that. Because it passes through the urethra, it usually heals faster than an American ampallang.

The apadravya is unique because this single placement incorporates multiple piercings: a Prince Albert on the lower portion and a reverse PA on the upper.

Initial jewelry for the apadravya is a barbell. Later, you could wear different pieces in various combinations: a ring in the PA plus a barbell through the entire glans, or separate jewelry in the PA and reverse PA segments, for example. The apadravya can be performed to work with a previous piercing: it is quite common to extend an existing PA up through the top. If you have a large enough Prince Albert, it might be possible to wear a shorter post by sizing the bottom ball to fit inside the PA hole. This is especially helpful for healing on those with a considerable difference between flaccid and erect dimensions. Alternatively, those extending an enlarged PA into an apadravya may prefer to wear a large ball, disc, or M&M to prevent the bottom of the jewelry from pulling into the piercing channel.

When you have the apadravya performed in one session, advantages include a single healing period and the assurance that the upper and lower parts of the piercing align nicely. If you already have a Prince Albert that is set well off to one side of your midline, it might be possible to make an apadravya on the other side and keep your PA as a separate piercing, if desired. However, the jewelry will pinch the sensitive tissue underneath if there is not enough space between the two holes.

APADRAVYA PIERCING: PROCEDURE

I usually perform the apadravya piercing using a freehand technique from the bottom up through the top, though different scenarios are possible. If the piercee already has the upper or lower portion of the apadravya, I carefully place the needle into the existing hole (sometimes with the assistance of a guidance tube that is like a short NRT) and pierce through the opposite side.

Depending on placement, jewelry choice, and previous Prince Albert size, some will elect to heal for a few days or weeks before reinserting PA jewelry. The channel might shrink, but it can't close—your new apadravya jewelry occupies the hole. If you have an enlarged PA, you might have room to put your jewelry back right away. Alternatively, you can drop to a thinner gauge in your PA or stretch up later to reinsert your usual jewelry.

APADRAVYA PIERCING: STRETCHING

A notable feature of the adaptable apadravya is that once it has healed, you have multiple piercings and the freedom to treat each section differently. For example, you can add a ring or other jewelry to stretch only the lower part of the piercing, leaving the top as is. You might want to do just that, because enlarging the upper side of the piercing is like stretching an ampallang: difficult. The bottom portion, however, is an easy-to-enlarge Prince Albert. It is reasonable to wait at least a year before attempting to stretch the upper portion.

APADRAVYA PIERCING: RETIRING

As with stretching, you have the same flexibility to keep part of the piercing and not the other. If you abandon it, the top will usually leave a divot or scar. The bottom may remain open, as a PA tends to, especially if it was stretched. Once you heal an apadravya, you probably have a permanent Prince Albert opening.

THE REVERSE PRINCE ALBERT PIERCING

- ○ **Healing time:** 4 to 6 months or longer
- ○ **Initial jewelry style:** Customized circular barbell (C-ring or U-ring) or curved bar; if extending a PA, a straight barbell
- ○ **Initial jewelry gauge:** Rarely 12, usually 10 gauge; some piercers will go larger
- ○ **Initial jewelry size:** Length or diameter anatomically dependent; 5/8-inch minimum curved barbell

This midline vertical piercing passes from the urethra to the top of the glans (see illustration, page 212). In essence, the reverse PA is the upper part of an apadravya. The procedure and initial jewelry depend on whether you have an existing Prince Albert. Just 44 percent of piercers in the survey perform this piercing.

REVERSE PA PIERCING: PLACEMENT AND CHOICE OF JEWELRY

Like the apadravya, the top may be positioned closer to the corona than to the urethral opening. It should span a *minimum* of a 9/16 inch of tissue from the top edge of the urethral opening when flaccid. Jewelry is worn from the top of your glans, through your urethra, and out the urinary meatus.

A curved bar or widened circular barbell is the preferred jewelry, since a hoop would subject the tissue to more trauma. If you already have a regular PA, it is best to extend it through the top using a straight barbell in the apadravya position, even if you plan to wear separate jewelry in the PA and reverse Prince Albert later.

REVERSE PA PIERCING: PROCEDURE

If you don't have a PA to extend, then the urethra is the avenue for piercing. A needle may be introduced gently into the urethral opening (possibly with the help of a guidance tube), and the piercing is made up through the glans. Alternatively, an NRT may be placed inside the urethra, and the piercing made from the top. The skin here is thick and tough, so this is significantly more challenging than performing a Prince Albert with the same technique. Regardless of the method, your piercing must be angled as vertically as possible for the jewelry to rest nicely.

When a Prince Albert is present, the piercing is the same as described for extending an existing piercing on page 213, "Apadravya Piercing: Procedure." During healing, you wear a barbell through the entire glans even though only the upper portion is newly pierced.

REVERSE PA PIERCING: HEALING AND TROUBLESHOOTING

The tissue of the reverse PA is much denser than that of the Prince Albert. You won't leak or drip urine because the skin remains tight around the jewelry and doesn't stretch on its own, as the PA does. Also, because the piercing is on the top of the penis, above the urethra, gravity works in your favor.

REVERSE PA PIERCING: CHANGING JEWELRY

You will find it easier to insert new jewelry from the outer surface of the piercing, rather than feed it in through your urethra. If you want to experiment with other jewelry styles after healing, one option is to wear a ring. Though if your piercing is very distant from the urethra, a large diameter hoop would be required.

REVERSE PA PIERCING: STRETCHING

Wait a year or longer before you attempt to expand your reverse PA. Do not expect the tissue to be anything like the highly elastic Prince Albert for which it is named. Stretching a reverse PA is much more akin to enlarging an ampallang or apadravya.

REVERSE PA PIERCING: RETIRING

If you remove a reverse PA piercing, you will be left with a mark, but it should not be disfiguring if you have not stretched to a thick gauge. Because the channel is relatively long and the tissue is solid, there is a strong likelihood that the piercing will close completely upon removal.

THE DYDOE PIERCING

- Healing time: 3 to 4 months or longer
- Initial jewelry style: Curved bar
- Initial jewelry gauge: 14 gauge; occasionally 12 gauge for those with full anatomy
- Initial jewelry size: Diameter anatomically dependent, with a ⅜-inch minimum

The *dydoe* piercing frames the rim of the corona (see illustration, page 212). It appears to be a modern innovation. Many builds do not have a defined enough flare to the glans to safely accommodate jewelry in this location. I've found that dydoes frequently migrate and reject, even on suitable candidates, so I generally decline to perform them.

THE CYPRIAN SOCIETY

The dydoe was ostensibly invented to increase the sensitivity diminished by foreskin removal in circumcision. The term was coined by piercing pioneer Doug Malloy as a free association for the word *doodad* (an added decoration). Doug claimed that after World War I, a group of men who called themselves the Cyprian Society opposed the indiscriminate circumcision of babies. Malloy reported that they carried out dydoe piercings to "heighten sexual pleasure . . . to offset the less sensitive skin which came with the loss of the foreskin." No evidence beyond Doug's claims has been found to confirm this tale.

DYDOE PIERCING: PLACEMENT AND CHOICE OF JEWELRY

An ample mushroom-shaped ridge at the rim of the glans is the ideal configuration for dydoe piercings. If the tissue is too minimal or the channel too superficial, migration and rejection are likely. Dydoes are traditionally done in pairs off to the sides, near two and ten o'clock, though sometimes narrower or wider. Others choose to wear a single piercing at the center. Generous anatomy might be crowned with multiple studs around the upper perimeter. If you are intact, you should wear this piercing only if you have a somewhat loose-fitting foreskin. If your glans is sheathed too tightly, excess pressure on the jewelry will cause trauma and healing difficulties.

The dydoe is the only penile piercing in which I use 14-gauge jewelry, due to the limited tissue of this location. A curved bar conforms well to the area to reduce catching and irritation. The ⅜-inch minimum bar diameter will accommodate enough tissue only if the corona is well defined. Jewelry may need to be 7/16 inch or longer, depending on individual build. Enough room must be left on the post to allow for growth during erections.

DYDOE PIERCING: PROCEDURE

I generally use a freehand procedure for dydoes. An NRT may also be used. Forceps could be applied if the area is pronounced enough, though they would pinch considerably in this spot.

Because the dydoe doesn't encompass a wide span of tissue, you might mistakenly believe that this is not a very intense piercing. However, most nerve endings are located close to the surface, as anyone who has had a rug burn or road rash that stings like mad will understand. You may be surprised to learn that a single ampallang is probably more comfortable to receive than a pair of dydoes.

DYDOE PIERCING: HEALING AND TROUBLESHOOTING

Be very gentle during sexual activities while healing because the dydoe generally frames the fullest part of the anatomy. Even once healed, dydoes may be too superficial to withstand the usual friction of sexual activities. Using a sterile gauze wrap around the glans when the piercing is fresh can diminish jewelry movement.

DYDOE PIERCING: CHANGING JEWELRY

The channel is short from entry to exit, so it shouldn't be difficult to change the jewelry on your own dydoes once you are healed. Just don't leave the holes empty for long, because this type of tissue is apt to shrink quickly.

DYDOE PIERCING: STRETCHING

The dydoe is situated in a minimal amount of skin close to the edge of the penis; therefore, large sizes are not desirable. These are seldom stretched.

DYDOE PIERCING: RETIRING

When you remove a dydoe piercing, you can expect to have some visible marks left on your glans. Even if the channel doesn't close entirely, it usually shrinks, and you will probably find it difficult and tender to reinsert jewelry.

THE FORESKIN PIERCING

- ○ **Healing time:** 2 to 3 months or longer
- ○ **Initial jewelry style:** Ring, barbell, or curved bar
- ○ **Initial jewelry gauge:** 12 or 10 gauge
- ○ **Initial jewelry size:** Minimum ½ inch length or diameter; commonly ⅝ inch

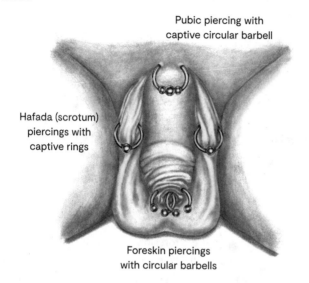

Pubic piercing with
captive circular barbell

Hafada (scrotum)
piercings with
captive rings

Foreskin piercings
with circular barbells

Foreskin piercing is not especially popular in the United States, where most were deprived of the possibility in infancy due to circumcision. However, those who engage in successful foreskin restoration[14] may be able to rebuild enough tissue to pierce. In turn, the piercing (once healed) can assist in the process by providing better purchase on the area for further tissue expansion.

The foreskin is one of the genital piercings with significant historical precedent, mostly for *infibulation* (the enforcement of chastity through physical means). Some piercees engage in consensual infibulation nowadays using multiple foreskin piercings (see "Infibulation," page 316), but this placement is primarily used to enhance sensation. Only 44 percent of piercers surveyed perform foreskin piercings.

FORESKIN PIERCING: PLACEMENT AND CHOICE OF JEWELRY

This thin skin could be damaged by wiry jewelry; so 12 gauge is a minimum, but 10 gauge is more common. A length or diameter of ⅝ inch should be large enough to accommodate sufficient tissue for a safe piercing. Let your piercer know during marking if you plan to stretch later or use your piercings for infibulation so they can be placed a little farther back.

When the foreskin is fully retracted, this piercing rests like a vertical frenum, generally near the mid-shaft of the penis. This highly elastic region changes dramatically, and your piercer must scrutinize these impressive alterations while marking. Even though your foreskin will remain over the glans most of the time, the jewelry must not pinch excessively when you retract it.

Standard procedure is to mark a reference line at the edge of the foreskin as it rests down naturally. The piercing will go on either side of this border so that jewelry frames the rim evenly. Marking for the piercing when your foreskin is in the retracted position assures placement that will fit with the size of your chosen jewelry. However, when your foreskin is covering the glans, it may appear that the piercing will be very near the edge of the rim. The marks must be double-checked with your tissue in both positions.

You can wear a single piercing, a pair, or multiples, depending on your personal preference. Sets of piercings at three and nine o'clock, or twelve and six o'clock, are popular. Anywhere around the perimeter of your foreskin is acceptable as long as you have enough space in between. Depending on your anatomy and the jewelry size and style, you might be able to wear four or more piercings in your foreskin, though certainly no more than that should be performed in a single session.

FORESKIN PIERCING: PROCEDURE

I use forceps to secure and spread the foreskin because the tissue stretches, rolls, and slides. Illumination demonstrates where your veins are located so they can be avoided. Bleeding in this region is usually minor. For comfort and ease of healing, I perform the piercing when your tissue is in its flaccid position to straddle the fold naturally. This placement is similar to the frenum piercing, and most would describe the sensation as fairly minor. Bear in mind that doctors routinely remove this tissue from infants sans anesthetic.

FORESKIN PIERCING: HEALING AND TROUBLESHOOTING

Be gentle and try to retract your foreskin as little as possible while maintaining sound hygiene during initial healing. Apply a moist warm compress, rinse, or do other maintenance to remove crusted matter beforehand. Since urine may pass over the area, you can follow the suggestions under "Urinating," page 168, and "Penis Region Piercings: Urinating," page 193.

FORESKIN PIERCING: CHANGING JEWELRY

Later you can wear a ring or bar smaller than the initial diameter, but jewelry must be large enough to allow you to retract your foreskin comfortably. Because of the membranous nature of the tissue, you might want assistance with changes. If you plan to swap it yourself, use an insertion taper, at least initially. Change jewelry when your foreskin is down, and the piercing is at its most compact.

FORESKIN PIERCING: STRETCHING
Foreskin piercings can be stretched to larger sizes, even though the tissue is relatively fine. If you engage in heavy play or wear weights, it might be possible to safely skip a gauge, as these activities expand the hole naturally. Wait six months or more before enlarging.

FORESKIN PIERCING: RETIRING
Evidence from only one of the holes will usually be visible if you remove the jewelry. The second mark will be exposed when you retract your foreskin. Due to the mobile nature of the tissue, finding the channel might be challenging if you try to reinsert jewelry in an abandoned hole.

THE POINT
Because of the private nature of the area, intimate piercings are a viable option for adults who do not have the freedom or desire to wear visible piercings. Many derive intense enjoyment and satisfaction from genital piercings. If you are attracted to one, take the plunge. Genital piercing can provide an extraordinary way of celebrating your body's beauty and the freedom to enjoy your sexuality to its fullest.

PART 5

HEALING, AFTERCARE, AND TROUBLESHOOTING

ESSENTIAL GUIDE TO HEALING
AND AFTERCARE..............................222

TROUBLE AND
TROUBLESHOOTING 246

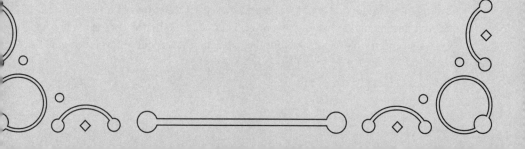

15

ESSENTIAL GUIDE TO HEALING AND AFTERCARE

Disclaimer: These care guidelines and suggestions are based on decades of professional experience, common sense, extensive research, and vast clinical practice; they are not to be considered a substitute for advice from a medical professional.

A piercing is a wound, albeit a fairly unique one, because it is created intentionally and meant to heal with a foreign object present in the body. Even so, when we refer to "aftercare," we're really discussing *wound care,*[1] which includes:
- Minimizing factors that inhibit healing
- Enhancing the healing process
- Reducing the risk of infection

Aftercare is not just about applying a particular product to a piercing. Much of it relates to behavior: what you should do, and what you should avoid.

THE EVOLUTION OF AFTERCARE

Many years ago, the standard treatment for a healing piercing involved applying alcohol twice daily and frequently turning the jewelry so it "wouldn't get stuck." This antiquated method is now viewed as a brutal abuse of a piercing.

Most over-the-counter wound-care remedies are not appropriate because they are not intended for the long-term use piercings require, nor are they meant for puncture wounds. Initially, piercers and piercees had to improvise because nobody knew what was best for healing piercings. Over the past few decades, piercers advocated an assortment of products, including Betadine, Hibiclens, alcohol, hydrogen peroxide, Neosporin, and antibacterial soap. Yet today these are all considered detrimental to healing piercings. Bactine and other pierced-ear solutions were also commonly suggested, but they also have fallen out of favor. See details in "What Not to Use on Your Piercings," page 238.

The methods of cleaning and caring for piercings have developed over time through trial and error. New regimens have come about through a better understanding of how piercings heal, and access to more suitable products.

Consider the experience of an unfortunate man who got his nipple pierced in 1986:

> "That piercing took six or seven years (yes, *years*) to properly heal . . . I would attribute that to the 'aftercare' we practiced back then. The usual choices were washing with Betadine (iodine scrub) or Hibiclens, a (possibly carcinogenic) surgical scrub. Yup, way too harsh. I cut the Hibiclens to half-strength a few years into it. See, aftercare was evolving even then . . . "—C.

Countless piercees have healed well using the commonsense aftercare advice offered below. That said, there is one fundamental principle about healing: *human bodies vary*. Not everyone will respond equally to the same products and procedures. Effort and patience are sometimes needed to figure out what works best for your piercing. You may even find that what functioned well in the past does not have the same effect on a subsequent piercing. Variations in climate, water quality, health status, and many other factors impact the healing course.

AFTERCARE ADVICE: THE GOOD, THE BAD, AND THE UGLY

Understandably, you may feel confused if you hear conflicting aftercare advice from different piercers, friends, and medical professionals. Some methods are obsolete, and others are bizarre or downright harmful. Individuals may swear by off-the-wall substances like wart remover, perfume, or hemorrhoid cream, but beware of wacky care regimes or a strict no-cleaning approach.

A wide array of products designed for piercing care is available. Many are touted as the best, so it can be confusing to decide which to buy, if any. In general, it is prudent to follow a straightforward healing regimen that emphasizes sound health habits and hygiene rather than miracle products.

Your primary resource for care instructions should be a competent piercer. Most professionals will provide information that is similar to what is advised below, though in less detail. (No piercer has the time to go into this amount of depth!) Other care regimens might work, but if your piercer's advice differs radically from everything discussed in this book, use caution and common sense.

The aftercare guidelines should be conveyed to you at the piercing studio both verbally and in writing. Some laws governing piercing mandate this dual approach because the information is so important. A piercer who does not make sure that you are versed in the required care and cleaning is doing an unprofessional job, regardless of whether their implements are sterile and piercings well placed.

THE WOUND-HEALING PROCESS

To care for a piercing properly, it helps if you understand the basic process your body goes through as it heals. The piercing follows a progression from a new wound to a healed piercing, during which the *fistula* (flesh tunnel) that holds the jewelry forms, seals up, and toughens. The stages described overlap during the healing process. Below is a simplified overview of the fundamentals:

During stage 1, or the *inflammatory phase*, a piercing is a fresh, open wound. Bleeding, swelling, and tenderness are all normal. Over the first few days, blood clots, platelets, and plasma infiltrate the wound to achieve *hemostasis* (stoppage of bleeding). As the wound begins to heal, the body forms and lays down *basal* (base) cells—the foundation layer of the *epidermis* (surface skin).

Stage 2, or the *growth* or *proliferative phase*, lasts several weeks for most wounds. However, this stage routinely takes several more weeks, months, or even longer when you get a piercing, because these processes must take place around jewelry present in the wound. This phase includes both *granulation*, during which your body produces cells, including *collagen* (proteins), to heal and strengthen the wound, and *contraction*, during which the edges of the injury usually pull together. Contraction, however, is impeded in piercing because of the jewelry. This is the stage when "crusties" regularly form (see "Normal Piercing Secretions," below).

During this phase, new skin cells, called *epithelials*, begin to grow from the edges of the wound inward, building upon the base layer. In a process called *epithelialization*, these cells grow together and thicken, and finally, they line the wound completely, merging from end to end across the piercing, creating a sealed channel. The new skin is delicate and can still be damaged or torn quite easily at this stage. By the end of this phase, initial healing is considered complete, and a piercing is no longer an open wound.

Stage 3 is called *maturation* or *remodeling*. During this phase, the collagen becomes more organized. For a piercing, it takes months to years for the cells that have lined the interior of the channel—essentially, scar tissue—to strengthen and stabilize after the fistula has formed from end to end. Piercings commonly go through a series of cycles between the second and third stages.[2]

When one or more of these phases is disrupted or delayed, complications frequently occur. This is why healing piercings can be challenging: keeping a foreign object inside a wound predisposes each stage to take longer than usual.

NORMAL PIERCING SECRETIONS

During stage one, as a response to the injury just hours after piercing, an *inflammatory serous exudate* (red and white blood cells, proteins, and other components) fills the wound to help with clotting, prevent infection, and begin the repair process.

Throughout much of the healing course, it is routine to experience "crusties," a nonmedical term used to describe the discharge that comes from a healing wound.

A small amount of clear or straw-colored fluid seeps from the channel, dries, and forms some crust around your piercing. It is composed of *serous exudate* (lymph, dead cells, and *interstitial fluid*, the liquid from between cells). Never pick at it! This secretion still forms in wet areas where it can't dry and form a crust; so you might notice some normal discharge emerging from such piercings.

This secretion is distinguished from *pus*, which is a yellowish-white, thick, often foul-smelling fluid. It is made primarily of white blood cells, bacteria, and dead cells. Pus is secreted in response to inflammation or infection. You may see a small amount early in the initial stage due to inflammation; after that, this is not a normal piercing secretion. Compounds produced by certain microbes cause it to have a yellowish, grayish, or greenish appearance. Colored pus is indicative of infection.

Sebum is a substance from your oil glands that collects in healed piercing channels. It is a naturally occurring product of the body, containing fat, *keratin* (a fibrous protein), and cellular material.[3] The purpose of sebum is to protect your skin and hair, keep it moisturized, and to inhibit the growth of microorganisms. People sometimes mistake it for pus, but it is more solid and cheeselike and has a distinctive rotten odor that reflects the dead cellular debris it contains. See "Regular Maintenance," page 268, for information.

WHAT TO EXPECT

Immediately after being pierced, some bleeding, swelling, and tenderness or pain are standard consequences. Bleeding may continue—usually intermittently—for a few days. Localized bruising is normal, though not typical, for most piercings. Heavy blood flow or bleeding that persists for longer than a few days may be cause for concern, and you should contact your piercer or physician. The placements that routinely bleed freely are discussed in chapters 11–14.

If a piercing bleeds, bruises, and/or swells substantially right after the procedure, ice should be applied as soon as possible. Prepared piercers keep disposable instant cold packs ready for use. They can be wrapped in a clean dental bib or paper towel, and sterile gauze placed between the piercing and the ice pack to maintain hygiene. Occasionally, a piercing will swell so much that your piercer needs to swap out your jewelry for a larger piece before you leave the studio. An adept technician will use an insertion taper to change it for you without causing pain or trauma to the area. Internally threaded or threadless jewelry is safer to deal with than the externally threaded type in these situations.

On occasion, some localized swelling of a fresh piercing can impinge upon a nerve, causing temporary numbness or tingling, loss of taste in oral piercings, or diminished hearing in ear piercings (rare). However, barring an unusual placement or healing complications, these are transient troubles.

You can expect slight swelling, redness, and oozing of fluid to persist for a prolonged period. Sometimes a piercing will have a *flare-up* and become inflamed, feel tender, and/or secrete after weeks or months of stability. This can be normal, and in the absence of other problems, there is no cause for concern. Any time a piercing has a flare-up, treat it like a fresh piercing and resume or accelerate your aftercare regimen.

HEALING VS. HEALED

Unfortunately, there's no way to know whether a piercing is fully healed just by having it for a certain number of weeks or months, or by how it looks or feels. Just because it isn't sore doesn't mean it has healed! Your piercing has passed through the first two healing stages when there is no tenderness, crusting, or discoloration. The openings look smooth and sealed, not raw or ragged. If sebum is present in your piercing, this usually indicates that you no longer have an open wound. Your piercing has passed through the initial healing and entered the final stage, maturation.

After the channel forms and seals, you are still in the third stage, as the *scar* (interior surface) matures over an extended period. A piercing that has only recently healed is more delicate than a seasoned one. The skin can be broken, turning your piercing into an open wound again. Just because a piercing has made it through initial healing doesn't mean that it can't regress if you mistreat it.

TIGHTNESS IS NORMAL

Many piercees worry that something is wrong because their jewelry won't move freely. The tissue in many parts of the body is naturally tight; the jewelry may not swing or slide unless wet or lubricated, even in a well-healed piercing. Pay attention to your body; if a piercing feels unyielding, go easy on it. See "Catching the Tube," page 262, to learn about the damage that can result from forcing jewelry to move.

MINIMUM HEALING TIMES

The healing time ranges listed in this book are estimates only. They represent the typical amount of time you can expect your piercing to take to reach the end of the second stage of healing (when you no longer have an open wound) and begin the final phase. This varies considerably from person to person, and yours may take longer. You should keep up with your care routine for the entire minimum time, even if you believe you have healed faster than usual. You must also continue being gentle with your piercing for longer than that. Wait until it has settled and been stable for months before you attempt any heavy play or stretching.

BASIC AFTERCARE

The sensible suggestions in this chapter are the result of years of informal research and clinical experience; they reflect and expand upon the current industry standard. Safe and appropriate piercing aftercare consists of the following:

- Upholding hygiene
- Maintaining good health habits
- Avoiding trauma
- Cleaning your piercing
- Applying warm compresses (optional)

You may have noticed that the act of cleaning is only one of several aspects. Caring for your healing piercing is not mysterious or complicated, but you must be consistent and committed. In-depth details here will equip you to facilitate your piercing's smooth passage through each healing phase.

HYGIENE

Hygiene involves keeping your piercing and your environment clean. If you go to a reputable professional who uses sterile implements and follows proper aseptic techniques, your chances of getting an infection at the studio are incredibly slim. However, if you expose the wound to bacteria by playing with it, swimming in dirty water, or not washing your clothes or body, you risk contracting an infection.

The Golden Rule of Hygiene to avoid infection is this: *do not touch your piercing with unwashed hands.* Unless you have just washed your hands (and not touched anything else, including the tap), you should keep them far away from the jewelry. Some bacteria exhibit *motility*, which means they can move on their own.[4] Therefore, you could deposit disease-causing microorganisms by merely touching your body *near* the piercing. I suggest keeping about six inches (15 centimeters) away from the piercing in every direction. For ear and facial piercings, don't touch yourself above the neck. Of course, the same goes for anybody else's hands. Optimally you should leave your piercing alone except when you're caring for it.

These hygiene precautions minimize your risk of infection during healing:

- *Properly* wash your hands before touching your jewelry and the surrounding area (see "Handwashing Technique," page 228).
- Change your linens (bedding and towels) at least once a week.
- Don't let pets sleep in your bed unless the piercing is well protected.
- Regularly clean objects that rest close to your piercing, such as phones, audio accessories, or eyeglasses.
- Avoid the exchange of bodily fluids, even with a monogamous partner: no oral sex, kissing, or intimate contact without barrier protection (e.g., condoms, dental dams, or waterproof bandages) through the third stage of healing. Details are in "Safer Sex," page 312.
- Keep personal care products such as sprays, lotions, and cosmetics away from your piercing.
- Disposable paper products (tissues, paper towels, cotton swabs, or gauze) are safer and more hygienic than cloth for drying piercings. Sterile products

are optimal, if available. Pointed makeup swabs are excellent for drying hard-to-access spots. Some piercers claim that cotton swabs are dangerous, but I've seen no corroborating scientific evidence.

o Your own sweat and bodily fluids won't harm your piercing if you clean according to instructions (but avoid everyone else's).

o Showering is safer, but if you must bathe in a tub, follow this process throughout healing to minimize hygiene risks:

  • Before filling the tub, wash it with a bleach solution (⅓ cup to a gallon of water) and rinse thoroughly.

  • After a bath, rinse your piercing under a faucet or douse with several large cups of clean water.

Be aware that your piercing is a vulnerable, open wound. Assess your environment and lifestyle for threats to the cleanliness of your piercing. Take all steps necessary to preserve hygiene at home, work, and play.

HANDWASHING TECHNIQUE

Handwashing has long been recognized as one of the simplest and most effective practices to prevent the spread of germs and disease. According to the Centers for Disease Control (CDC), "Hand washing is the single most effective way of preventing the spread of infection."

Always wash your hands before and after handling a piercing. The proper method is simple:

Wet your hands with running water, add soap, and rub your hands together to create lather. The friction is crucial to dislodge dirt and germs.

- Wash every part of your hands thoroughly—including wrists, palms, between your fingers, and fingernails—for at least twenty seconds.
- Liquid soaps are more hygienic than bars.[5] Avoid antibacterial products (see "The Antibacterial Issue," page 235).
- Rinse and dry your hands thoroughly with a paper towel; this friction also removes bacteria from fingertips.[6]
- After handwashing, it is vital to avoid touching anything that may harbor bacteria until after you have dealt with your piercing. Use paper towels to turn off the faucet. Since you just turned it on with dirty hands, touching it will render them unclean again.

THE T-SHIRT TRICK

Before you go to sleep the first night after you get an above-the-neck piercing, put a fresh pillowcase on your pillow, and then dress it in a clean t-shirt. If you have concerns about bleeding, use a black shirt or an old one. This soft surface helps you avoid staining your bedding.

Then, on the following night, flip the pillow over and use the second clean surface. On the third night, turn the T-shirt inside out; the fourth night, flip it again. Replace the shirt every four nights. If you're a pillow flipper, you may want to change it every other night.

HEALTHY HABITS FOR RAPID HEALING

Healthy people heal faster than those who are stressed, run-down, or unwell; therefore, your first line of defense during the healing period is to take care of yourself.[7] Here are some things you can do to encourage a speedy and smooth healing experience.

- Eat a balanced diet of nutritious whole foods, including complex carbohydrates, protein, and healthy fats such as avocados, nuts, and seeds. A variety of fresh fruits and vegetables in an array of colors should be a staple each day. Cut back on fast food, refined sugar, and processed junk. Vitamins A, B complex, C, E, and K, and the minerals zinc, copper, and iron are essential for wound healing.[8]
- Get plenty of sleep. Adults need seven to nine hours per night for optimal immune function and healing.[9] Studies show that rest is at least as vital as nutrition.[10]
- Drink lots of water every day, as hydration is essential for healing and tissue health.[11]
- Avoid or minimize emotional stress. It can increase healing times by 40 percent.[12]
- Don't ingest excessive alcohol or caffeine, and stay away from recreational drugs.
- Do not smoke! The nicotine causes *vasoconstriction* (narrowing of the blood vessels), which inhibits oxygen circulation in the blood and negatively impacts healing ability. Smoking also suppresses immune function. These are a few reasons doctors advise patients to cut down or quit smoking before surgery. Try not to smoke for a week before you get pierced. At the very least, avoid smoking for ninety minutes before your piercing; a single cigarette can cause vasoconstriction for that long.

These suggestions may sound so elementary that you fail to give them more than a passing glance, but *do not underestimate the power of healthful habits to boost your immune system and healing capacity*. Taking good care of your body is one of the most effective "treatments," whether you are healing normally or experiencing complications. These factors form the basis of your body's ability to heal.

RUBBING YOU THE WRONG WAY: FRICTION AND TRAUMA

Physical trauma is one of the biggest dangers to your new piercing, whether caused by mechanical stress from the movement of your body, accidental impacts, or pressure and chafing from clothing. Repeated trauma leads to inflammation and *edema* (excess fluid in the tissues that causes swelling), which interferes with local oxygen supply. This reduces your ability to process the wound effectively. Over the long term, friction on your healing piercing will cause complications, including irritation, delayed healing, and ultimately excess scar tissue or other types of bumps, and possibly migration or rejection. To minimize trauma to your healing piercing, follow these guidelines:

- Resist the temptation to play with your new piercing, for the sake of hygiene as well as trauma.
- Wear jewelry of the proper size and style to minimize motion and friction.
- If your jewelry fits well and is high quality, leave it in during the entire healing time. Changing it can damage the fragile tissue.
- If your jewelry causes problems due to its quality, material, style, or fit, visit a piercer to replace it right away—even during healing.
- Do not handle your piercing roughly during cleaning, or at any other time.
- Avoid cloth towels, terry washcloths, and loofah sponges. The little loops can catch jewelry and cause damage.
- Make sure your sleeping position doesn't put pressure against your piercing. If you are a stomach sleeper, you might need to temporarily change to your back or side to protect a navel or nipple piercing. You may have to adjust the way you rest your head on the pillow for an ear or facial piercing. A doughnut-shaped cushion might help to diminish physical stress and irritation.
- To avoid accidentally catching or pulling your jewelry, be aware of your actions and your piercing's presence.
- Take care not to bump or snag your jewelry when dressing or donning hats, eyeglasses, or sunglasses.
- For below-the-neck piercings, try to wear clothing or underwear that provides support and reduces friction.

PHYSICAL ACTIVITY AND EXERCISE

Generally, you can exercise during healing if you avoid extremes of motion and prevent impact to the pierced area. Still, your activities will need to be modified—at least for a while—if they create problems with your piercing.

A direct blow can cause delayed healing, excessive scarring, or traumatic tearing. Especially in exposed areas like the ear and face, jewelry could be snagged or possibly torn out during rough play. Soiled, sweaty equipment such as helmets can expose piercings to bacteria, resulting in infection. Friction from body motion or protective gear can cause irritation and migration. Before wear, thoroughly clean any sports apparatus that comes near your piercing. Regular workouts enhance overall health, which has a positive effect on the healing process.[13] Don't stop all fitness endeavors; discover what works for you, listen to your body, and take extra care during healing.

PROTECTIVE PATCH
Even piercings concealed beneath clothes can be at risk unless you take extra precautions. A hard plastic, vented eye patch secured over the area can shield a nipple or navel from impact. Hold it in place with snug, stretchy workout clothing, or by winding a length of elastic bandage around your torso. Add a few sterile gauze squares between your skin and the plastic guard for a comfortable layer of clean, absorbent padding. These supplies are readily available at any drugstore or pharmacy. You can use a patch for a range of circumstances, from shielding a navel piercing against snug leggings or stockings to protecting a nipple piercing from a bulletproof vest.

WATERPROOF PROTECTION
Swimming is downright dangerous when you have an open wound! Do not expose your healing piercing to a hot tub, pool, lake, ocean, or any body of water, even if it seems clean. The chemicals in heavily chlorinated pools could be as damaging as the microorganisms and dirt in natural bodies of water. You can protect some areas with a Nexcare waterproof bandage, Tegaderm transparent dressing, or similar covering. If you don't use a sealant bandage, then you should avoid submerging (or even splashing) your healing piercing. You can also use these dressings to protect nipple and certain genital piercings from contact with bodily fluids during sexual activities.

TANNING
Tanning during healing can cause the tissue around your piercing to become darker or lighter than your normal skin tone, and the discoloration can be permanent. Some doctors recommend keeping scars out of the sun for a year. Once healed, you can apply sunscreen to the area to limit your exposure. This is particularly important if you heal with visible scar tissue surrounding your piercing.

Extreme temperatures can disrupt the delicate new cells of a healing piercing. The concentrated heat of a tanning bed could be even worse than the sun. Jewelry that gets burning hot will not feel good on your piercing and could damage fragile cells. Gold is the most temperature-reactive body jewelry metal, and it can overheat quickly during tanning. Do not get tanning lotion or oil inside your piercing.

SKIN IS SENSITIVE

Avoid exposing your healing piercing to harsh chemicals. Hair spray and dye, deodorant, bug repellent, and other products can irritate or damage your piercing. Stay away from laundry detergents that contain stain-fighting enzymes. These biological molecules influence chemical processes, and they include bioengineered products designed to break down proteins and other components of fabric stains. They may impede healing by destroying epithelial cells, so check the label on your detergent.

Soaps also have the potential to bring on an allergic reaction that manifests as *contact dermatitis*, a skin rash from contact with an allergen or irritant (see "Contact Dermatitis," page 260). Depending on the sensitivity of your skin, nearly any product or substance can cause such a reaction. Typically, if you discontinue using an offending product, your problem will resolve. Medical treatment will rarely be needed. Unless you've used something exceedingly strong or caused yourself a secondary infection by scratching an itchy rash, the piercing should not be set back too much by such an incident.

IRRIGATION: SALINE

Wound irrigation is described as the "steady flow of a solution across a wound surface." In the case of piercings, you can irrigate to hydrate, gently cleanse, and soften and remove debris, including secretions and crusted matter.[14]

Brief irrigation with saline spray (0.9 percent sodium chloride solution) is the current industry standard aftercare practice, suggested by 95 percent of piercers surveyed. This saline is mild, *isotonic* (has the salt concentration of human fluids), and will not harm healthy tissue, unlike many potent antiseptics. Lots of piercers sell or supply saline spray in their studios. Some products are plain sterile saline in a clean delivery can, and others contain enzymes or additives. Barring an inappropriate ingredient or an overly forceful stream, these products are safe and convenient. Use spray according to package instructions, or as directed by your piercer. Generally, it is applied one to three times daily.

Bottled saline for contact lenses and ear or nasal irrigation often contains substances that may not be suited to healing piercings. For safety, a saline solution marketed for a purpose other than wound care should be used only if the label confirms that the container holds "isotonic saline," or 0.9 percent sterile saline without added ingredients.

Soaking your piercing in a warm saline solution used to be routine for aftercare and troubleshooting; however, the practice has fallen out of favor due to potential issues with homemade mixtures. Now that sterile saline sprays are preferred, piercees are likely to miss out on the benefits of applying warmth to a wound. To accelerate healing or soothe an irritated piercing, try warm compresses. See "Running Cold and Hot," page 236.

IRRIGATION: WHAT'S ON TAP

In place of saline, other types of water can be used for irrigation. Perhaps surprisingly, substantial medical research has shown that rinsing with potable (drinkable) water is as safe and effective as irrigating with sterile saline for cleansing wounds.[15] Depending on the water quality in your area, you may need to rinse off your piercing with something cleaner. You can irrigate with distilled, purified, or spring water from a bottle; or tap water that has been filtered or brought to a rolling boil for at least a full minute and then cooled. Even if you believe your source is suitable, should you experience healing difficulties, use cleaner water for final rinses. This is also important if you travel while healing and stay in areas with water unfamiliar to your body.

In the shower, use warm running water to irrigate and help soften and loosen any crusties. Shield the pierced area from forceful spray if you have high water pressure. It is critical to avoid damaging the delicate healing tissue as you wash. If you live in a hot or humid climate or engage in sweaty activities, then a second daily clean-water rinse of your piercing is a good idea, if this is your chosen method of aftercare.

DEBRIDEMENT

Wound debridement is the process of removing dead, contaminated, or adherent tissue or foreign material.[16] In the case of piercings, you should gently detach any stubborn matter that remains after spraying, washing, or rinsing. If you do not remove crust and debris regularly, it can impede healing. Use moistened cotton swabs or gauze pads. Wet them with hypochlorous acid spray (see "Aftercare: My Professional Advice," page 235), sterile saline, or clean water, and keep at it until all secretions are gone. *Never* pick at matter with your fingers or nails.

CLEANSERS AND SOAPS

Overcleaning a piercing can be as problematic as not keeping it clean enough, but either can be damaging. Using the wrong product or too many of them can delay healing or cause other issues. Anything you apply to your piercing must help more than it harms. As healing takes place, new cells grow to form the skin tunnel from the openings on either side. But if cells are killed each day by harsh products (or trauma), the piercing will take longer and be more challenging to heal. Lots of cleansers and soaps contain parabens, sulfates, and other ingredients that can dry or irritate your skin and negatively impact your piercing.

More than half of the piercers surveyed don't advise the use of soaps, but some still suggest antimicrobial or germicidal cleansers. The Association of Professional

Piercers has removed soaps from their care guidelines, and I support this decision. However, if your skin is oily or soiled, soap will help to release dirt and grease, and water will rinse it away. Any piercer advising the use of a strong product (like Dial) is not keeping up with industry standards—and you would be wise to find a better-educated practitioner. The organization has never suggested such harsh cleansers. If you do elect to use soap for piercing care, make sure it is *mild*, fragrance- and dye-free, and low pH or pH balanced. Products with a pH greater than 7 are alkaline and tend to be irritating to the skin.[17]

If you wish to cleanse with soap, which may be appropriate if you work or play in dirty environments, a castile-based liquid such as Dr. Bronner's Baby Unscented formula would be preferable. It is gentle, natural, and made from vegetable oils. Adhere to package instructions for diluting your product. Another mild option is a foaming cleanser formulated for use on piercings called Naked Natural Alternative Soap. Simply lather the jewelry and piercing and rinse thoroughly, once daily.

When you bathe, you may continue to use regular soap on the rest of your body, but do not apply it directly to your piercing unless it is suitably mild. You don't want runoff or residue from personal care products to remain, so at the end of your shower, rinse your piercing gently but thoroughly as described in "Irrigation: What's on Tap," page 233.

THE SPIN ON ROTATION

Piercers used to advise rotating jewelry to work soap into and out of the channel. It was believed that this was required to clean the interior. This action can damage the delicate healing tissue—and I do not suggest using soap on even the *exterior* under normal circumstances. It was also thought that moving the jewelry was necessary to prevent it from becoming stuck, but this reasoning is faulty: sutures are not rotated, yet they don't become stuck. Jewelry should never be turned just for fun, either. There are, however, a few situations in which it is appropriate to rotate jewelry:

- **During healing**: To clean the interior of the piercing channel *if* soap, dirt, or other foreign matter has gotten inside it. A small amount of gentle rotation while rinsing is reasonable to ensure that you remove all undesirable substances from the interior.
- **After healing**: Under certain circumstances. See "Regular Maintenance," page 268.

Advice, trends, and products used for aftercare come and go, but rough handling of a healing piercing is never helpful; do not force your jewelry to move. To learn about the severe consequences that you could suffer, see "Catching the Tube," page 262.

DRYING

After your piercing gets wet, it is essential to dry it thoroughly. When kept too moist, there is a tendency toward complications, including the formation of excess granulation tissue. Gently pat dry the jewelry and surrounding area with clean disposables such as tissues, paper towels, or toilet tissue. Swabs or gauze squares are useful for drying ears, navels, and other spots with nooks and crannies. Some piercers suggest the use of a blow dryer on a cool setting. Based on research about bathroom hand dryers, don't keep one anywhere near a toilet, due to risks of bacterial contamination.[18] Hold the blow dryer about eight inches from the piercing and be cautious to avoid overheating metal jewelry and burning your skin.

THE ANTIBACTERIAL ISSUE

Antibacterial (also called antimicrobial or antiseptic) soaps—especially those containing Triclosan—used to be everywhere. Due to suspected risks to human health and the environment, the FDA launched an investigation. Ultimately, manufacturers failed to prove that soaps containing Triclosan and eighteen similar antibacterial chemicals were safe or effective, so the FDA has prohibited their inclusion in consumer soaps and body washes. Long-term frequent exposure is also suspected in the proliferation of ultra-strong, antibiotic-resistant microbes.[19]

Soaps with different antimicrobial ingredients are still available, but they are not suggested. Many studies show that regular soaps kill the same amounts of germs as antibacterial products, without their dangers.[20] Because these soaps tend to be harsh and appear to have health risks, they should be avoided, *especially* on open wounds, including piercings.

AFTERCARE: MY PROFESSIONAL ADVICE

Following extensive research, for aftercare I advocate using Briotech or other pure, stable hypochlorous acid (HOCl) solution sprayed on three to five times daily. The active ingredient is the same broad-spectrum antimicrobial and anti-inflammatory substance that is naturally produced by the white blood cells as part of the body's immune response. Hypochlorous acid rapidly inactivates bacteria, viruses, and fungi—even antibiotic-resistant "superbug" strains. At the proper concentration (100–200 ppm) and pH (4.0–5.5) it is benign, nonirritating, nondrying, and *noncytotoxic* (doesn't kill cells), unlike most soaps and other products that clean more effectively than saline. Though deadly to pathogens, it is so biocompatible and mild to the human body that it can safely be sprayed in the nose, mouth, and eyes. It is frequently used in ocular care.

HOCl has long been utilized in the medical field, and numerous scientific studies attest to its safety and effectiveness for wound healing. It stimulates the body's cells that are involved in tissue repair,[21] increases oxygenation of the site, and decreases the incidence of scarring complications in wounds.[22]

Produced using the controlled application of electrical energy, and with the sole inactive ingredient of saline, HOCl is vegan, natural, and environmentally friendly. Since it actually fosters wound repair, unlike saline or soaps, my clients are healing more quickly and easily than ever using this spray. Learn more on page 245.

RUNNING COLD AND HOT

In addition to any care products you may choose to use, ice packs and warm compresses can increase comfort, decrease post-piercing symptoms, and facilitate healing. Always place a barrier such as a clean cloth, paper towel, or sterile gauze between your piercing and the compress to maintain hygiene and protect your skin. Use only fresh disposable products or launder your linens with bleach between uses and store them carefully to avoid contamination. Place compresses onto your piercing gently to avoid injuring it.

- Ice packs (cryotherapy): Apply ice during the first forty-eight hours to help reduce the discomfort, swelling, bleeding, and bruising that can accompany a fresh piercing. Use a clean zip-top bag containing chipped ice, cubes, or frozen peas or blueberries. You can add a bit of water inside to help the contents conform to your body more comfortably. Wrap the baggie in a clean paper or cloth towel and replace soggy coverings with dry ones as condensation wets them. Too much moisture can disrupt a fresh scab, resulting in prolonged bleeding. Place the ice pack on your piercing for ten minutes and remove it for forty-five minutes to an hour before reapplying. Follow instructions carefully; icing too long can cause tissue damage (ice burn) and reduced blood flow, which slow the healing process.

- Warm compresses (thermotherapy): After the first forty-eight hours, if initial bleeding has stopped, you may begin using warm compresses. They can feel soothing, diminish swelling, and stimulate circulation. Heat causes an influx of oxygenated blood, which brings in more nutrients to help repair injured tissues and flush out debris. Warm compresses can be dry or moist.

- Moist (or wet) compress: Wash your hands and soak a clean washcloth, paper towel, or lint-free gauze in hot—but not scalding—water. Use a sterile saline spray or any of the suitable water types mentioned in "Irrigation: What's on Tap," page 233. Heating it in a microwave is fine. If possible, check the water temperature with a thermometer. It should be no hotter than 105F° for children or 120F° for adults (like hot tap water). Wring out the compress and apply it until it no longer feels warm, then reheat and reapply. Repeat for fifteen to twenty minutes, up to three times daily.[23]

o A simple option is to spray saline onto gauze squares, heat until warm to the touch in a microwave, and apply. Research shows that a moist healing environment helps prevent cell dehydration and death and improves the rate of epithelialization (skin cell growth) and other aspects of wound healing, along with the cosmetic outcome.[24] Another method is to use a foil-wrapped sterile saline wipe, run the sealed packet under hot water, remove the warm pad, and apply it.

o **Dry compress**: Pop a paper-wrapped packet of two sterile gauze squares in the microwave for about thirty seconds, open carefully, and apply. Alternatively, place a wet compress inside a zip-top baggie. You can also use a hot water bottle, microwavable heating bag, electric heating pad, or another type of commercially available hot pack. Follow package instructions for use.

o Whether moist or dry, cover your compress with a folded dry towel to help maintain the warmth longer.

Following the application of heat or cold, your skin should look pink, not bright red, and never blistered! When finished, gently pat the area dry with a clean paper towel, tissue, or gauze.

COMPRESS EXTRAS
Certain natural substances can be added to moist compresses. You may find that these further aid healing and serve other functions, though scientific research is not conclusive. Finish with a clean-water rinse afterward if you include any of the following in a compress.

o Add a tablespoon of white or apple cider vinegar to one cup of water and use this mixture to wet your compress. The acetic acid in vinegar is antimicrobial, and there is some evidence that it may also help promote wound healing.[25]

o Add chamomile tea or use a warm, wet chamomile tea bag as your compress to minimize irritation and inflammation. Avoid this if you have an allergy to any of chamomile's cousins: ragweed, marigolds, daisies, or chrysanthemums.

- ○ Add lavender tea to your compress to facilitate healing. You may also find its scent to be relaxing. Boil three tablespoons of flowers in one liter (a quart) of water for ten minutes, then strain.

- ○ Add witch hazel tea to your compress. Boil two to three grams of witch hazel leaves, twigs, and bark in a cup of water for about fifteen minutes, then strain. This may soothe and reduce inflammation, minimize bleeding, and support healing.[26] Do not apply commercial witch hazel; it is distilled and contains alcohol, which is harsh and drying.

- ○ Add four to five drops of any of the suggested essential oils (see "Herbal Remedies" on page 241) to a cup of water and use this water to make your compress.

DON'T TRY THIS AT HOME

An alternate approach that I do not advocate is referred to as *dry wound care* or *anti-care*, in which the crust is left undisturbed. There is no wetting or washing of the area for weeks or months, and all care and cleaning products are avoided.

The health care community is in widespread agreement that regular irrigation or cleansing with water or saline and removal of secretions (*debridement*) is appropriate in the presence of broken skin.[27] Further, medical research suggests that a moist wound will heal more quickly and easily than one that is kept continuously dry.[28]

ANOTHER OPTION

Less risky is the "Leave It the Heck Alone" (LITHA) philosophy. This undemanding "method" is effortless because it involves doing nothing to your piercing other than providing regular daily bathing or routine oral hygiene, depending on placement. No sprays, soaps, oral rinses, or other such products are used. This lends itself well to oral and certain genital piercings because the mucosal tissues have faster rates of regeneration than other areas. Critical elements to the LITHA way, as with all aftercare, are sound overall health habits and good hygiene. If you work or play in dirty environments or live in a hot, humid climate, this laissez-faire approach is probably not a wise choice for you.

WHAT NOT TO USE ON YOUR PIERCINGS

The products listed below were used on healing piercings in the past, but they are no longer considered suitable. Piercers or friends who do not keep up with industry standards, and sometimes even uninformed medical professionals, might suggest them. None of these things, however, is advisable for use on fresh puncture wounds, including piercings.

o **Alcohol**: Shown to be *cytotoxic* (kills cells), too strong, and drying.[29]

o **Hydrogen peroxide** (over-the-counter strength): Too strong and also cytotoxic.[30]

o **Bactine, pierced ear care solutions, and products containing benzalkonium chloride (BZK) and benzethonium chloride (BZT)**: These antimicrobials are not intended for long-term wound care and have a short shelf life once opened. Such solutions can cause dry, flaky skin, but if you dilute them, you diminish their effectiveness and can contaminate the container. Further, some of these products contain alcohol, fragrance, or numbing agents such as lidocaine (xylocaine), which can irritate your piercing. The manufacturer of Bactine explicitly states that it is not for use on piercings or other puncture wounds.[31]

o **A+D Original Ointment, Neosporin, bacitracin, and other ointments**: Labels advise against use on puncture wounds. Particularly with triple antibiotic products, many people are sensitive to at least one of the three active ingredients. Further, ointments tend to occlude a wound, thereby preventing oxygen from reaching it.[32] Because these petroleum-based products are not water-soluble, when cleaning a piercing coated in such salves, you could be washing the ointment rather than your healing tissue beneath the greasy coating.

o **Full-strength tea tree oil**: Irritation, dryness, rash, and itching are possible effects, and many piercers report frequent adverse reactions and healing issues. You should *never* apply tea tree oil (or any other essential oil) to a wound without significant dilution of at least 90–95 percent.

o **Betadine and other povidone-iodine products**: Studies show that iodine is not suited to wound care, as it can damage new cell walls, causing cellular material to leak out.[33] Packaged pads or swabs are excellent for prep *before* piercing or other procedures in which skin will be broken, but iodine stored in plastic (PVC) bottles is susceptible to the growth of infectious organisms once opened.[34]

o **Dial liquid or bar, or any antibacterial soap**: Again, too harsh and drying, and possibly harmful. If you elect to use soap on your piercing, there are plenty of more suitable, milder options.

o **Listerine and other alcohol-containing mouthwash or whitening rinses**: Alcohol is damaging to the new cell growth of healing tongue, lip, or other piercings. Overuse can upset healthy flora, leading to thrush, an oral yeast infection. Whitening rinses usually contain hydrogen peroxide, which is too harsh on delicate healing tissue.

INNOVATIONS AND ALTERNATIVES

The aftercare guidelines described above follow accepted principles of wound care, and they are safe and effective for most piercees under ordinary circumstances. However, there isn't only one correct method or even a single best way to clean and care for all piercings; each body is unique and responds differently.

Some piercers make honest attempts to discover new and better ways to facilitate healing. Others, however, have less honorable motivations for deviating from the typical care routine, including:

- A lack of familiarity with industry-standard guidelines
- The conventional advice doesn't help to heal their bungled piercings—but nothing will
- A desire to do things differently simply to make a name for themselves as innovators

Unless the suggestions are genuinely horrid, at least some piercees will probably have success with even the most unconventional of treatments. I had a client who managed to heal more than a few piercings by topically applying Bacardi 151 rum! Still, beware of being a human test case. If you don't feel convinced that a proposed departure from more traditional care sounds superior in some way, abide by the commonsense principles in this chapter.

Several alternative healing methods and products are outlined below, including those specifically designed for piercing care. Just because something is *natural* (unprocessed or minimally processed) does not necessarily mean it is safe or effective to use on your piercing.

SPECIALTY PRODUCTS

In response to increased consumer demand and sometimes in the name of making a buck, companies manufacture an array of products designed specifically to care for healing piercings. Some of them are safe and convenient. Among the options are liquid-filled swabs, powders, gels, individually packaged pads or towelettes, and sprays.

Consider whether the manufacturer's claims seem reasonable, and assess the following:

- **Ingredients**: Does the label provide clear information about the active ingredients and other components? Are there potential allergens, irritants such as alcohol or peroxide, or other undesirable or unfamiliar substances?

- o **Application**: Do you have to mix something yourself? (This allows for possible user error.) Consider the delivery system; if a spray is too forceful, it can damage healing tissue.[35]

- o **Cost**: Some specialty goods are quite pricey. Weigh the cost and convenience and consider your piercer's opinion.

ALTERNATIVE HEALING METHODS

Below is a brief introduction to a few alternative aftercare regimens that diverge from the standard guidelines. Many piercees have successfully used these and other approaches. This is far from an in-depth investigation of all the possibilities. If you are interested in pursuing alternatives, there is a great deal of information available online, but stick to scientific research studies, not sales pitches or opinion pieces.

THE BETTER OPTIONS

These methods and products are generally accepted as being among the safest and least controversial of the alternatives:

- o **Lubrication**: Dab a small amount of almond, jojoba, olive, coconut, or other natural oil around the holes of the piercing several times daily. Naked Natural Alternative Oil is formulated for use on piercings and is among the most popular in the industry. Apply it only on the surface, without getting it inside the channel. Oils might help to minimize dryness and crusting and reduce damage when the jewelry is bumped or moved. Do not use Vaseline or other petroleum-based products. Lubrication can also be done in conjunction with the standard care regimen.

- o **Herbal remedies**: Herbs have been used in medicine for thousands of years. Though tested by time, few herbs have been researched as rigorously as more modern treatments. It is believed that when used correctly, certain herbs can be beneficial to healing. You can apply them in several ways: make a warm wet compress with an *infusion* (a tea that is steeped longer than usual) or topically apply diluted *essential oils* (concentrated liquid compounds from plants).

- o Lavender,[36] chamomile, and comfrey[37] are herbs commonly used for healing wounds. Select one at a time unless you are a skilled herbalist or receive advice from one.

- o Add one to two teaspoons of dried herb per cup of boiling water to make an infusion. Let it steep for at least ten minutes before you strain it. Some herbalists recommend infusing for hours. Keep the mixture covered in the refrigerator for two to three days. Heat the tea (a microwave is fine) and use it as the liquid in a warm moist compress.

o Essential oils are much too harsh for full-strength application on piercings; they *must* be diluted first. Be aware this carries risks of user error and product contamination. Since they vary significantly in quality and concentration, seek guidance from a knowledgeable supplier before putting this type of product on a piercing. Most preparations are far too strong and drying. Diluted tea tree,[38] lavender, rosemary, or ylang-ylang[39] essential oils may be used for healing wounds by adding a few drops to the water used for warm moist compresses.

o An *infused herbal oil* (an essential oil that is mixed into a carrier oil base) is milder and can often be used topically on a piercing at full strength. This can be used for lubrication.

THE JURY IS OUT

o **Aloe vera gel**: This plant has been used medicinally for thousands of years, including for wound healing. The gel—best taken from the living leaves—can be applied to the exterior of the piercing several times a day. Some studies on the use of aloe for wound healing report positive results, but others show no benefit, or negative effects.[40]

o **Colloidal silver**: Controversial at best, its many touted benefits have not been medically proven. The FDA issued a ruling declaring that all over-the-counter drug products containing colloidal silver or silver salts are not recognized as safe or effective for internal or external use. There are documented cases of unexpected side effects.[41]

o **Honey**: According to some evidence, certain types of honey are beneficial for wound healing and have antibacterial properties.[42] No research has been done regarding its use on piercings, so take this sweetness with a grain of salt. I can't imagine putting anything so sticky on a healing piercing, and as an ethical vegan, I do not advocate using any animal products.

o **Additional natural remedies**: Many other preparations and plants have been recommended for wound care, including turmeric (curcumin), calendula, marshmallow root, gotu kola, echinacea, plantain, banana peel extract, garlic, ginkgo, and seaweed, among others. More research is needed for these to be considered advisable for piercing care.

AFTERCARE FOR ORAL PIERCINGS

The same principles of avoiding trauma and maintaining sound health habits also apply to healing oral piercings. However, lip and tongue piercings need some additional care on the inside of the mouth. For labret piercings, it is necessary to care for the exterior the same as any other part of the body; additionally, you should follow the guidelines in this section to care for the interior.

See the tips in "Tongue Piercing: Healing and Troubleshooting," page 137. Below are several additional things you can do to minimize swelling and discomfort during the first few days:

o **Rest:** Don't speak or move your jewelry unless necessary.

o **Ice:** *Gently* suck on chipped or shaved ice made from clean water, or small cubes of frozen chamomile tea (big cubes can be uncomfortable and irritating). Sipping iced chamomile tea may be helpful.

o **Elevation:** Sleep with your head propped up on an extra pillow the first few nights; keeping your head above your heart helps to minimize overnight swelling.

CLEANING AND HYGIENE

Your primary aftercare for oral piercings (including tongue, labret, and lip piercings) consists of providing good hygiene and rinsing your mouth. You can use clean water (see options in "Irrigation: What's on Tap," page 233), or normal saline. Some piercers suggest twice-daily rinsing; others advise it after eating or drinking anything other than water. Alternatively, you can swish with a mouth rinse containing HOCl, such as Briotech's SOS (Super Oxidizing Saline), or an alcohol-free mouthwash according to package instructions, if you ordinarily use one. Natural rinses with mint or other essential oils may be suitable if they are mild. There is no need to purposely move your jewelry while rinsing—oral piercings get an abundance of motion, no matter how diligently you try to avoid it.

Rinsing too frequently or using harsh mouthwash can cause complications by diminishing your healthy, protective oral flora. Products that contain alcohol are still recommended by piercers who are not keeping up with industry standards. Avoid whitening toothpaste and rinse products. These include ingredients such as abrasives and forms of peroxide, which can irritate a healing piercing and may destroy new cells.

Brush your teeth normally after each meal (before rinsing), floss, and use a tongue scraper daily. Take care not to irritate the piercing, and rinse thoroughly after scraping. Pay attention to what you put in your mouth while you are healing an oral piercing. Don't chew on pens, sunglasses, fingernails, or other foreign objects; they are likely to harbor germs. Dirty cups, plates, and eating utensils can expose you to pathogens, so keep all kitchenware clean and don't share during healing. Avoid having your teeth cleaned or getting nonurgent dental work when your piercing is new. It can irritate the piercing and may increase your risk of infection.

Throughout healing, your piercing is an open wound, so you must avoid others' bodily fluids, including saliva: this means no unprotected oral sexual contact and no French (wet) kissing. Failing to comply brings risks, including STIs, HIV, and hepatitis B and C. Even if you have a long-term partner, you must still abstain due to the possibility of infection. Performing oral sex is also inadvisable during the first few weeks of healing. This is true even if you use barrier protection for hygiene, as vigorous activity can damage the delicate cells.

Smoking and drinking alcoholic beverages should be minimized or eliminated initially. Chewing tobacco is not safe while you are healing an oral piercing.

TOOTHBRUSH HYGIENE

It is wise to use a new toothbrush when you get an oral piercing. Keep it hygienic: store it in a clean area separate from anyone else's toothbrush—and well away from your toilet. Studies show that "toilet plume," aerosols containing bacterial and viral spray from flushing, can land on surfaces (including a toothbrush) up to eight feet away![43] Closing the lid helps, but does not entirely prevent the spread of microbes.[44]

THE POINT

Caring for your piercing can be confusing if you receive different advice from multiple sources. New information and aftercare products are always surfacing, so the current suggestions may be modified again. Regardless of how many other people have had success with a method or product, the ultimate test rests with your own body. Unless negative results are apparent, it is reasonable to stick with a routine for a few weeks before deciding it isn't working for you.

You're most likely to heal successfully if you get a well-placed piercing with quality jewelry, and rely primarily on sensible health habits, responsible behavior, and gentle treatment. Ultimately, you must listen to your body and trust your instincts, bolstered by knowledge, research, and common sense. Should your efforts cause problems or fail to foster healing, there are other options to try. And if you run into trouble, read the next chapter.

HYPOCHLOROUS ACID (HOCL)

HOCl is not a new invention, but piercing aftercare is a new application for a substance that has been widely used in the medical field. Until recently, it wasn't possible to stabilize HOCl, but an innovative, shelf-stable HOCl product has been developed and is available to the public. It promotes powerful local stimulants of wound healing and germ killing:

HOCl causes blood to coagulate faster and allows the clot to last longer.

HOCl alters several key components of human blood to increase local clot formation and inhibit dissolution of the clot. HOCl helps stop bleeding by making blood clot in wounds.[45]

HOCl boosts the body's immune reaction to infectious microbes and disrupts biofilm.

HOCl is an *adjuvant* (a substance that enhances the immune system) that hypes up the body's responses by increasing T-cell function, improving immunity to germs.[46] It also eradicates *biofilm* (a slimy adherent layer of microbes), which can be a serious problem causing infections in healing wounds. Biofilm forms when microorganisms collect, proliferate, and generate a protective shell. Most of the antiseptics that can penetrate it impair healing.[47]

HOCl promotes new skin cell growth on wounds.

Keratinocytes are the cells of the outer layer of skin; they move in and close wounds, and lay down new, outer skin layers. HOCl stimulates the migration of keratinocytes and other cellular growth factors, and also increases oxygenation to improve healing.[48]

HOCl is a known anti-inflammatory.

HOCl is widely known for its effectiveness as an anti-inflammatory agent. It is believed to prevent inflammation by reducing or blocking chemical signals that activate an inflammatory response.

HOCl stimulates enzymes that reduce or improve scarring.

Collagenase enzymes affect the behavior of the fibroblast cells that lay down fibrous scar tissue. By activating these enzymes, HOCl reorganizes scar fibers, reduces the risk of scarring, and lightens/softens existing fibrous scar tissue.

This all sounded too good to be true when I was first introduced to HOCl, so I embarked on my own research. I was intrigued to learn of HOCl's hundred-year history in the medical field, and about more recent studies, especially. The evidence was incredibly persuasive: multiple hundreds of peer-reviewed, published papers demonstrate its safety and efficacy in wound healing and disinfection. HOCl (at the right strength and pH) works as well on piercings as I thought it would, based on the existing science.

16

TROUBLE AND TROUBLESHOOTING

Disclaimer: The suggestions in this book are not to be considered a substitute for advice from a medical professional.

Occasionally things go awry with piercings, even when they are performed by a qualified professional according to accepted practice and cared for properly. Depending on what is wrong, the solution might be as simple as changing your care regimen or jewelry. Sometimes minor complications improve spontaneously, while other times, an over-the-counter remedy may be helpful. In more serious cases, doctor visits and medical treatments are called for; on occasion, jewelry removal is the ultimate result. Fortunately, grave situations are rare, but it is crucial to ascertain precisely what is wrong so that you can take appropriate steps to resolve the issue.

If you need to see a physician, your piercer may be able to refer you to a piercing-friendly practitioner. Rapid intervention can prevent more severe consequences, so it is vital to address problems quickly. If you have a history of health conditions or experience any critical symptoms, seek *immediate* medical attention.

Some medical terminology is included below for clarity, especially in situations when health care services will be rendered. Piercers in a studio setting do not ordinarily use the same vocabulary. As with the different names used for various piercings, try not to get too caught up in the linguistics.

ANXIETY

If you are concerned about the state of your piercing, take action instead of just worrying. Certain piercings typically become discolored, irritated, and oozy during healing. This can be worrisome if you are not familiar with their usual appearance. Piercees sometimes experience panic over piercings that look perfectly normal to a trained eye. Fortunately, all that's needed is some reassurance. Have a piercer examine you, and they will be able to determine whether your healing course seems to be progressing normally. Most piercers are happy to check your progress, and some schedule routine follow-ups.

Excess nervousness and anxiety *are* healing problems—even if they aren't based on the condition of your wound. If you are particularly stressed out, your healing is apt to be delayed.[1] Not all medical professionals are familiar with the way healing piercings present. Whether you simply want a little support or urgently need expert troubleshooting, an experienced piercer is an excellent resource.

SEVERE PROBLEMS

Scientific data on this topic is limited, and few research studies include large populations of piercees. Surveys on the incidence of complications often use geographic samplings of participants. These reveal more about the quality of piercing in a given region than about industry practices in general. One study adds redness, swelling, drainage, and bleeding to the list of "complications," along with infection and trauma. The first four are common consequences of piercing and do not generally belong in the category of "problems."

The available literature confirms that the majority of piercing problems are relatively minor and that conditions grave enough to require hospitalization or surgery are rare. However, the frequency of infected piercings reported in the research is as high as 35 percent.[2] This does not reflect my clinical experience, which demonstrates very few infections in piercings that are performed and cared for responsibly. Studies support my assertion that the quality of both aftercare and piercer, including "experience level of the clinician," affects the rate of infection.[3]

The most severe conditions (including the few deaths attributed to piercing) appear to have been impacted by one or more of the following circumstances. The piercee:

- Did not have the piercing performed in a hygienic, professional setting
- Neglected to follow suggested aftercare protocols
- Failed to respond promptly to infection or other complications
- Had a preexisting health problem such as a heart condition or diabetes[4]

WHAT TO DO

At the first indication something is amiss, visit a piercer for assistance. If you were not impressed with your own practitioner, seek out one with more expertise. They should evaluate:

- Your suitability for the piercing
- The placement and angle of the piercing for your anatomy
- Jewelry style, material, quality, condition, and fit
- Your care practices, including lifestyle factors (health habits, avoidance of trauma, nutritional intake, substance use/abuse, stress levels, recent injury, illness, or allergy, medication, travel, water quality, and more)

The majority of piercing problems can be resolved by proper handling of these critical aspects. If your piercer finds that the first three points above are satisfactory, study the aftercare techniques in chapter 15 and apply yourself to diligently following the suggestions.

IF YOU STILL HAVE PROBLEMS

This chapter contains information intended to help you deal with the most common piercing complications that are not resolved by proper practices and care. I describe the usual signs and complaints to help you figure out precisely what type of problem you are having, possibly with the assistance of your piercer or doctor. And I provide suggestions on the most effective ways to handle them. Try to be patient and understand that everyone is different; frequently, some experimentation is needed to figure out what works best for you.

LEAVE JEWELRY IN!

Try to discover what is wrong before taking out your jewelry. Chances are there is no need for such a drastic measure. In any case, simply removing your jewelry and giving up on your piercing may not be the best approach to your problem. It is not always preferable to take out your jewelry now and try to get it reinserted or redone later. Delayed healing and other issues can occur from repiercing the same spot after unnecessarily abandoning a hole.

When you seek medical care for an ailing piercing, some physicians will immediately ask (or order) you to take out your jewelry, though that isn't always medically necessary. If an infection is suspected or diagnosed, leaving jewelry or an appropriate, inert alternative in place will keep the channel open and allow for drainage. If the piercing is left empty, it is possible that the surface cells could close up, sealing the infection inside, theoretically resulting in an abscess. Discuss this with your doctor. Of course, if removal truly is required, then you must comply with your physician's advice.

If you leave metal jewelry in a troubled piercing, it must be a high-quality piece in perfect condition and made of a suitable, inert material. An appropriate style and good fit are crucial. Problem piercings frequently swell and may require a larger size. If you aren't sure what is causing your complication, a jewelry swap is often a good idea. Have a piercer help you when your piercing is distressed.

An inert polymer retainer is a good substitute for metal jewelry; you can obtain one from a piercer or online. Their flexibility makes them more comfortable to wear in a tender piercing, and an adverse reaction to metal will quickly be ruled out or resolved. If a retainer is not readily available, microbore extension tubing, thick suture material, or an epidural catheter (found in medical settings) can suffice in an urgent situation.[5] Details can be found in "Medical and Dental Emergencies and Appointments," page 303, and "Retainers," page 305.

LOCALIZED INFECTION

When a piercing acts up, a common assumption is that *infection* (invasion and multiplication of disease-causing microorganisms that have a detrimental effect) is to blame. However, not everything that is wrong with a piercing is caused by pathogens. When piercings are performed and cared for according to accepted practice, infections are not prevalent; other complications, such as irritation, are far more common. However, when a piercing is infected, prompt care is required. If left untreated, it can worsen to become extremely dangerous and, in rare cases, life-threatening.

Many minor (or *self-limiting*) soft tissue infections resolve spontaneously or are successfully treated at home. If your condition is recent, mild, and you do not take steroids or have a chronic illness or other health condition, you can try the suggestions listed below for a few days. Numerous products are readily available in drugstores to treat minor skin infections. If your piercing is visible to the public, show it to a pharmacist. Ask for their suggestion on the best over-the-counter product, or whether they think you need to see a doctor. Note that if you suspect an infection in a piercing of the ear cartilage or nose, you should seek help right away.

IDENTIFYING MINOR LOCALIZED INFECTION

- Pinkish or reddish skin, swollen, and warm to the touch
- Localized tenderness, burning, and/or itching
- A small amount of pus
- Swollen lymph nodes

You can have an infection even if you don't have all of the symptoms above. Conversely, having several of them doesn't guarantee that your piercing is infected. Some redness, swelling, and tenderness are normal in fresh piercings, especially during the first two weeks. You are susceptible to infection throughout the healing period. Once the wound has sealed and settled, it is unlikely to become infected unless the piercing experiences a flare-up or gets injured, and the tissue is open again.

WHAT TO DO FOR A MINOR LOCALIZED INFECTION

The following suggestions are for *minor* infections only:

- Keep the area clean and wash the skin around the piercing daily with a mild fragrance-free soap, but don't get it inside the channel. Rinse gently but thoroughly, and dry with fresh, disposable paper products.
- Apply warm, moist compresses to stimulate circulation, encourage drainage, and relieve discomfort (see the information on warm compresses in "Running Cold and Hot," page 236).

- Apply topical over-the-counter antibiotic cream or gel (not ointment) according to package instructions. While this type of product is *not* suggested for routine aftercare, this is the time to use it. Topical antibiotics usually contain bacitracin, neomycin, or polymyxin B, individually or in combination, to fight different types of microorganisms. Combinations of these ingredients work against a broader spectrum of bacteria, but allergic reactions to neomycin are common.[6] Stop using it if you notice redness, itching, or skin eruptions, and consult your physician.

See a doctor right away if you experience the following:
- Your symptoms last more than a few days or markedly worsen.
- You experience a fever, chills, nausea, vomiting, dizziness, or disorientation.
- The piercing is very painful, swollen, has red streaks emanating from it, or there is a loss of function in the region.
- You have copious pus discharge that is greenish, yellowish, or grayish.

For topical treatment, a cream called *Bactroban* (mupirocin antibiotic, available only by prescription) is recognized as an effective medication for localized bacterial infections in piercings.[7] A doctor unfamiliar with piercings may be unsure what to recommend, so you can inform them this is commonly prescribed. *Never* try to self-treat an infection with leftover medication or someone else's prescription.

INFECTION: ABSCESSES

An *abscess* is a pocket of infection containing pus, trapped under the skin, surrounded by inflamed tissue. Medical research shows that they usually occur long after the initial piercing—on average, from four to twelve months later.[8] It is believed that an abscess could be created by removing jewelry from an infected piercing, thus eliminating the pathway for pus and matter to leave the body. Though anecdotal evidence exists, there has been no research to substantiate the theory. There have also been several reports of abscesses forming after the jewelry was removed from unhealed piercings. The individuals went swimming or engaged in other risky behaviors before the wounds had closed and healed completely.

An infection will occur occasionally, and an abscess will form adjacent to a piercing when jewelry is in place. This is more apt to happen if your jewelry constricts the tissue because the initial size was too small, or because of an unexpected amount of post-piercing swelling. Due to the duct system in the breasts, an abscess can form inches away from a nipple piercing.

IDENTIFYING AN ABSCESS
- Tenderness, pain, inflammation, heat, and swelling at the site of a hard, localized mass (feels like a marble under the skin).

- Redness or darkening of the skin (if the abscess is closer to the surface, rather than very deep underneath).
- Worsens over time and may cause nausea, fever, and chills if severe.
- Infections caused by the bacterium *Mycobacterium abscessus* have been described as *cold abscesses* because of the absence of tenderness and inflammation. This means you could have an abscess when a hard mass is present, even if you don't have any of the other symptoms.

WHAT TO DO FOR AN ABSCESS

- For milder cases (a small localized abscess of less than ½ inch or 1 centimeter, without systemic symptoms such as fever or nausea), the application of warm compresses for twenty minutes, four times daily, might cause spontaneous drainage.

- Switching to jewelry of a thinner gauge may also help to encourage drainage if the mass is right next to an opening of the piercing.

- If possible, keep the area elevated to improve comfort.

If the abscess does not drain within forty-eight hours as a result of these steps, or if symptoms worsen, a visit to the doctor is urgent. Infection can spread to deeper tissue or the bloodstream if untreated. This is serious!

- If red streaks emanate from the site, the lump is larger than ½ inch across, or a fever is present, you *must* visit the emergency room or urgent care right away, as the infection may have spread and become cellulitis (discussed next).

- An incision and drainage procedure to empty the pus-filled cavity is commonly needed. If the abscess is close to the piercing, the channel may be lost (cut) in the process.

- Antibiotics alone will not necessarily resolve an abscess. It usually must be physically cleared out as well. In fact, doctors sometimes drain an abscess without prescribing antibiotics.[9]

CELLULITIS

Cellulitis is a common type of bacterial skin infection. When it spreads beyond a localized area throughout the deeper layers of the skin and surrounding tissue, immediate medical attention is required. **Without proper care, this can enter the bloodstream and lymph nodes and become *septicemia* (a severe total body infection), which is potentially deadly.**

IDENTIFYING CELLULITIS
- Inflammation and redness of the skin more than ½ inch from the wound, possibly including broad areas of redness, or red streaking
- Tight, glossy, stretched appearance of the skin, or dimpling like an orange peel
- Warmth, tenderness, and swelling
- Drainage of clear yellow fluid or pus from the skin

Emergency medical care is required immediately if:
- The rash is changing rapidly, or a large area is already involved.
- Fever, pain, chills, weakness, vomiting, body aches, swollen lymph nodes, or mental confusion accompany the other symptoms.
- The infection is on your face, especially near the eye.
- You are immunocompromised (HIV/AIDS, diabetes, or lupus) or have other medical history of concern, including a heart condition.

WHAT TO DO FOR CELLULITIS
You must visit a doctor for treatment; do not delay. Cellulitis is not a condition that can be handled with home care. If the infection is deemed severe, you may need to be hospitalized for intravenous antibiotics or surgical intervention.

THE "IRRITATION BUMP"
Many piercers refer to a variety of healing issues as an "irritation bump," "pressure bump," or the even more vague "piercing bump." Some also call them a "piercing blister." Avoiding the use of medical terminology in the studio is appropriate, as piercers are not to diagnose or treat any health conditions. That said, I believe different complications call for particular interventions, so this chapter takes a deeper dive into the specifics. The types of bumps addressed below include an overgrowth of granulation tissue, the localized piercing pimple, and excess scar tissue. Keloids are far more than a bump, but they're discussed too, along with other piercing problems.

ANGLE-RELATED BUMP
A common kind of bump around a piercing is caused by the angle of the channel not resting at a perfect 90 degrees. This isn't necessarily a failure on the part of your piercer, as aesthetics and individual anatomy often require that a piercing be positioned at an angle that isn't quite perpendicular to the tissue.

You can identify an angle-related bump because it *always* happens on the obtuse (wider) angle of the piercing. In fact, an experienced professional can point out which side of the jewelry an angle-related bump is likely to occur just by looking at a new piercing.

IDENTIFYING AN ANGLE-RELATED BUMP

- ○ Raised fleshy bump right next to the piercing
- ○ Located to one side of the jewelry, rather than surrounding the entire opening
- ○ Usually red, pink, or darker than your regular skin tone
- ○ Does not seep or secrete pus, blood, or matter (unless you also have an infection, in addition to this issue)

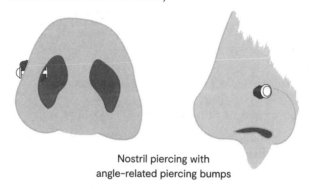

Nostril piercing with
angle-related piercing bumps

WHAT TO DO FOR AN ANGLE-RELATED BUMP

Apply plenty of warm compresses. Continue them for two weeks after the problem seems resolved.

Attempt to redistribute the pressure caused by the angle of the piercing. Switch a ball or small ornamental end to a broad (3 millimeters or larger), flat-bottomed piece, such as a disc or cabochon gem. This will sometimes reduce the size of an angle-related bump.

If unsuccessful, have your piercer remove the jewelry and repierce at a later date with an angle that better suits your anatomy.

HYPERGRANULATION (EXCESS GRANULATION) TISSUE

The terms *hypergranulation tissue, granuloma,* and *pyogenic granuloma* are all fancy words for certain *benign* (noncancerous) growths that form on wounds. These can simply be a consequence of injuring the body, or they can be caused by excessive trauma, moisture, or infection. If you use Accutane or take certain birth control pills or other medications, you are at increased risk for this complication. Your piercing may improve if you lower the dosage or discontinue taking it.[10] Discuss any proposed alterations to your medication with your doctor, and always take it as prescribed.

These bumps are comprised of cells that are a standard part of wound healing, but they overgrow, often quite rapidly. These unsightly lumps are most common on piercings of the navel, outer labia, nostril, and the inside of the lip, though they may also occur elsewhere. In some cases, they can successfully be treated, and the piercing may be maintained, though healing is suspended while excess granulation tissue is present.[11] You may need to be patient and try different treatments or combinations of remedies to achieve a satisfactory resolution.

IDENTIFYING HYPERGRANULATION TISSUE
- Bump of red tissue protrudes above the surface of your skin
- Looks similar to raw hamburger or like the inside of the piercing is on the outside of your body
- Oozing clear or yellow sticky drainage
- Bleeds easily
- Usually looks worse than it feels, though it can be tender

WHAT TO DO FOR HYPERGRANULATION TISSUE
Keep the area as dry and free from friction and irritation as possible. This is critical, and often the only way to resolve the issue. Try only one product at a time, and keep a careful watch on the area to monitor your response.
- Aggressive sodium chloride treatment using a *hypertonic* product (contains more salt than the body's fluids do), such as Curasalt (20 percent sodium chloride–impregnated gauze), or Hypergel Hypertonic Gel (20 percent hypertonic saline gel). Apply according to the package directions, but be careful to cover *only* the affected tissue, or you will cause drying and irritation to the healthy skin surrounding the problem.[12]

- Topical application of over-the-counter cortisone cream according to package instructions.

If home treatment doesn't help your condition or it worsens, visit a doctor. They have a variety of therapeutic options to offer. Excess granulation tissue often recurs, especially when a problem with moisture, jewelry fit, or friction is not resolved. If the condition proves intractable, you will need to abandon the piercing. The bumps ordinarily diminish significantly or entirely disappear when you remove your jewelry.

THE "LOCALIZED PIERCING PIMPLE"
This complication is somewhat common, but the piercing-friendly medical professionals I polled failed to reach a consensus on a diagnosis or suggested treatment. Therefore, I've named it based on its appearance and address it below using professional piercing experience in conjunction with accepted health care principles. Overall, the symptoms are similar to those of *folliculitis*, inflammation and infection in or around a hair follicle.[13] However, this type of problem routinely occurs near the openings of nipple piercings, where hair follicles are not plentiful.

Sometimes a *pustule* (a small round area of inflamed skin filled with pus) will appear under the skin near the opening of a piercing. It may be caused by trauma or a mild infection that remains contained locally. A small pocket forms close to the surface and repeatedly fills and drains. Sometimes it seems to be gone for good, but then the cycle begins once again, weeks or months later. The best way to resolve the problem appears to be by helping your body to break down and absorb the sac or pocket that has formed. You may be tempted to pop this pimple-like eruption yourself, but never lance your skin with nonsterile implements; use warm compresses to encourage drainage. If you have a localized pustule that won't open or drain and needs to be lanced, seek medical assistance.

IDENTIFYING A PIERCING PIMPLE

o Small, slightly elevated pus-filled bump or pimple adjacent to the piercing
o Red and inflamed but contained locally
o May be tender, itch, or burn, though some are painless
o Usually secretes pus and/or blood when drained (or popped)

WHAT TO DO FOR A PIERCING PIMPLE

o Follow the suggestions under "What to Do for a Minor Localized Infection," page 249.

o Over-the-counter antihistamines taken according to package instructions may diminish itching and inflammation.

o Do plenty of warm compresses. *Continue them* for two weeks after the problem seems resolved.

o When it looks improved, manually break up the pocket to prevent refilling by rolling the tissue surrounding it between your fingers.

o If you do not respond to treatment, lab analysis for an invading microorganism may be needed to determine if the cause is fungal or bacterial so your doctor can prescribe appropriate medication to target the problem.[14]

o You must see a doctor if you have increased pain, a temperature of 100°F (37.8°C), or the infection worsens or spreads.[15]

o If you have a verified diagnosis of folliculitis, laser hair removal can destroy the problematic hair follicle, prevent future episodes, and reduce the scarring of repeated eruptions.

SCARRING

A *scar* is defined as "a mark left on the skin after the healing of a cut, burn, or other area of wounded tissue."[16] Scar formation is a natural process following any breach in the tissue, including piercing. Unfortunately, however, the body sometimes fails to perform this job properly, and complications occur. Below are some of the most common scarring problems, with suggestions on how to handle them.

ATROPHIC SCARRING

Atrophic scarring, a depression or pitting below the normal skin level, sometimes occurs when a piercing migrates. A visible divot or pit is also frequently left when healed piercings are retired. Unfortunately, this type of scarring is usually perma-nent. Navel and facial piercings are the most common sites to find this type of pockmark. There are no easy fixes, but a dermatologist can provide treatments that might be effective, such as glycolic acid peels, dermabrasion, or laser resurfac-ing. If the piercing is viable, the best option is to leave jewelry in place to mask the scar—or at least part of it.

EXCESSIVE SCARRING

Keloids and hypertrophic scars are the types of bumps and lumps commonly found on ear cartilage piercings, though other pierced sites also fall victim to these conditions. The presence of a foreign object (jewelry) causes prolonged healing and predisposes the wound to chronic inflammation. Both of these conditions increase the likelihood of excessive scar formation, along with genetic, systemic, and local factors, including wound depth and skin tension.[17] Both types of scar-ring are caused by an overproduction of collagen.

A *keloid* is an exceedingly large, dense mound of fibrous scar tissue that becomes significantly bigger than your original wound. They can be extremely unsightly, and some grow to shocking dimensions. Unfortunately, once you have formed a keloid, they are often challenging to get rid of, even with medical treatment. They are approximately fifteen times more prevalent in those with darker complexions and often run in families, though anyone can get them. Keloids occur in about 5 to 15 percent of wounds, with the average age of onset from ten to thirty years of age.[18]

A *hypertrophic scar* is the smaller and far more common type of bump that forms around a piercing. They can extend several millimeters above the skin's surface. These scars are not as massive or severe as keloids, respond better to treatment, and are more easily resolved. Sometimes they go away spontaneously or may recur and recede in cycles for an extended period before improving sub-stantially or disappearing. Friction and trauma are common causes that you must minimize for a successful resolution. Hypertrophic scars are frequently misla-beled as keloids—sometimes even by doctors—possibly because both are types of excessive scar tissue.

IDENTIFYING HYPERTROPHIC SCARRING

o Thickening of the tissue resulting in a raised fleshy bump surrounding a piercing

o Stays within the bounds of the injury

o Usually somewhat pink or red, at least initially, though can turn lighter or whitish over time

o Not tender; may itch

o Tends to form during the healing period or following injury of a healed piercing

o No pus or other drainage

WHAT TO DO FOR HYPERTROPHIC SCARRING

There are many scar-reduction products on the market. (You can try them on any type of scar, but they are not likely to help with bulbous keloids or atrophic depressions.) Unfortunately, even with consistent compliance, scar treatments are not successful for all users. Some products have guarantees, however, so check before making a purchase. Listed below is a sampling of the available options. Try one method at a time. Many should not be used on a wound that is still healing, so read packaging information carefully and always follow instructions diligently. Read customer reviews to assist with your selection of any commercial products.

o Mederma, Derma E Scar Gel, and other products containing *allicin* (onion or garlic extract). This is intended to act as an anti-inflammatory and may inhibit the overproduction of collagen in a scar. These need to be rubbed in several times daily for months.

o Celsus, PuriDerma, and other creams, oils, and lotions with natural ingredients such as cocoa butter, shea butter, aloe vera, calendula, lavender, green tea, ginseng, camphor, and many other botanical compounds.

o ReJuveness, Epi-Derm, and other silicone strips and sheets; and Aroamas, Xeragel, and other silicone gel systems. It is believed that silicone helps scars heal by trapping moisture to increase hydration, and by suppressing overactivity of scar-related cells and normalizing their activity. Some strips are washable and reusable, so they may be among the more economical options.

o *Compression* is the continuous mechanical pressure on a scar to flatten it.[19] It can minimize the formation of scars by preventing tension on the tissue.[20] Medical paper tape (such as 3M Micropore) can be placed onto the area and continuously worn to diminish excess scarring. Use clean scissors to cut a circle or shape that will cover the affected zone completely, or use a disinfected hole punch for a small bump. Snip a slit to the center and slide the piece around the jewelry; stick it down over the affected tissue. (Do not apply it like a Band-Aid over the whole area.) Replace the tape as needed and wear it for at least six weeks for maximum effect. On a piercing that is still healing, carefully change the tape daily. Discontinue if you experience skin irritation.

o Wear a disc of autoclavable, medical-grade silicone in gentle, direct contact with the affected tissue. A piercing disc combines the accepted scar-reduction techniques of compression therapy with silicone. Your jewelry may need to be resized to allow for the disc(s) to apply light pressure. These can be used on any piercing with an overgrowth of scar tissue *if* the jewelry can keep it in continuous contact with the bump. Some studios stock them, and they're available online. This safe, inexpensive method is often successful at resolving excess scar tissue. Discontinue use if you do not see improvement in two to three months.

o Over-the-counter glycolic acid or another alpha hydroxy acid (AHA) product, used according to package instructions. These exfoliate the skin and may diminish scar tissue over time. Use only products containing less than 10 percent AHAs. This concentration promotes exfoliation but is not potent enough to generate collagen production, increasing the size of a hypertrophic scar. AHAs can cause sun sensitivity.

o Daily gentle massage with a nonirritating oil or lotion to increase circulation, and soften and hydrate the tissue.[21] See "Lubrication," page 241.

o Topical treatment with an over-the-counter corticosteroid cream according to the package instructions. Corticosteroid injections are known to be more effective, but some piercees have positive results with cream, and it is a less invasive option.

o Steroid injections, laser revision, cryosurgery, or other medical interventions may be able to reduce or eliminate hypertrophic scars if home care is unsuccessful. See a dermatologist for evaluation and treatment.

IDENTIFYING KELOIDS
o Bulbous and large, extending well beyond the boundaries of the original wound; they may continue growing for years
o Sometimes tender, painful, or itchy
o Usually red or hyperpigmented (dark) and vascular, containing broad bundles of collagen, which are absent in hypertrophic scars
o Can develop over many months, or even up to a year following the piercing

WHAT TO DO FOR KELOIDS

Prevention is best; avoid piercings if you or a member of your immediate family has had keloids. You can try any of the scar-reduction options discussed above, but medical intervention is usually necessary. Even then, treatments are often ineffective, and recurrence is common. Combination approaches are standard, using multiple modalities as suggested by a doctor.

HYPERPIGMENTATION (DISCOLORATION)

Hyperpigmentation is when the skin turns a deeper or darker shade than usual. Discoloration about the size of a pea extending from your piercing can be a regular part of the healing process on a variety of placements. This is common with the navel, and it can remain for months. Shades described as purplish, pinkish, reddish, or brownish are typical, depending on the individual complexion. This issue is apt to diminish over time; still, a mark beyond your piercing's borders could be permanent. Related factors include skin type, healing course, and the location of your piercing. Tanning during healing can also cause this to occur.

Hyperpigmentation is more probable with darker skin tones,[22] or when problems or trauma are experienced during healing. It often dissipates or disappears over time without intervention. After your piercing is no longer an open wound, try one of the scar-reduction product options described on page 257, to minimize residual discoloration. Many over-the-counter lightening and bleaching creams and serums are available, but they should be avoided until your piercing is well-healed and settled (at least a year). Sometimes the best resolution is to wear jewelry with a ball, gemstone, or another ornament that obscures the discolored area.

DRY SKIN

If the area around your piercing is dry, chapped, or cracked, this can cause discomfort, delay healing, and increase your risk of infection. To keep your skin moisturized and in good condition, follow the instructions under "Lubrication," page 241, or apply a fragrance-free, water-based, nonirritating moisturizing cream (with clean hands) to the exterior of the piercing, two to three times daily.

There are some ways to minimize dryness:

o Avoid harsh products; use only *mild* soap and rinse thoroughly at the end of your shower. Keep lather away from your piercing unless it is necessary because your work or leisure activities take place in a dirty environment.

o Limit bathing to ten minutes, once daily in water that is cool or warm, not hot, and avoid soaking in a tub.

o Moisturize immediately after bathing when your skin is still damp.

o Use fragrance-free, dye-free laundry detergent without stain-fighting enzymes.

"TARNISH TATTOO"

No, this isn't a new type of body art; it's a complication caused by inappropriate jewelry. If you wear sterling silver in a piercing, especially during healing, a residue can turn the interior of the hole dark blue, gray, or black. The technical term is *localized argyria*, and it is caused by skin exposure to silver or silver salts. Stains can also be left by wearing low-karat or poorly alloyed gold, or other unsuitable metal. In the absence of irritation, this kind of dark blotch is largely a cosmetic issue. But once the discoloration sets in, it is permanent without medical intervention. Avoid wearing silver or "mystery metal" (junk jewelry) in nostril and facial piercings, where a tarnish tattoo can be particularly unbecoming.

CONTACT DERMATITIS

Contact dermatitis is a skin rash caused by an allergen or irritant. When it appears near your healing piercing, it is usually from a care product or poor-quality jewelry containing unsuitable materials. Harsh soaps and cleansers are apt to cause irritation, inflammation, and sometimes dermatitis in the adjacent tissue (in addition to killing off some of the delicate new skin cells that form during healing). When you have sensitive skin, problems can develop even from mild soap.

A red rash that surrounds your piercing or one that covers a large area (without pain and swelling) usually indicates contact dermatitis from your cleaning product or jewelry. Skin eruptions below your piercing, where soap suds run during bathing, obviously demonstrate contact dermatitis caused by your cleaning product.

Many people are sensitive to nickel, one of the top causes of allergic contact dermatitis.[23] Unfortunately, it is used in cheap jewelry of all sorts, including some made for piercings. A nickel allergy may develop after your initial exposure to an item containing it or after repeated or prolonged exposure. Even a piece that seems acceptable initially can cause trouble over time if the nickel content is too high. A lasting allergy can form that has ramifications for many aspects of daily life. If you become highly sensitized to nickel, you should not eat foods that contain traces of it, including nuts, chocolate, beer, tea, coffee, and apricots. Skin contact with metal, including watches and other jewelry and clothing with metal snaps, buttons, rivets, or zippers, can all cause localized itchy rashes that could spread to other areas of your body.[24] Treatments, whether prescribed by a doctor or over-the-counter, are temporary solutions to deal with an outbreak, but they cannot desensitize you or cure an allergy. Do not use clear nail polish to coat offending jewelry, because it contains chemicals including toluene, formaldehyde, or dibutyl phthalate, which can cause dermatitis in nickel-sensitive individuals.[25]

IDENTIFYING CONTACT DERMATITIS

- Redness, rash (multiple pimple- or blister-like eruptions, or hives), and inflammation; sometimes cracking, flaking, or peeling skin follow the initial outbreak
- Localized swelling, tenderness, and possible warmth
- Oozing clear fluid
- Itching and possibly burning (not present in local infection or cellulitis, which share some of the same symptoms)
- The hole of your healing piercing becomes visibly bigger than the jewelry in it (the skin appears to be receding from the ornament)

WHAT TO DO FOR CONTACT DERMATITIS

- Replace your jewelry with a more inert material[26] or stop using an offending care product. This usually results in rapid improvement, with clear skin within one to three weeks; no other action may be required.

- Apply cold compresses for fifteen to thirty minutes several times a day to diminish itching.

- Ease symptoms with over-the-counter topical hydrocortisone, allergy-relief medications such as Benadryl (diphenhydramine), and/or topical anti-itch products.

- Do not scratch an itchy rash with dirty fingers, as you can cause a secondary infection.

- If your allergy is severe, visit a doctor for evaluation and, possibly, prescription medication.

EMBEDDED JEWELRY

When you fail to change out jewelry that is too short, it can become embedded under your skin. It is much easier to prevent this from happening than to treat it after it does. If your jewelry is starting to sink into your tissue, see your piercer for a longer piece *right away.*

Tongue and lip jewelry commonly *nest* (sink a millimeter or two) into the soft oral tissues, but if more than half of a ball has disappeared into your piercing or the skin appears to be growing over your jewelry, visit your piercer immediately. Oral tissue regenerates exceptionally quickly, and jewelry can end up embedded overnight. You can try elevation, rest, ice, and possibly an over-the-counter anti-inflammatory to minimize swelling as temporary measures until you can get to your piercer and have the jewelry changed.

In the unfortunate event that the tissue completely grows over the jewelry and you or your piercer cannot push it back through the surface, you must seek medical care. A small incision will be made (generally under local anesthesia) to remove your unintentional implant. If you want to preserve the hole, obtain jewelry of the proper size beforehand, as it might be possible to insert it after the embedded piece has been liberated. Ask your piercer about the size and style of jewelry that might be suitable following such an incident.

TRAUMATIC TEAR

Skin is pretty tough, so a severe snag is needed to cause real damage. When you wear jewelry of the suggested minimum thickness and exercise some awareness of your piercing, this type of unfortunate event seldom occurs. But accidents can happen, and piercings occasionally catch and tear. If your jewelry is ripped through your piercing, control the bleeding and clean the gash. Seek medical help right away if you cannot join the edges of the split tissue together properly or if direct pressure does not stop bleeding within fifteen minutes, which is rare.

If the jewelry was not completely torn out, it *might* be possible to preserve your piercing, depending on the original placement and the extent of the damage. Place the jewelry or an inert polymer retainer in the original location as close to the body as possible and use medical tape such as Micropore to secure it. Resume your care regimen as if you have a brand-new piercing, and replace the tape as needed. If the tissue heals satisfactorily, you should be able to maintain the piercing, though it may permanently require extra gentle handling following a tear because scar tissue is only about 80 percent as strong as normal skin.[27]

CATCHING THE TUBE

This isn't about surfing; it's a type of trauma that can happen when you force your jewelry to move, and a tube of skin adheres to it that used to be the lining of your piercing. Forcibly removing the interior of a piercing may cause tenderness or bleeding. It also sets back your healing, as your body repeats the process of generating new cells to line the channel. You are starting over at the beginning and must initiate aftercare practices all over again. Multiple episodes can result in excess scar tissue. Be gentle!

DEALING WITH REJECTION AND MIGRATION

When your jewelry moves closer to the surface and your tissue gets thinner, or narrower between the openings of a piercing, you are experiencing migration. The piercing may move only a little and then settle and stay in a different position. On piercings that rest parallel to the body (such as nipple or frenum), if the tissue at an opening suddenly has a V-shape, trouble looms.

For safety and longevity, a piercing should encompass at least 5/16 inch (8 millimeters) between the entrance and exit holes. If your piercing is narrower than that, there is a strong possibility you will lose it. Do not allow jewelry to come through to the surface, or an unsightly split scar will often remain—unless you undergo plastic surgery. Future repiercing could be more difficult or impossible if you permit the jewelry to be expelled from your body.

You should abandon the piercing if the tissue between the entry and exit gets progressively smaller or thinner over time and any of the following happen:

o   Only ¼ inch or less of skin remains between the openings.

o   It is flaking and peeling, red and inflamed, or hard and calloused looking.

o   Just a thin filament of nearly transparent tissue is left, and you can virtually see the jewelry right through your skin.

These issues can arise long after healing. I know of piercings that remained stable for ten or twenty years, and then migration or rejection occurred without any indication as to why. This is especially distressing when you've had a piercing for a long time because it feels like you are losing a part of yourself. Whether your piercing is old or new, immediate intervention is needed when migration is detected.

If friction or trauma is responsible, this must be corrected right away. Check the fit, quality, and condition of your jewelry. Wearing inferior metal or a piece with a scratched finish can wreak havoc. Even if the jewelry seems satisfactory, swapping it for a different style, size, or material is sometimes all you need to stop the movement of your piercing. Switching to an inert polymer retainer may calm a piercing that has started to migrate, whether jewelry was the apparent cause or not.

If ring-style jewelry won't rest flat against your body after the first few weeks of healing, or barbell ends sink into your tissue at all, these are clear indications that your jewelry is too small. Inserting a piece that fits well may halt migration that has been caused by constriction if you make the change while sufficient tissue remains.

REPIERCING AFTER LOSS

When trauma, migration, or rejection results in the loss of a piercing, you can often be repierced—unless you were unsuited to begin with or end up with excessive scarring or a lack of tissue pliability. After losing or abandoning your piercing under problematic circumstances, it is prudent to wait a year or more before trying again. Your piercer will usually position the new piercing behind any scar tissue. However, this does not assure success, because scars are weaker than regular skin, contrary to what many piercers believe. If the area remains hard, tight, or dense, it should be left unadorned.

If you repeat exactly what you did before, you can expect the same results. Consider what caused your problem and what you can do differently so that it doesn't happen again. When you do get repierced, try a different approach with the jewelry or care regimen if you are not sure what went wrong previously. In cases of migration or rejection, ask yourself relevant questions: Did I sleep on the piercing? Was I experiencing an unusual amount of physical or emotional stress? Did I care for the piercing properly? Was my jewelry suitable?

Sometimes a migrated piercing that is too shallow to support jewelry will remain an open channel long after you abandon it. When it comes to repiercing, an old hole might become inflamed or infected after a new one is made nearby. Due to continuous secretion or irritation from the previous piercing, occasionally these situations cannot be resolved satisfactorily, and you will not be able to wear jewelry in the site.

CHOKING

Although not a common occurrence, it is theoretically possible to accidentally choke on body jewelry, which could be very serious. Most oral body jewelry, however, is too small to become stuck or cause an obstruction in the throat if it becomes unfastened.

What to do for jewelry caught in the throat:

- o *Immediate* emergency medical care is required if you cannot breathe. Dial 911 or have someone call for you, if possible.
- o If you cannot speak or cough, the *Heimlich maneuver* (upward abdominal thrusts) may be used to force air from your lungs in an attempt to dislodge the obstruction. You may be able to perform the procedure on yourself using the back of a chair or other object, if you are alone.
- o If you can breathe but feel jewelry lodged in your throat, cough vigorously to attempt to bring up the piece. If this is ineffective, seek emergency medical attention.

SWALLOWED JEWELRY

Much more frequently, jewelry is swallowed and passed through to the digestive tract and out the other end. This seldom causes any negative consequences. The aftermath may include anxiety, loss of your adornment, and the expense of buying a replacement.

If you swallow jewelry, do not attempt to induce vomiting. A lost ball will simply move on through; a ring or barbell post usually will, too. If you were wearing a treasured ornament, whether precious in price or sentiment, you might wish to hunt for it over the next few days by checking your stool. A strainer is helpful for this process. An advantage of finding a lost item is that you will know it is not stuck inside.

It is doubtful that a piece of jewelry smooth enough to be worn safely in your mouth will cause internal damage on the way through. Also unlikely is swallowing jewelry large enough to obstruct your digestive tract. Barbell posts are less apt to be ingested, but could be more dangerous. A worst-case scenario would be perforation of the bowel or intestine. Of all accidentally swallowed foreign bodies, 80 percent pass naturally, and surgical intervention is indicated in less than 1 percent of cases.[28] The remainder are removed via *endoscopy* (a small tube inserted down the throat with a camera and instrument port for retrieving the object).

IDENTIFYING INTESTINAL DAMAGE FROM SWALLOWED JEWELRY
o   Abdominal tenderness, pain, or vomiting
o   Abnormal bowel sounds emanating from your abdomen
o   Dark stool containing blood

Jewelry can pass through the digestive system, all the way to the end, where you might encounter a rare (perhaps hypothetical) complication: it gets lodged on the way out.

IDENTIFYING JEWELRY STUCK IN THE RECTUM
o   Sudden, sharp pain when eliminating
o   Fresh red blood in your stool or the toilet bowl

Should you experience any of the above symptoms after swallowing jewelry, *seek immediate medical attention*. Diagnostic tools such as X-rays can determine the position of a lodged item, and a variety of methods are available to remove it, depending on its location. Prevention is best: wear quality jewelry and regularly check to ensure that it is securely fastened.

ASPIRATED JEWELRY
It could be life-threatening if you should manage to *aspirate* (inhale into your airway) any part of your jewelry. Though this dire consequence is frequently cited in warnings about piercing risks, I could locate no verified cases in the literature on piercing complications.[29] If you do manage to inhale jewelry, you must *seek medical attention immediately*. A foreign object that remains in the lungs typically causes inflammation and infection, including pneumonia.

THE POINT
If a complication occurs, the best chance you have to resolve it is to identify what is wrong and follow the suggestions accordingly. Prompt attention and optimal handling of problems can prevent more severe conditions. Seek assistance from a qualified piercer or health care provider when you need it. If a piercing must be removed, you won't win by fighting. The good news is that with appropriate action, you can achieve a positive outcome most of the time.

PART 6

LIVING WITH YOUR PIERCINGS

UPKEEP AND STRETCHING...............268

ADVANCED JEWELRY
AND PRACTICES 285

SPECIAL SITUATIONS 302

SEX! 311

17

UPKEEP AND STRETCHING

After your piercing has healed, it still requires routine maintenance, however minimal, for life. This chapter covers necessary upkeep and activities such as changing your jewelry, stretching to larger gauges, and retiring your piercing.

REGULAR MAINTENANCE

Attending to your healed piercings should be part of your personal hygiene routine. Simply wash your jewelry and the exterior of your piercing with your usual soap and water. It is not necessary to rotate the jewelry unless your piercing has an odor from sebum buildup. If so, lather it up, gently move the piece to cleanse the interior, and rinse well using the same motion to remove soap and residue. This keeps the area clean and free of matter and eliminates the normal (and smelly) secretions that can coat jewelry and lodge in a healed piercing.

Check regularly to make sure hair does not become tangled around your jewelry. A single coiled strand that remains next to your tissue can cause an accumulation of secretions and lead to irritation and even infection.

You do not necessarily need to remove jewelry for regular upkeep. It can often be left in place for maintenance and worn for years on end. However, once you are healed, if your ornament looks or feels dirty and you've done everything you can while wearing it, then you will need to take it out for more scrupulous attention. Snug-fitting styles may require at least brief removal for thorough cleaning.

Body jewelry metals lose their luster when coated with personal care products or natural body oils and secretions. Gold may tarnish (it is the other metals in the alloy that discolor) when worn in a piercing. This can happen even to high-karat, quality pieces; it is not necessarily a sign of cheap jewelry.

If the ornamental end on your piercing is broad and flat, such as a cabochon gemstone, debris can accumulate underneath it without being noticed. You can use dental floss to scrape the underside of the jewelry. Pre-threaded Y-shaped flossing picks work wonderfully for this purpose. Thorough maintenance is especially crucial on surface piercings and anchors.

Commercial jewelry-polishing cloths can help return the shine to your adornment. Different types are available, so use one made for the metal you're wearing; a gold-polishing cloth, for example, will not be useful on steel or titanium. Keep harsh cleaning products away from your skin. Many chemicals that are suitable for rings and necklaces could be dangerous if put on jewelry that will be returned to your body or mouth. Toothpaste on a firm toothbrush makes an excellent jewelry polish whether your ornament is in an oral piercing or not. Pieces that contain durable gems (like diamonds, rubies, and sapphires) can get the toothbrush treatment, too; it will keep settings clean and stones sparkly.

Inexpensive jewelry cleaning machines that use steam or ultrasonic technology do a more thorough job than polishing cloths, but all require temporary removal of your ornament. The steam units use distilled water, and an ultrasonic unit will work with a mild soap solution or plain water in place of strong chemical detergents. Check with your jeweler/piercer before using such equipment if your jewelry contains genuine or synthetic gemstones. Certain setting styles and stones, such as opals and emeralds, are too fragile for this treatment.

If you don't have a spare ring or bar to wear during cleanings, buy a retainer to keep the channel open, and/or a taper to facilitate the reinsertion. Many piercings shrink so quickly that you may not be able to put your jewelry back after it has been out for just a few minutes—even if you have had it for years.

REGULAR MAINTENANCE: ORAL PIERCINGS

Any jewelry worn continuously in your mouth is subject to plaque formation, just like your teeth. Most people don't take their teeth out to clean them, and if you are highly conscientious, you may be able to perform sufficient upkeep without removing your oral jewelry either. However, it is challenging.

Regular use of an antiplaque oral rinse can help keep jewelry clean. Still, there is no substitute for a vigorous scrub. Meticulously scour each end of a bar with a firm toothbrush as you hold the other side between your fingers. The hard-bristle brush that is best for use on jewelry may be firmer than your dentist recommends for your teeth. Use a loop of dental floss to clean the junctures where your barbell ends connect to the post. Regular scrubbing of the in-the-mouth part of lip and labret jewelry is as necessary as brushing your teeth. The ball or disc on the underside of your tongue is particularly susceptible to collecting plaque.

If brushing, flossing, and rinsing don't do a thorough enough job, jewelry can be removed and submerged in hydrogen peroxide, a mixture of equal parts white vinegar and water, or a denture-cleaning soak according to the manufacturer's directions.

CHANGING JEWELRY

Quality body jewelry can be left in a piercing indefinitely. If you like what you're wearing and it fits properly, there is no need to change it. Most piercees don't have the requisite know-how, dexterity, or aseptic technique to safely insert a new ornament into a healing piercing at home. A clumsy attempt to swap out jewelry can cause irritation, delayed healing, and infection. See a piercer if you experience problems; otherwise, your original piece should remain in place until the piercing has made it through the healing process.

After that, however, it should be safe to replace your jewelry when you meet all of the following conditions:

- Your piercing is no longer secreting and getting crusty.
- It is not tender or experiencing any issues or flare-ups.
- The minimum healing time has passed (see "Minimum Healing Times Chart," page 333).

Many piercees prefer to have a professional change their jewelry, especially the first time. Depending on placement and whether you can see and access your piercing, you may be able to perform the job yourself. Studios generally charge a nominal fee or offer free jewelry insertions when you purchase something new. Ask for a lesson on how to deal with your own jewelry; good piercers are amenable to educating their clients.

INSERTION TAPERS FOR JEWELRY CHANGES

If you are a novice and wish to swap out your jewelry, an insertion taper is invaluable for keeping the channel open and avoiding excess trauma. Its tapered shape helps to slide the existing ornament out and ease the new one into place.

A taper that does not correspond to the gauge and style of the jewelry you are putting in can be worse than not having one. Internally threaded pieces use a *threaded-pin* taper (the end screws into the jewelry), or a *pin-coupling* taper (the back end is formed into a pin that fits into the hole that is tapped in the post). The pin type is also used for threadless jewelry. Fixed and captive bead rings, and most clickers and seam rings, use a *concave taper*. The bowl-shaped end of the taper connects with the convex end of the jewelry. See "Insertion Tapers," page 76. To avoid an unpleasant surprise, check the fit of your taper with your new jewelry before removing what you're wearing.

If you feel confident that you can follow the old jewelry with the new (and you are not stretching up), then a taper is not required. But if your old jewelry comes out before the new piece passes through, finding the exit hole can be harder than you think. Trying to shove jewelry through a channel that has shrunk is not only painful, but it is also traumatic to the tissue, especially for a recently healed piercing. Piercings can be injured or lost due to inept attempts at changing jewelry at home.

JEWELRY CHANGE PROCEDURE

I've had far too many piercees show me an inflamed or empty piercing and recount a painful tale of trying to change jewelry at home for "over an hour." When properly handled, the procedure should take only a few moments. Learning what to do and using the correct tools will ensure your comfort and safety.

o **Prepare yourself**: Swap out your jewelry after a shower when your skin is clean, and the tissue is looser. Your hands must be washed and dried.

o **Prepare your work area**: If you are near a sink, plug it carefully. Pieces of small body jewelry can easily be lost down a drain. Thick carpeting and home jewelry changes don't mix. Select an area where it will be easy to locate and retrieve dropped items.

o Assemble everything you will need for the process from beginning to end:

☐ Jewelry: Clean or sterile and open, ready for insertion

☐ Lubricant: A water-based product such as K-Y Jelly

☐ Tissues or paper towels: To keep your fingers dry and wipe off the jewelry after insertion

☐ Clean zip-top bags: To store your jewelry after removal

☐ Tight-fitting medical gloves, possibly with textured fingertips

☐ An insertion taper that connects with your new jewelry (optional)

☐ Jewelry tools (discussed on page 273) such as ROPs, RCPs, hemostats, and/or brass-jaw pliers (optional)

o **Choose the right jewelry:** Purchase only from a reputable source. New jewelry is often sold in individual packages, but you can't tell if it is sterile by looking—you have to ask (and you must trust your supplier). If you are unsure, have a piercer sterilize the jewelry in an autoclave before you wear it.

o **Prepare the jewelry if you wore it before:** If stored in a clean environment, you could wash jewelry with soap and water, but autoclaving it is preferable. If you did not keep it in a hygienic location, it must be sterilized before reinsertion. Many piercers will autoclave jewelry for free, or charge a small fee. It is not advisable to share worn jewelry with others, as certain proteins can remain, even after appropriate decontamination and sterilization processes. [1]

o **Open the jewelry:** Unscrew a threaded end, remove a ball from a captive, twist open a fixed-bead ring, and so on. Rings must be spread wide enough to clear your tissue without pinching your skin. If a piercer sterilized your jewelry, they should have taken it apart for the process.

o **Assemble the right tools:** If your hands aren't strong enough for the job, you will require tools to help. They must be appropriate, or they can damage you or your jewelry (see "Jewelry Tools," page 273). Regular workbench pliers are not suitable. If you scratch the metal (which is easy to do, even with the proper implements), your jewelry will be unwearable. If you have to use regular tools in an emergency, clean them thoroughly and wrap each tip with a strip of cloth tape or adhesive bandages to form a protective cushion. Be sure you have a very firm grasp before attempting to bend jewelry that is in your body.

o **Lubricate:** Apply a small amount of lubricant to the jewelry you are wearing and work it into the piercing channel. Apply some to the end of your new jewelry or taper, but keep it off your fingers.

o **Make the swap:** Try to keep something in the piercing at all times. Support the tissue on the exit side to facilitate the transfer. Push out the old jewelry using your new jewelry (or a taper). If you're using a taper, chase your old jewelry out with the thin tip. Or, if the taper matches the size and style that you're wearing, you can use the thicker end of the taper to back your old piece out. Next, connect your new jewelry to the back end of the taper and use it to push the tool out of the piercing.

o **Close the jewelry:** Wipe off the lubricant with a clean tissue and fasten your jewelry.

o **Clean up:** Wash your worn jewelry and insertion tapers with soap and water and dry well with clean paper towels. Store the items in clean zip-top bags or another hygienic location, keeping jewelry made of different metals in separate containers to avoid scratches.

JEWELRY HYGIENE

Any retailer who permits customers to try on body jewelry, including ornaments worn on rings or bars, and puts unwanted items back in stock without sterilizing them first is a menace. One who handles worn jewelry without gloves is also a hazard. Do not buy or touch anything there! I've been in studios where piercers are so lax or uninformed that they allow customers to try on body jewelry and then return it straight to the showcase. If you wouldn't willingly share bodily fluids with a total stranger, don't insert anything from a display counter or bulk inventory without having it sterilized.

JEWELRY TOOLS

Your piercer may use these during a piercing procedure or jewelry insertion, and you can purchase them for home jewelry changes, if necessary. If you have personal implements that you do not share, washing them with soap and water between uses should be sufficient if you keep them stored in clean zip-top bags.

Large-gauge, small-diameter, or unannealed captive rings usually require tools for removal and insertion. Using them frequently for swapping out jewelry will cause some unavoidable damage, even if not readily noticeable. You will likely need to replace the piece as wear and tear add up.

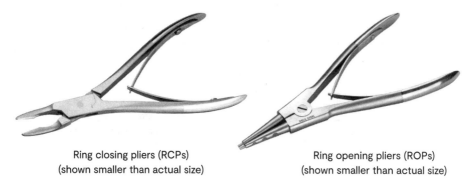

Ring closing pliers (RCPs)
(shown smaller than actual size)

Ring opening pliers (ROPs)
(shown smaller than actual size)

RING OPENING (OR EXPANDING) PLIERS (ROPs)

ROPs are reverse pliers, with tips that spread apart when you squeeze the handles. ROPs help widen the gap on a captive ring so you can insert or remove the bead. Make sure that there is no tissue between the tool and the jewelry, or you will suffer a mighty pinch. It is equally essential to be cautious when releasing the handles to avoid nipping your skin as the pliers close.

ROPs are generally needed only when the metal is too hard or thick to bend by hand or when you are inserting a bead that is delicate, or larger than usual. Squeeze the handles *slowly*, to engage the spring tension. Do not spread the gap any more than necessary to insert or remove the bead. If you do open the ring too wide, then you'll need the next jewelry tool, ring closing pliers.

Tip: When removing a bead, grasp it in your fingers to pull it from the ring as you use the tool to spread the hoop just enough. Don't enlarge the gap of the ring so far that the bead simply falls out. ROPs can also be used to widen a circular barbell to modify its shape and diameter.

RING CLOSING PLIERS (RCPs)

These pliers have a grooved rounded head that is used to close the gap on captive rings. If a hoop has been opened too far by ROPs or you are inserting a smaller bead than the one previously in the ring, this tool is indispensable. Some small RCPs also have a grooved end that can be used to unscrew barbell balls that are affixed too tightly to open by hand.

Tip: Whenever possible, use RCPs to make adjustments to your ring when it is not in your piercing. If you are wearing the hoop when you use the tool, exercise extreme caution to ensure that the pliers do not slip and pinch your skin.

HEMOSTATS (HEMOS)

This multipurpose tool can be used to bend small rings open and closed, adjust nostril screws, and hold jewelry or a bead during insertion and closure. Hemostats used on metal body jewelry must have smooth jaws, never serrations. Brass-jaw hemostats, ROPs, RCPs, and pliers diminish the risk of damaging jewelry because brass is softer than the metals that are worn in the body.

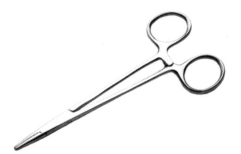

Only smooth-jaw hemostats should be used on body jewelry (shown smaller than actual size)

JEWELRY EMERGENCIES

Loss occurs on occasion, even with quality pieces. To minimize the likelihood of losing your jewelry (and avoid the mishaps described in the previous chapter), regularly check ends for tightness, and see to it that captive pieces are seated correctly. Purchase an extra bead, ball, or end so you will always have the parts needed to keep your ornament where it belongs. If you lose a ball or other closure and have no spare on hand, there are temporary measures to prevent your jewelry from falling out. Try one of the following until you can obtain a replacement:

- **Eraser:** Use a small, clean piece of a pencil eraser and cut it to the desired size and shape. Press it onto the end of a barbell post or between the tips of your empty captive ring to keep jewelry in place.

- **Band-Aid or medical tape:** Apply it to your jewelry and/or body to keep the piece from falling out.

Here are some tips:

- Never assume that a piece of jewelry will fit because it looks like what you have at home. Jewelry made by different manufacturers, especially threaded items, may not be interchangeable. Variables include the size and depth of the threads and thread counts per inch. Captive rings have different size gaps, and so on. Bring your jewelry with you when shopping for replacement parts, but do not handle it at a body art studio. Keep it in a baggie to maintain hygiene on the premises.

- Other than your take-along spare, don't carry jewelry around unless you are transporting it for assistance with an insertion or some other purpose. Keep any jewelry you're not wearing in a secure place at home.

- Don't underestimate the ability of a piercing to shrink quickly. Plenty of piercees have learned the hard way that it was a bad idea to leave even an old hole empty for "just one night."

NEW JEWELRY

To be assured of a good fit when you shop for new jewelry—especially for your first change—buy from a studio where a piercer can do the insertion for you. Jewelry for some piercings comes in increments as small as 1/32 inch or fractions of a millimeter. A piece that appears to be the right size might not fit.

It's helpful to keep accurate records. Write down the style, gauge, and length or diameter with other pertinent details. When you go to purchase new jewelry, you will know exactly what you're wearing. This is useful whether you would like to get a duplicate of a piece you already have, obtain a different style in your current size, or if you intend to stretch. Record all changes, and you will always have an up-to-date list.

POST-HEALING UPS AND DOWNS

After putting in new jewelry, you might experience some irritation. This can occur from swapping it out, even if your piercing is well healed, and the process handled smoothly. Or your body may be adjusting (or objecting) to the new ornament. If you do not improve within a week or so, you may need to return to your previous jewelry. Visit your piercer for advice if your condition worsens.

On occasion, tenderness, secretion, or other symptoms of a fresh piercing occur long after your healing period. These flare-ups can result from physical or emotional stress or hormonal changes, but sometimes no cause is apparent. Whenever a piercing acts up, it is always best to treat it like it is healing and resume aftercare. If you believe something is wrong beyond routine ups and downs, seek assistance from your piercer or doctor.

STRETCHING

If you've seen photographs of African women with enormous plates in their lips, you have witnessed the astounding elasticity of the human body. The practice of stretching piercings (sometimes referred to as *gauging up* or simply *gauging*) to wear larger jewelry has gained acceptability, much like piercing itself. Some modern stretching harkens back to the appearance of tribesmen and women with enlarged ear, septum, or lip piercings. There are people who expand their nipple or genital piercings for increased sensation. You may want to go up only one size from your initial jewelry, or you might yearn for a gigantic perforation in your body. Regardless of your motives or goals, the method is the same: stretch piercings slowly and gradually. The process requires patience and restraint; without it, tissue damage is likely.

Typically, even old piercings can't go up more than one size at a time, barring heavy play, wearing weights, or tearing from trauma. You must allow a sufficient interval of time between each enlargement for your tissue to fully regain its suppleness and integrity; only then is it safe to go further. Skin is remarkably resilient if not abused, but if you become impatient and try to force your piercing, the consequences can be severe. Overstretching tends to result in a buildup of scar tissue and reduction of flexibility, which can limit your capacity to stretch in the future—or shrink back to normal, if desired. Failure to adhere to appropriate procedures can cause the destruction and loss of your piercing from tissue *necrosis* (death).

Many factors affect whether the alterations are irreversible, including your age, piercing placement, sun exposure, and the speed and extent of your stretches. The slower you go, the better you will preserve your tissue elasticity, which increases the chances that the hole will shrink back down if the jewelry is removed. Quick, brutal expansion to a modest 8 gauge could result in a void that daylight can be seen through, and an unhurried stretch to a much larger size might contract to leave a mere dimple. There are no guarantees, so think before you stretch.

At the sight of a noticeably enlarged piercing, some people think, "Ouch! That had to hurt." But the process should be close to painless, if not entirely without some sensations. Safe stretching involves paying careful attention to the responses of your body and heeding warning signals.

ANCIENT PRACTICE
A 5,300-year-old naturally mummified body found in an Austrian glacier in 1991 had earlobe piercings that were enlarged to a hefty 7 to 11 millimeters in diameter.

WHEN TO STRETCH

Human tissue varies considerably, so there is no established timetable for stretching each type of piercing. In fact, it is possible to have a matched pair with one side that expands easily and the other that just won't give.

Before attempting any enlargement, it is safest to wait a minimum of two to three times the duration your piercing took to heal. For quick-mending areas, doubling the healing period is sometimes sufficient; but piercings that are slow to heal will require an extended delay before you should try to stretch.

After moving up to a thicker gauge, you generally need to let the tissue recuperate and stabilize for a minimum of several months before attempting to fit in the next size. The gauges become progressively larger. So, the stretch from 14 to 12 gauge is minor (.43 millimeters), but from 4 to 2 gauge is a significant jump (1.36 millimeters). The bigger you go, the longer you usually need to wait between stretches. The size differences escalate between gauges, and the tissue often becomes more difficult to expand as you strain its capacity.

The type of jewelry you wear is another factor to consider. A metal ring or any style with added weight helps you by passively enlarging the hole—though this can put extra stress on the bottom of your piercing. Plugs, eyelets, and other lightweight jewelry styles do not cause any stretching over time, so you may need to wait longer before you are ready to increase the gauge.

HOW TO STRETCH

Many people go to a piercer for help, which is advisable if you are not acquainted with the process. If you have the right equipment and can see and access the area, you should be able to stretch your own piercing at home. When your piercing is ready to go up, use the technique explained in "Jewelry Change Procedure," page 271, but with a taper of the next larger size (smaller gauge number).

When you change jewelry with a lubricated insertion taper, the tool glides right through because it is the same size as the channel. However, when stretching tissue with a larger taper, you will feel resistance, so you must push the tool through. You have to know how much pressure you can exert before causing damage to your tissue (not much!). If a taper the next size slides in without any force and results in only slight warmth or pressure, you may be able to safely stretch to the next gauge. Only Prince Albert, inner labia, fourchette, and ear lobe piercings routinely expand that quickly and easily. You are clearly not ready for the bigger size any time you push quite firmly but the tool won't progress further, or if only the tip of a taper fits in comfortably. Agony is *not* a part of safe stretching; if it hurts that much, you are applying excessive force and causing damage.

Enlarging a piercing should never cause visible tearing or bleeding, but it is routine for stretching to weaken the skin and cause micro-tears. This invisible damage makes you susceptible to infection, so always handle fresh stretches gently and hygienically.

GAUGING THEIR REACTION

To a piercer, the term "gauge" is a unit of measure for the thickness of body jewelry. Over time, the word morphed into a noun for stretched holes and the jewelry worn in such piercings. "Gauging" is also used as a verb for stretching a piercing. Piercers fought a valiant battle to keep this variant out of the vocabulary, but we seem to have lost the war. To impress and delight your piercer, reserve "gauge" to refer to the thickness of jewelry.

STRETCHING TIPS

o Do not attempt to stretch shallow piercings without consulting a piercer.

o Do not expand piercings that are irritated, inflamed, or infected.

o Take a shower or perform a warm compress to loosen the tissue first.

o Use plenty of lubricant, working some throughout the channel using the existing jewelry or tip of a taper before attempting to stretch.

o Keep lubricant off the surfaces you need to hold for the jewelry transfer.

o An oil-based product such as bacitracin ointment is acceptable for stretching, even though it is not suggested for use on fresh piercings. Some piercers use liquid soap as a lubricant, but this is not advisable.

o   Don't use cheap tapers that aren't smoothly graduated. Some are too bullet-shaped and can cause damage as they pass through the tissue, especially if your skin is tight. An evenly sloped taper is imperative for safety and comfort. Some plugs and eyelets that are popular for enlarged ear piercings require specific styles of tapers for smooth jewelry transfers.

o   Support the tissue at the exit (where the taper comes out) with a two- or three-finger grasp. This helps to increase the comfort and evenness of the stretch.

o   Don't rush! Stretching should be done in a slow, controlled manner. Never jam the taper through.

o   Don't screw the taper in, though a slight bit of rotation or twisting is sometimes helpful.

o   As the tissue expands, you may feel discomfort in the form of tightness, warmth or burning, or pinching. It should not be excruciating, nor should you experience sensations of tearing or splitting.

o   Don't force it! It should not require much muscle to work the tool through. If it does, stop pushing and go back to your previous size. See the next sections for ways to help you enlarge your piercing more gradually.

o   Insert jewelry of an appropriate material and style. Many large ornaments are not suited to a fresh stretch. It is best to choose one of the options approved for new piercings and to wear an alternative only after the area has settled.

WEIGHTS

Stretching with a taper is the traditional method, but there are other approaches. One is to add weights or wear hefty jewelry so that the piercing enlarges itself over time. Some people affix additional weight for a specified duration daily. Others attempt to wear something heavier full time. It is crucial to pay attention to your body's responses. Soreness, redness, or inflammation indicate a problem. Lighten the load for a while and try again later with less weight, wear it for shorter intervals, or wait longer between additions.

To supplement the weight, you can add multiple rings onto a hoop worn through a piercing (rather than adding them through your tissue). This affords control of the added load, is a creative way to use surplus jewelry, and looks attractive, too. Another method is to wear an eyelet through the hole (once it is large enough to accommodate one) and add weight through the aperture. Eyelets help to distribute the burden over a somewhat larger area.

Note that using weights or wearing heavy jewelry sometimes causes thinning or irritation of the tissue at the bottom of the hole due to excessive pressure. And, of course, wearing a weighty adornment may enlarge your piercing whether you want it to stretch or not.

IN-BETWEEN SIZES

It can be advantageous to wear jewelry in odd sizes as you stretch larger. The jump from one full gauge to the next may simply be too vast. Jewelry of intermediate dimensions is sometimes available in natural materials, such as wood and horn.

In the American Wire Gauge (AWG) standard used for metal jewelry, each gauge size is progressively larger. Single-flared glass plugs, however, are manufactured in both metric and AWG sizes. They are available in thicknesses that don't exist in the body jewelry metals to provide more smoothly graduated increments, which is considerably safer and more comfortable. Glass jewelry for stretching is limited primarily to earlobes, as the styles don't lend themselves well to other parts of the body.

A product called SnapPlugs works on the small-gradations principle and can be used for safely stretching earlobes at home—if you follow the instructions. It comes as a set of ten different graduated sizes of plugs made of an implant-grade polymer. The ends are slightly tapered, and they connect securely to move from one piece to the next.

DEAD STRETCHING

Dead stretching is the term used for simply pushing a larger object into a piercing. This is safe only when the tissue is ready, and what you're inserting is no bigger than your piercing can handle; otherwise, damage will occur. Adding multiple thin rings into a piercing over time is one relatively safe way to accomplish dead stretching, but this sometimes results in a piercing that isn't smooth and round.

PIERCE AND STRETCH

This technique is relatively common, but it is even less advisable than dead stretching. A piercing is made with a needle and then immediately expanded with a taper to a larger gauge. This takes a wound that was neatly formed by a sharp instrument and distorts it, which can make it more challenging for your body to form the base layer of cells, the literal basis of tissue healing. Doing immediate damage in this way can also predispose the piercing to trouble, including delayed healing or excess scar tissue formation.

TAPERED JEWELRY: CAUTION

Many graduated jewelry styles come in metal, glass, and an array of natural materials. One type is called a *stretching crescent* or stretching ring, and these are curved or circular insertion tapers. Variations include hooked talons, spirals, and straight pieces that look just like insertion tapers. These can be dangerous because wearers tend to cause tissue damage by stretching too quickly with them. Also, when tapered jewelry is used for enlarging, the O-rings required to keep the ornament in place can irritate due to excessive pressure against the skin. Wear tapered jewelry only in holes that have already been stretched.

MAINTENANCE OF STRETCHED PIERCINGS

Because a stretched piercing has an increased surface area, the amount of sebum may also be amplified. Be especially vigilant with your hygiene routine to get rid of these deposits. After your stretch has settled, if your jewelry is easy to remove, slip it out daily to wash it and the inside of the channel. Many piercees with enlarged holes find that wearing jewelry made of natural materials helps to diminish sebum formation. Some can easily swap back and forth between two jewelry gauges; others can fit only one size because their piercing shrinks too quickly.

RESTING

A technique called *resting* or *relaxing* is the practice of removing large-gauge jewelry (approximately 2 gauge and thicker) for a period of time each day or night. This is to relieve the tissue of the jewelry's weight and pressure. It may help to promote healthier skin by increasing circulation, especially at the bottom of the piercing, which supports most of the burden.

Experiment to determine the amount of time you can leave the hole empty without it shrinking too much. Generally, the longer you have worn a particular size, the easier this becomes. Some individuals take their jewelry out overnight and slide it right back in the next morning. Others can leave the channel empty for only an hour or so before the hole starts to feel uncomfortably tight during reinsertion. Try removing your jewelry for increasingly longer periods until you find a comfortable interval. Ideally, you want to leave it out for as long as possible but reinsert it before the hole shrinks enough to cause discomfort or irritation during reinsertion. If you run into trouble getting your jewelry back in, try a warm compress, some lubricant and possibly a taper. After reinsertion, wait until the tissue has fully recovered before attempting to rest your piercing again.

TISSUE MASSAGE

Daily massage of stretched piercings can be a tremendous help in maintaining elasticity and vascularity, keeping your tissue in top condition, and facilitating future stretching. Use a biocompatible emollient such as shea or cocoa butter or other skin lotion. Wash your hands, apply a small amount of emollient, and massage the tissue firmly for a few minutes during your rest period, especially on the bottom of the piercing. Roll and rub the skin between your fingers to work in the lotion. If the piercing is large enough to fit a cotton swab or fingertip inside, massage the interior of the hole particularly well. This treatment moisturizes the skin, which is essential; dryness can result in brittleness, weakness, and tears. The manipulation also helps to break down scar tissue, stimulate circulation, and promote healthy, vital skin.

TROUBLE AND TROUBLESHOOTING

Although *some* tenderness, secretion, or redness is not unusual for a few days after a stretch, if it is excessive, you have enlarged too fast. You will need to regress to your previous jewelry size, or possibly even smaller, depending on the extent of the damage. Do not wear heavy jewelry in an irritated stretch, and stick to the materials that are suited to new piercings.

If you end up with a painful weeping wound from overzealous expansion, you may decide to give up and abandon the piercing completely. Be aware that tissue inflamed by overstretching sometimes responds even more poorly to being left empty than it does to having smaller jewelry in place.

Treat an overstretched piercing like a brand-new one and follow appropriate care and cleaning. Failure to do so can result in severe consequences, including infection and tissue loss. If you make the mistake of stretching until your skin thins and splits in two, the piercing is lost; reconstructive surgery will be needed to repair the deformity to your bifurcated tissue.

Another nasty consequence of stretching too quickly is a *blowout*, in which some skin pushes out from the channel's interior. In essence, the piercing twists itself inside out due to excessive pressure. The most common location for a blowout is the back of the earlobe. It may not be as painful as it looks, but it clearly indicates a problem. You must immediately remove the offending ornament, try to realign the tissue, back down at least one gauge, and resume aftercare procedures. If the skin is allowed to remain distorted, it will generally stay that way. A blowout might be improved by doing your next stretch from the opposite direction to force the tissue back inside the channel. Another option is treatment with a compression technique. Wear tube- or plug-style jewelry with an inert silicone disc right up against the body on each side to compact the blowout back into place. Use O-rings to hold everything firmly together. Remove the jewelry to massage the tissue daily with lotion, and you can try resting the piercing at night.

If you overstretch, wait a few additional months before attempting further expansion. Slow down! Whatever method you choose, being patient and heeding the signals from your body are vital elements for success.

RETIRING A PIERCING

Retiring a piercing is permanently removing your jewelry and abandoning the hole. Though a piercing has the potential to be a lifelong adornment, there is no doubt that it is easier to be rid of than most body modifications, especially if you haven't stretched it too fast or made it too large.

It is best to retire your piercing when it is in good health. A notable exception is when a piercing is rejecting and has migrated too close to the surface. A potential risk of removing jewelry is whether this might trap matter inside. If there is any purulent drainage (pus), pain, inflammation, or suspected infection, discuss jewelry removal with your doctor. See "Leave Jewelry In!" page 248, and subsequent sections for more information.

If your piercing is healed and doing fine, but you have decided you no longer want it, wash your hands and the area, unclasp your jewelry, and remove it. A little bit of water-based lubricant such as K-Y Jelly can help make the transition smooth. Wash the area daily when you bathe. Abandoning a piercing is that simple.

WILL IT CLOSE?

Depending on the size, age, and location of a healed piercing, as well as the course of stretching, if any, it may not seal up completely. Most holes contract quite rapidly and can continue to shrink over time. During the ensuing weeks, the area will stabilize, and the channel is apt to remain in whatever state it has achieved within a month or two—smaller, or fully closed.

It is nearly impossible for a foreign object to accidentally enter a vacant piercing channel of average size after the jewelry is out and the tissue has shrunk. You will not have an open pathway into your body if the piercing is fully healed before removal. A piercing that has formed a healed tube (fistula) is sealed off and separate from the rest of you. If you retire a piercing before healing concludes, your cells will continue to grow together and seal the wound up completely. Neither is harmful or dangerous.

A fully healed piercing that is abandoned but does not seal up may excrete sebum. A simple test can be done to see if a channel might still be open: squeeze the tissue as if trying to push something out of it. If a thick white secretion of sebum comes from the hole(s), there is a strong possibility the channel is intact. This is not harmful and does not indicate a problem. The area will stabilize, and you can ignore it if you have no itching, swelling, or inflammation. Should your empty piercing discharge sebum spontaneously, you may wish to assist with expressing it periodically. One method is to squeeze the tissue in an attempt to release the matter from each side. Another is to use a small, clean insertion taper (usually 18 or 16 gauge, depending on how tight the channel shrinks) and run it through periodically to clear out the hole's interior. The taper should fit snugly but pass through without irritating the tissue. Beyond this annoyance, there is seldom any problem from retired piercings.

The only way to be entirely rid of all traces of a previous piercing is by having the residual fistula removed by surgical excision. There is seldom a need to go to that extreme, and, of course, such surgery will leave some scarring of its own.

Many regretful piercees who have abandoned their piercings return to have their jewelry reinserted or to be repierced. Carefully consider whether you are genuinely done with a piercing before removing your jewelry. Reinserting it in a channel that has shrunk can be much more painful than the original procedure—but if a hole is still present and can be stretched, then repiercing is not usually appropriate. If the initial placement was correct, relocating the piercing is undesirable. However, if your piercing closes and leaves you with diminished tissue pliability or excess scar tissue, repiercing the original location might not be possible. Additionally, there is potential for complications when piercing near an open channel. See "Repiercing after Loss," page 263, for details. If you think there is any chance you might want to put your jewelry back in later, don't take it out in the first place.

THE POINT

For many body art enthusiasts, part of the attraction to piercings is their versatility. Not only does a piercing change your body, but you can also change your piercing. You have the option of swapping out the jewelry, and also the possibility of stretching. Whether you own a collection of ornaments that you change daily with your mood, or you replace your jewelry infrequently, the choice is yours.

18

ADVANCED JEWELRY
AND PRACTICES

This chapter delves into advanced jewelry, including natural and human-made materials, for healed and stretched piercings. It also describes certain advanced piercings, more extreme modifications, and alternative practices.

JEWELRY FOR HEALED AND STRETCHED PIERCINGS

The form and function of initial body jewelry is primarily about safety, so relatively few materials and styles are suitable; however, after your piercing has healed, a bounty of beautiful ornaments can be yours for a price. They come in myriad materials, sizes, and styles. These factors, along with the weight and finish, determine whether jewelry is suited for daily wear.

Many pieces are safe and comfortable for continuous wear, but others are tolerable for just a few hours of dress-up fun. And, unfortunately, some designs are best left in a display case, solely for viewing enjoyment. Extremely heavy adornments will seldom be appropriate for everyday use. Anything with an uneven, etched, twisted, or matte finish could irritate your tissue. Quickly replace jewelry that does not agree with your piercing, no matter how much you like the way it looks.

NATURAL MATERIALS

After your piercing has healed, it may tolerate (or even thrive with) jewelry crafted of alternative—though traditional—materials, including horn, bone, wood, bamboo, amber, stone, and other substances created by Mother Nature.[1] Often referred to as *organics*, people have worn these materials in piercings throughout the ages and around the globe. Some modern piercees favor natural jewelry options, especially for enlarged piercings in the ear, septum, or lip, though you should not wear them in recent stretches—or new holes.

Some body jewelry is produced with consideration to avoid harming the earth and its creatures. Socially and environmentally conscious piercees can obtain natural ornaments made from ecological or renewable resources, including sustainably harvested or scrap woods, and seasonally shed antler.

Like all body jewelry, these products vary in quality and wearability. Natural materials are very fragile compared to metal. In thin gauges, jewelry with pointy or narrow areas can easily be broken. Many alternative materials and styles are not safe to wear during sports or sleep, and some organic pieces should be removed for bathing and swimming. Choose your jewelry to suit your lifestyle as well as your budget and aesthetic preferences.

These natural materials are too delicate to be autoclaved, so you must disinfect (rather than sterilize) them before insertion. Wash new items with soap, then rinse and dry thoroughly. A gentle product such as Dr. Bronner's liquid soap is recommended. If you prefer a more potent cleaner, use tea tree oil, though this can sometimes cause drying or cracking. Be vigilant to avoid exposing your jewelry to chemicals such as bleach, chlorinated swimming pools, strong soaps or cleansers, and harsh personal care products, including hair dye and straightener. These chemicals can be harmful to the jewelry and to you; in some cases, they may be absorbed and deposited into your body. Temperature extremes and overexposure to light and humidity can negatively affect natural materials; drying, splitting, or warping may result.

Naturally occurring cracks, pits, and uneven surfaces are common even in finely crafted organic pieces, though that shouldn't be an excuse for shoddy manufacturing or improperly selected and finished materials. Crevices and flaws may encourage the growth of microbes, so you must monitor the condition of both your jewelry and your piercing. Depending on the material, you will need to rub natural jewelry with oil or wax to preserve and maintain it properly. Some people use jojoba, vitamin E, or mineral oil, and others favor food-grade oils such as olive, coconut, or peanut oil, though these can become rancid over time.

Handle natural body jewelry only with washed or gloved hands, and clean and oil it before wear, as well as periodically, even if it is not being worn—including the pieces in a display case at a studio. Safeguard extras in a sealed baggie or airtight container to minimize changes in humidity. If your jewelry appears to be dry, oil it more frequently. Body jewelry made of natural materials needs to be removed and washed regularly with mild soap and water. It is standard for these substances to absorb moisture and skin oils.

Countless styles and variations of spirals, claws, tusks, crescents, and elaborately carved ornaments are fashioned of natural materials, though plugs and eyelets are among the more popular designs. Ears are unquestionably the most prevalent location for this type of jewelry.

A SAMPLING OF NATURAL MATERIALS

o **Wood:** This material's relative lightness (compared to metal) makes it functional for large jewelry. There are numerous varieties of wood, and some are suitable for body jewelry styles. Different species vary significantly in their biocompatibility. Many are tolerated by the body, but some can cause irritation, allergic reactions, or even *anaphylaxis* (life-threatening immune response). Others are toxic, so patronize a knowledgeable distributor. Particularly porous species can more readily harbor bacteria and other germs. Do not expose wood jewelry to excessive heat or humidity. Wood may not do well in damp areas of the body. Jewelry will need to be sanded periodically if the grain expands in response to dampness. High-quality pieces with a proper finish and smooth texture are less reactive to contact with moisture. Do not wear wood if you have irritated or sensitive skin.

o **Bamboo:** Unlike wood, bamboo is a species within the grass family. There are many different varieties of this lightweight material, and it comes in colors ranging from yellow to green and even close to black. It may be mottled or even in coloration. Because the bulk of it is hollow, bamboo is an ideal material for a natural eyelet design. Nonstandard sizes are common because the natural plant dimensions form the jewelry diameters. When the *cuticle* (smooth protective coating) is left on the surface, only the ends of the jewelry need finishing.

o **Bone and horn:** Even though these are different materials, they share many of the same properties: both are porous, semi-hard, and lightweight. Bone is white, while horn ranges from tan to black. Horn is *thermoplastic* (it can be heated and then shaped to some extent, and will retain its new form once cooled). Avoid exposing horn jewelry to very hot water, as it can cause the material to revert to its original shape.[2] Water buffalo horn is the type most often used for body jewelry.

o **Porcupine quills:** These are sometimes worn in septum piercings without alteration save for cleaning, and possibly waxing or oiling the surface.

o **Fresh ivory:** *Ivory* can be defined as the dentine portion of a mammal's tooth,[3] though a purist may say that it comes only from elephants. Unfortunately, these animals have become endangered due to the demand for their tusks. Worldwide restrictions are in place to protect their dwindling population, so you should avoid elephant ivory. Body jewelry can be crafted from the canines or incisors of boars and warthogs, which have been considered more acceptable sources of fresh (not fossilized) ivory;

purchase from a reputable distributor and make sure you know the source of any jewelry made from fresh ivory. Sunlight can bleach it or cause yellowing or brittleness, and ivory is also susceptible to damage from sudden changes in temperature and humidity.

o   **Fossilized ivory:** This ancient material comes from animals that lived during the Ice Age—walrus, mastodon, and mammoth. It is found in the tundra or permafrost of Alaska, Russia, and other frigid places, and colors vary from creamy-white to brown. This particularly sensitive material can also crack from rapid changes in temperature or humidity. A number of local and international governing bodies have banned the sale of both fossilized and fresh ivory, so laws should be heeded, and sources scrutinized carefully.[4]

o   **Antler:** More affordable and readily available, antler is composed of annually shed bone from a moose, deer, or elk. It comes in brown and gray, as well as lighter shades that can be an excellent substitute for ivory.

o   **Amber:** Amber is a lightweight fossilized tree resin. Although best known for its yellow and orange shades, it can range from nearly colorless to red, blue, brown, or black. It can be transparent or cloudy, and may contain visible inclusions of preserved insect or plant life. Amber is among the most delicate of natural body jewelry materials. Heat and chemicals can cause damage, including softening, chipping, and breaking. Make sure the amber is genuine, as faux products may not be sufficiently inert to wear safely in your body. Real amber is buoyant in saltwater, feels warm to the touch (compared to glass and gemstones), and when rubbed briskly with a cloth, emits a piney odor and creates static electricity. Low-priced pieces containing whole, clearly visible insects are imitations.

o   **Gemstone, semiprecious stone, and rock:** These materials are dense, so big pieces can be quite weighty. This category includes jade, obsidian, quartz, hematite, fluorite, agate, onyx, jasper, lapis lazuli, tiger eye, amethyst, turquoise, and many others in a full spectrum of colors. Some stones are more durable due to their structure, such as jade; others are more fragile and apt to crack. Expect any piece that you drop on a hard surface to chip or break. Some stones may fade from exposure to sunlight.

HUMAN-MADE MATERIALS

Body jewelry is fashioned from a variety of nonmetal materials, including plastic and glass. Some piercers use PTFE (Teflon) and other autoclavable, biocompatible polymers in new piercings, so they are discussed with the other jewelry materials in "Nontoxic Plastics," page 95.

o **Acrylic/plastic:** *Acrylic* is a general term for many varieties of plastic. Unfortunately, despite their prevalence, not all of these materials are safe to wear in the body. Acrylic's safety is a subject of fierce debate in the piercing industry. Though some are described as "FDA approved," none should be worn in healing piercings or fresh stretches. Unless the material is certified by the ASTM or ISO for implant use in the body, safety is uncertain. Chemical substances can leach out of plastic and cause allergic and cytotoxic reactions with local and systemic side effects, and this is the primary safety concern.

o Change your jewelry right away if your piercing becomes distressed or you experience localized irritation! Acrylic threaded ends and ornaments in which the material does not pass through the tissue *might* be safer to wear. Most plastics cannot withstand the pressure and high temperatures of an autoclave, so these items must be disinfected rather than sterilized.

- PMMA (polymethylmethacrylate) is a type of plastic used for many medical and dental applications, including bone cement, wrinkle fillers, and dentures. Some body jewelry of this material is referred to as dental acrylic. I've seen some of these products melt or warp at high temperatures even though they are marketed as capable of withstanding autoclave sterilization. Despite their pervasive use in the health care industry, some people are sensitive to this type of acrylic.

- Silicone is another type of polymer used in medical applications, including scar reduction, as discussed in chapter 16. It appears to be safer and more biocompatible than many others.[5] Silicone is a soft flexible material usually worn in piercings as eyelets, plugs, and retainers. It has also been used for ornaments like balls or beads. The softer the silicone, the stickier it will be, and this can be a source of irritation if it adheres to your tissue. Not everyone can tolerate it in piercings. Clean silicone jewelry regularly and carefully and keep it as dry as possible. A tight fit can trap secretions and cause irritation and infection. Your skin cannot breathe well with snug-fitting silicone occluding the tissue.

o **Glass:** Though there are many varieties, the two most popular types for wear in piercings are *borosilicate* and *soda-lime.* Borosilicate is a specialty glass used in laboratory beakers, and soda-lime is the more common type, used in art glass, most windows, and kitchen glassware. These types of glass are safe, inert, and biocompatible when they are lead-free. They are nonporous, stable, resistant to chemicals, and durable—but still potentially breakable, especially in small sizes. Glass doesn't get as cold as metal jewelry, and, unlike most of the alternative materials, it isn't harmed by the high heat of autoclaving. It has a very smooth surface, so insertion and removal are comfortable, and its nonporous nature makes it easy to clean. Glass is lighter than metal, transparent, and colorful. Countless color and design variations are possible.

- Store glass separately because steel and other metals and materials can scratch it. Ear and septum piercings are suitable sites to wear glass jewelry, but the risk of breakage is generally higher in nipple or genital piercings. Except for plug or eyelet styles, it is safest to avoid glass jewelry in 8 gauge or smaller. Removing glass jewelry is advisable when playing sports, sleeping, swimming, or showering. Because glass nostril screws cannot be custom fit like metal jewelry, it might be challenging to find a comfortable piece in this material.

- Obsidian is a naturally occurring volcanic substance, which is similar in composition to soda-lime glass. The majority is black, but it comes in a range of colors, including gray, green, golden, silversheen, snowflake, and rainbow. Obsidian is the glass with the longest history in body modification. It is still being carved into beautiful septum pieces and plug designs for ears and lips—like the Aztecs, and my neighbors the Maya, did for millennia.

o **PVD (physical vapor deposition):** These high-tech films represent a superior modern version of electroplating. In a sealed vacuum system, a machine applies layers of vaporized metal condensation on the surface of other materials, including metals. PVD coatings are used in everything from firearms to medical and dental appliances. Jewelry with a PVD coating has a shiny, metallic-looking surface. It comes in colors that are otherwise unavailable for body jewelry, such as deep black and shades corresponding to materials that are potentially harmful to wear in the body, like brass and copper. Gold-colored PVD jewelry can serve as an alternative to unsafe colored gold, potentially dangerous gold-plated pieces, or pricey high-quality 14- or 18-karat adornments. Some PVD coatings are certified biocompatible by a lab that tests medical devices that contact bone, skin tissue, or blood.[6] Not all piercings respond equally well to these finishes, and product quality varies. If PVD jewelry is bent, the coating could crack and flake off, causing damage and complications to your piercing.

ADVANCED PIERCINGS

To the uninitiated, all piercings may seem alike. However, certain placements, including surface piercings, industrial projects, and orbitals, call for a professional with a higher level of skill.

SURFACE PIERCINGS

As the name implies, *surface piercings* are situated on areas of the body where there is no fold or protrusion of tissue in which to place them. People wear jewelry in many nontraditional locations throughout the body. For a time, wrist and hip surface piercings were trendy, though neither turned out to be very practical. More recently, sideburn piercings have gained popularity. These are positioned vertically on the facial surface, in front of the tragus. (A vertical tragus piercing, however, goes through the nub of cartilage itself.) The nape of the neck is one of the spots most likely to heal well and remain indefinitely. The chest surface over the sternum is a fashionable site for ornamentation, though it is generally more subject to complications. The surface piercings in current vogue come and go, but most are apt to require some patience and dedication.

A specialized jewelry style called a *surface bar* (see "Surface Bars," page 90) is typically used, minimizing trauma and conforming well to the area when properly fitted. Flat discs or low-profile gems are the preferred ornaments, since they rest closer to the skin and help to diffuse pressure from swelling. Some piercers use a technique called *wound shaping*, which appears to be helpful and may improve the success rate of surface piercings. In this freehand procedure, the piercer shapes the channel like the jewelry, or as close to it as possible.

Surface piercings are often more challenging to heal and subject to more problems than traditional placements. Some last for weeks or months before they migrate and reject. Others do just fine, especially in stable areas that are subject to minimal movement, friction, or other trauma.

Seek a piercer who is skilled in surface piercings and check their qualifications carefully. If they can't show you photos of older, established surface piercings they have done, don't stay. There is a vast difference between just performing these piercings and placing them so that they heal well and remain in the body long term. A piercer who will puncture any area of the body without thoroughly examining it and giving due consideration to your anatomy and situation doesn't care whether your piercing will endure.

Some people are predisposed to healing surface piercings. If you are not among the lucky ones, then migration, rejection, and scarring are all probable consequences. If you can't live without attempting a surface piercing, be prepared for a lengthy healing period (usually six to nine months or longer) and the prospect that you will be wearing a scar instead of jewelry by the end of it all.

You may have an ambitious vision of being covered in rows of multiple surface piercings. Still, it is wise to try just one first to determine your body's willingness to accept foreign objects in unorthodox locations. Also, if you get overloaded with too many piercings at once, it is probable that none of them will heal well. If a qualified piercer counsels you against a piercing because they believe it would not be successful, heed their advice. Most of the piercers surveyed (68 percent) perform surface piercings.

O-NEEDLE SURFACE PIERCING

An O-needle (or a small *dermal punch*, described below) is sometimes used in an alternative technique to perform surface piercings. Each hole for the legs of the bar is created using a circular tool. The tissue in between is pierced with a regular needle at the correct depth for the jewelry post. A surface bar is inserted into this prepared channel. The concept is that there will be less pressure against the tissue because the piercing is made with angles that match the shape of the jewelry. This is another form of wound shaping. A small gauge is used, so this technique is not an extreme modification.

INDUSTRIAL PIERCINGS

The *industrial* or *scaffold piercing* is a single barbell that connects two or more piercings in the ear. The traditional configuration threads a long barbell through two holes in the upper cartilage from close to the head to the outer edge of the ear. A variation passes from the tragus through the conch. Another style pierces vertically behind the ear through the upper and lower edges of the conch so that a long span of barbell post is visible from the front. Possibilities are limited by your imagination, and more importantly, your anatomy—and the skills of your piercer. *Industrial projects* involve more than two piercings joined by specialized jewelry.

Many people are not good candidates; they simply lack sufficient supporting structures where the

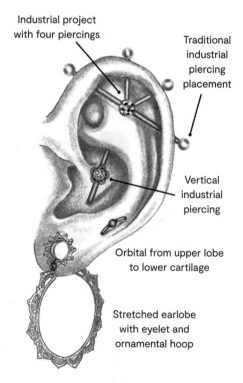

Industrial project with four piercings

Traditional industrial piercing placement

Vertical industrial piercing

Orbital from upper lobe to lower cartilage

Stretched earlobe with eyelet and ornamental hoop

piercings should be situated. Your configuration must be ideal so the piercings can be angled without distorting or causing stress on the tissue. Alternatively, your piercer must have the proper equipment and know-how to customize a barbell without damaging the metal. Attempting to cheat tissue into the piercing is common but injurious. Along with the grief of troubled healing, an ear cartilage piercing that is under constant pressure will feel downright agonizing.

Any piercing can swell during initial healing. Even minor inflammation in one or both wounds can be disastrous for an industrial because the piercings are connected. Excess scar tissue formation, migration, and rejection are typical in poorly placed industrials.

One technique is to determine the optimal position of the second hole while the back end of the needle is still in the initial piercing, directing the way to the perfect, natural angle.

In the event you experience swelling or scarring during healing, you can attempt to preserve your piercings by replacing a single long bar with two individual pieces of jewelry, such as short barbells. But, once released from their conjoined status, the piercings may heal at slightly different angles. Similarly, making two new cartilage piercings with separate jewelry and a plan to unite them later won't always work.

The subtle jewelry curves usually suited to industrial piercings are easier to create than the sharper bends of a surface bar. Some piercers are capable of safely modifying barbells in the studio, but they must use appropriate equipment. Bending jewelry, even a little bit, must not produce any burrs or scratches in the metal. It is highly advisable to repolish the piece after altering it, as the damaged surface finish should be restored to facilitate your healing process. If a piercer uses nonsterile tools to customize a bar post, they must autoclave the jewelry before inserting it into your new piercings.

A *nasallang* is the only industrial piercing that is ordinarily performed on an area other than the ear. It is discussed in "Alternative Nose Piercing Placements," page 127.

ORBITALS

Like the industrial, an *orbital* joins two piercings together, but with a ring instead of a barbell (see illustration, page 292). This style can connect two holes in the lobe, upper cartilage, or other regions such as the cartilage of the tragus and anti-tragus, or forward helix and rook. It is rarely used in other areas of the body. Unlike the industrial, it may be best to start the piercings with separate pieces of jewelry and insert one ring through them after healing, or to connect one piercing that is healed with one that is new. Depending on placement and ring diameter, it is sometimes possible to link two healed piercings.

One problem is the tendency for a hoop to rest unevenly between the holes and constrict one or both piercings. This causes the same issues as any ill-fitting jewelry. The piercings must be situated the correct distance apart to fit one of the standard ring sizes safely. Changing to a smaller or larger bead can adjust a captive ring's diameter to a limited extent. Otherwise, a widened circular barbell or custom jewelry is needed. Earlobe tissue is forgiving, and an imperfect fit may be tolerated, but the same is not true for cartilage piercings. Conch piercings with hoops have been dubbed "orbitals" on social media, but that is a misnomer.

SURFACE ANCHOR/DERMAL ANCHOR/MICRODERMAL

This technique with multiple names became explosively popular when it initially emerged. Their prevalence diminished over time as their generally temporary nature became evident. Still, about three-quarters of the piercers surveyed do perform them. During the procedure, a tiny ornament is inserted into an L-shaped opening formed in the tissue. Anchors are similar to surface piercings because they are done on flat areas. Placement options are greatly expanded all over the face, torso, and other locations of the body. Unlike the pairs always present in piercings, these have a single adornment per perforation. The embedded jewelry remains under the skin, while the visible threaded end can theoretically be changed. Multiple surface anchors are sometimes arranged in patterns.

The procedure is performed with a piercing needle, O-needle, or small dermal punch (see page 295) to make the opening. The jewelry is placed into a small pocket that is formed with a needle, taper or similar tool, or the jewelry itself. Surface anchors may bleed more than the average surface piercing, and they tend to heal more quickly. The average healing time is approximately three months.

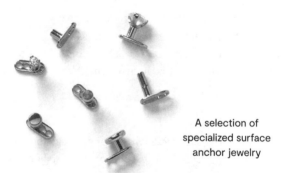

A selection of
specialized surface
anchor jewelry

The mini jewelry used in this procedure has a small, flat plate (only about ¼ inch long) that is inserted under the skin to affix it. The longer toe is placed in first, followed by the nub-like heel that helps to hold the piece in the tissue. A short upright threaded post passes through the skin and extends to the surface where a gem, disc, or other threaded ornament screws onto it. Changing the end can be very difficult and problematic, even after successful healing. When inserted correctly, the jewelry appears glued onto the skin. Some of the plates are drilled with holes, so tissue grows into the base. The intention is that this helps to secure the piece in place. Any benefit is debatable, but there is no doubt that it complicates removal. Ultimately, migration and rejection are the most frequent result. However, due to the diminutive size of the wound, scars are apt to be fairly minimal—especially when compared to failed surface piercings.

For removal, the surrounding area is held steady, the jewelry is grasped firmly, and the ornament is taken from its pocket. Massage is often helpful, though brute force is sometimes necessary. If scar tissue has grown to the plate, a needle may be needed to free the piece. *Single-point piercing* (yet another name for this piercing) is often short-lived compared to the traditional variety. Unfortunately, it is not the miracle we hoped to find for potentially permanent ornamentation all over the body.

EXTREME MODIFICATIONS

You would expect to find piercing or tattooing within a body art studio, but some techniques take altering the human form significantly further. Several of these processes are much more intense than traditional piercings. Body modifications such as branding, cutting, tongue splitting, and ear pointing are not covered here; only those involving an ornament (or implant) are discussed below.

THE DERMAL PUNCH

A *dermal punch* or *biopsy punch* (medical tool designed for use in tissue biopsies) is sometimes used to create a piercing. The device has a razor-sharp circular blade on a handle. Unlike a piercing needle, these do remove tissue during a procedure. The risks of small punches (1.5 millimeter and 2 millimeter) are similar to those of an ordinary piercing. Larger holes are commonly created with them, however, and with increased sizes come elevated risks.

Before you decide to have a piercer/puncher remove a substantial chunk of your tissue, you must feel confident that they are proficient. If they make a mistake with the angle of a big punch, or you abandon one (over 6 or 4 gauge, or 4 or 5 millimeters), you may be stuck with a void people can see through, unless you get reconstructive surgery.

If you remove the jewelry during healing, there is a chance that your skin could grow over and seal the hole, depending on size. Any cartilage that has been removed, however, is gone forever.

The process and the equipment may seem frightening, but most "punchees" report that a skillful procedure causes only a brief, intense sensation of pressure. Some describe it as similar to a regular cartilage piercing. Perhaps the most disturbing element of being dermal punched is the sound. Since the action often takes place on your ear, the *c-r-r-runch* of cartilage can be quite loud. The nostril and nasal septum are also sometimes punched with this tool.

The punch is usually performed with a sterile backing on the exit side to support the tissue. Some piercers use a thick stack of gauze. Even though the tool is razor sharp, it can take a fair amount of force to get through. Unlike a piercing needle, this instrument might be rotated as well as pushed to make the perforation. Even when your piercer uses illumination to map and avoid visible vessels, heavy bleeding is expected from a large punch. It could last for several days, so prepare by purchasing sterile gauze in advance.

If you are a dedicated body art enthusiast and you desire a cartilage piercing that is bigger than usual, you may find the dermal punch is a viable option. This tool is not commonly used for ear lobe piercings or other soft areas that are amenable to stretching. Cartilage piercings are notoriously challenging to enlarge, but making a hole with a needle 10 gauge or larger can result in excessive damage to the dense tissue. After stretching my conch from 10 gauge—the size it was pierced—to 2 gauge, I have painful personal knowledge (and professional experience) to support those assertions.

Some piercers feel that dermal punches are superior to needles for all ear cartilage piercings, and use them routinely instead of a traditional needle. In certain regions of the United States, nonmedical personnel are forbidden to use dermal punches. However, O-needles or *chamfer needles* are similar options, being circular at the tip rather than pointed, but lacking a handle. They are available only in the usual initial piercing sizes.

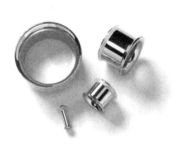

A selection of single-flare eyelets with clear silicone O-rings

For comfort and safety, the jewelry placed in a punched hole must be lightweight and minimal (no large rings). A single-flare plug or eyelet that secures with one O-ring, or a tube that uses two O-rings, are suitable styles. Dermal punches are sized by millimeter, but American body jewelry is generally measured by gauge or fractions of an inch, so an exact size match might not be available. The glass plugs made in metric sizes are commonly used as initial jewelry in dermal-punched holes for this reason. If the jewelry is even slightly smaller than the punch, the void will be inadequately plugged, so extra bleeding is likely. There is also a higher risk of jewelry falling out if the flares or O-rings, which normally keep the piece in place, aren't large enough. But unlike a piercing made with a needle, the dermal punch removes the hard cartilage, so the opening is looser. This makes it easy to slide in jewelry that is marginally larger than the punch without damaging the wound.

Before leaving the studio, your piercer should give you sufficient time to recover and be sure that bleeding is under control. Both can take a little longer, especially when you get a sizable dermal punch rather than a regular piercing with a traditional needle.

SCALPELLING

Scalpelling is the technique of using the familiar razor-sharp instrument for creating or enlarging a piercing. Nonmedical personnel are prohibited from using this tool in some parts of the United States and abroad. Once the incision is made, the opening is generally stretched (or at least shaped) with a taper to make it round and facilitate jewelry insertion. This procedure can be more extreme and create larger openings than dermal punching. The relative safety of this method is undocumented, but excessive bleeding is an obvious risk, even in the hands of an expert. **This act should not be undertaken lightly; mishaps may require medical attention and could conceivably result in the loss of a body part such as a nipple or earlobe.**

When a needle or dermal punch is used, the instrument's size automatically limits the dimensions of the aperture. However, during a scalpel procedure, your cutter/piercer must have the skill to use the blade to create an opening of the desired size in the correct spot. Enclosing the area in unslotted forceps provides a solid perimeter to limit the extent of a cut.

Proponents explain that the scalpel method for enlarging existing piercings offers greater control than traditional stretching. For example, a low placement or thinning spot at the bottom of an earlobe can be "fixed" by cutting upward, effecting a minor repositioning of the piercing. Another possibility includes merging adjacent ear piercings into a single expanded hole by cutting the tissue that divides them.

IMPLANTS

Implants are similar to piercings because foreign objects are placed within the body, and because piercers and body modification artists perform them. There are, however, notable differences. In *subdermal implants* (as opposed to *transdermal implants*, described next), no portion of the object remains outside the body, as jewelry does in a piercing. The procedure is also different from piercing. A scalpel cuts to the subcutaneous layer, and the tissue is lifted to form a pocket. An object is placed in this cavity, and the skin is closed with sutures or medical tape. Sometimes several implants are inserted through a single incision. Generally, they are made of silicone or Teflon, though metal is sometimes used. Hearts, stars, and other shapes are implanted to create a textured, 3-D effect of the object(s) under the skin.

This procedure is surprisingly widespread, given the risks involved. After insertion, the implant is often taped or bandaged to encourage it to heal in the desired position. The object may shift under the skin and remain crooked, after which it cannot be adjusted. To fix it, the implant must be removed and then, if desired, reinserted in another location or at another time. Rejection and loss sometimes occur with implants, as with piercings. These complications are minor when compared to some of the other dangers.

One critical hazard is the potential for tissue damage in the area beneath the implant due to stress, friction, and diminished blood supply. Over time, the continuous pressure of an implant rubbing on bone or cartilage can cause *resorption* (erosion). This can ultimately result in bone loss beneath an implant. Soft tissues may also be affected, as an implant can press into muscles, tendons, or nerves, resulting in pain and impairment of the affected structures. Implants made of softer materials such as silicone may help to slow this process, but some damage is likely, and perhaps inevitable, over an extended period.[7] **In an area such as the skull, where horn implants are sometimes embedded, bone resorption can result in an implant wearing through the cranium.**

Infection is a severe risk because the wound is closed following the implantation. Drainage cannot readily exit to the surface as it does with a piercing, so an infection could spread to deeper tissues more quickly. This has the potential to be quite grave. Regrettably, at least one life has been lost due to sepsis from an implant gone wrong. **If an infection is suspected, immediate medical attention is required.**

Reversing an implant is also much more challenging than removing a piercing because it requires another incision. This is often done at the site of the original cut, or a new opening will be made. If tissues encapsulate or adhere to the implant during healing, removing it can be considerably more challenging than inserting it. Even if a body artist puts in an implant, you may need a doctor or surgeon to remove it.

Insertion of small magnets into the fingers is not quite as risky. These allow wearers to sense magnetic fields, pick up diminutive metal objects, and determine whether metals are ferrous. Magnetic implants are generally quite tiny (just a few millimeters) and are placed a bit to the side of the fingertip's padding. For safety, the magnet is encased in silicone or another biocompatible material. The incision is so small that a single stitch can close it. Implanted magnets will need to be removed if you require an MRI; therefore, they could be problematic in an emergency. Fortunately, this doesn't seem to be an issue with the tiny radio-frequency identification (RFID) chips that are sometimes inserted in the body, usually in the fleshy part of the palm, near the thumb.[8] Though these are not nearly as invasive, infection and rejection remain risks.

GENITAL BEADING AND GENITAL RIBS

Genital beading is a modification in which beads are implanted within the genital tissue, generally to add sensation. It is more popular to place them in a penis, but these can be performed on vulvas as well. The procedure is the same as for a regular implant, or it may be done with a pierce-and-taper method. A large piercing is made with a needle, and then a taper is used to expand the hole. A bead is left in the channel, and sutures or surgical tape close the wound. *Genital ribs* are a variation in which rod-shaped pieces are inserted for a different sensation and appearance. Beads and rods may be used in combination as preferred by the wearer.

TRANSDERMAL IMPLANTS

Transdermal implants use a procedure similar to the one described for subdermal implants. However, an opening is made apart from the incision, which is closed after insertion. This allows an ornament above the surface to attach to the implant via screw threads or a magnetic connection. Larger pieces are sometimes implanted, and multiple holes made for rows of spikes or other adornments. These are subject to the dangers of resorption, like the subdermal implants, and are reported to have a long-term success rate as low as 20 percent.[9] Rejection is a possible complication; alternatively, the whole implant can become unintentionally embedded.

UNPROVEN TERRITORY

Some experimental practitioners test the limits of the human body in an active effort to invent new techniques and modifications. Risks and failures are common consequences when you enter unproven territory or when anyone other than a licensed medical professional performs invasive procedures. If you are considering a modification beyond the scope of traditional body piercing, exercise extreme caution and use common sense. If the technician does not astonish you with their skill and experience and cannot demonstrate successful, fully healed examples of radical body modifications, it is safest to walk away.

ALTERNATIVE PRACTICES

Some practices are related to piercing but are not traditionally performed within a piercing studio. They include play piercing, which is frequently done by laypersons rather than professional piercers, and different types of pulls and suspensions, for which a piercer with more knowledge is required.

PLAY PIERCING

Play piercing is the temporary insertion of a needle or needles for a ritual, performance, or BDSM or erotic scene; it frequently takes place between intimate partners. The piercing or piercings are made in the skin (usually surface-to-surface), but jewelry may not be inserted. When the session or event is over, nothing will remain in the body, as it does in permanent piercings. Play piercing routinely involves multiple punctures (sometimes many of them), which may be as thin as acupuncture needles or as thick as those used in body piercing. The needles can be placed nearly anywhere, including the face, arms, legs, torso, and genitals. Sterility and hygiene are imperative, as always, because the skin is broken. All types of people engage in play piercing, and they may not have access to the sterilization equipment required in piercing studios. Therefore, disposable packaged products such as sterile hypodermic tips should be used and then discarded carefully. Of course, needles must *never* be reused or shared.

If you find yourself getting pierced because you enjoy the experience but don't desire to heal piercings and wear jewelry in them, then play piercing may be a good alternative for you. It is possible to do this safely in the privacy of your home, but you must seek input and guidance from an experienced mentor before attempting it. A book on the subject by Deborah Addington, simply titled *Play Piercing*, can provide you with additional information.[10]

THE PULL

Other types of impermanent piercings require more knowledge and expertise. The *pull* (or *energy pull*) involves temporary piercings in which needles or hooks are inserted, usually in the chest or back, and two or more people tethered together by these piercings pull in opposite directions. This is not an all-out tug-of-war, but a cooperative shared experience. A solo pull is possible if the rope or cord is attached to an immovable object. Multiple people can engage in a pull when joined to a central point. Pulls are enacted using a wide variety of materials, from thin 18-gauge hypodermic needles lassoed with dental floss or suture material to large hooks. The individual(s) involved control the intensity and extent of the pull, and motivations can include seeking a physical rush or trance state, facing fears, or connecting people in body and spirit.

SUSPENSION

Suspension is another form of temporary piercing that is practiced privately for a variety of reasons, such as personal exploration and transformation, or ritual purposes. They are also performed publicly for entertainment. During a suspension, large, sterile hooks are temporarily inserted through the flesh of the back or other areas of the body, and specialized rigging is used to lift the individual so that they are suspended from these hooks for a (usually brief) period. Expert knowledge about the size, number, and placement of the hooks is required. Skill regarding the mechanics of the rigging is also imperative for safety.

Do not attempt a pull or suspension on your own. If you want to undertake such experiences, you must seek qualified assistance. These activities are not for everyone, but those who have pulled or suspended usually describe achieving profound effects: enhanced self-confidence, altered states of consciousness, and spiritual awakening among them.

CORSET PIERCING

Corset piercing is another temporary practice that is sometimes done for dress-up or exhibition. A professional piercer typically performs this type of creation. They will make rows of aligned piercings on the torso, limbs, or other areas of the body. Jewelry is inserted, then the "corset" design is laced up with ribbon, cord, or chain. Such projects are meant to be temporary, as they are generally done with jewelry that is not suited to permanent surface piercings, in regions of the body that are unlikely to heal successfully.

THE POINT

From common ear piercings to advanced modification techniques and alternative activities, the world of body art is vast and varied. A fantastic array of jewelry styles and materials is available to wear in piercings. Depending on your desire and level of involvement, changing your jewelry for the first time can be as exciting as getting a new dermal punch or trying out suspension. Each person is unique, so follow your own path, do it safely, and enjoy yourself along the way. Respect others who make choices different from yours, including the decision to be heavily pierced, or to remain unpierced.

19

SPECIAL SITUATIONS

Various facets of your life are noticeably affected when you coexist with a piercing. I've worn most of my own for over a quarter century; we have endured some piercing-related ups and downs together. Dealing with daily activities can sometimes be a challenge for a pierced person. For instance, there is a unique set of considerations for piercings in relation to pregnancy, childbirth, and breastfeeding. Whether you are wearing body jewelry while traveling or dealing with planned or emergency medical care, life is just a little more interesting with a few extra holes. This chapter addresses some everyday situations and concerns.

FITNESS AND SPORTS

If you are involved in athletics or physical fitness endeavors, evaluate the impact of your activities on your piercing, literally and figuratively. Participation in rough sports can be dangerous to a piercing, regardless of how long you have had it. Wear close-fitting jewelry to minimize the risk of catching accidents, or consider changing to a flexible polymer retainer, which can be more forgiving if bumped or struck.

Use protective gear such as athletic cups or chest protectors to shield genital and nipple piercings during heavy contact sports. Note, however, that the equipment itself can sometimes cause problems. Wearing a helmet for football, bicycling, or other pursuits can exert pressure on above-the-neck piercings. Mechanical stress increases the likelihood of irritation and complications, even if you're well healed.

Certain physical activities and piercings just don't mix. Try all the different jewelry options and protection possibilities you can find. Ultimately, you still might decide that your piercing hinders your game, or your sport gets in the way of your piercing. Regardless of profound dedication to both, you may need to decide which to sacrifice.

WEIGHT LOSS OR GAIN

Most piercings are not at all affected by a modest weight gain or loss. Even a significant change will have a negligible impact, if any, on above-the-neck placements. Piercings in or near areas with a lot of adipose tissue, such as the abdomen, breasts, and thighs, are more apt to experience effects from a substantial change in weight. An alteration in the size or shape of your chest or breasts can have cosmetic consequences, such as a shift in the angle of your nipple piercings, but this will not be harmful.

Adding inches to your waistline might cause a navel piercing to become irritated, even if it is well established. Genital piercings can be subject to extra pressure or friction from weight gain due to a substantial pubic mound or proximity to the inner thighs. Swapping your jewelry for a different size or style may help alleviate these issues.

MEDICAL AND DENTAL EMERGENCIES AND APPOINTMENTS

If you are rushed to the hospital in an emergency, your body jewelry might be cut off along with your clothes. Some medical professionals have learned the proper way to open popular body jewelry designs. Still, paramedics and emergency room personnel will be more focused on handling your urgent situation than preserving your personal property, and rightly so. When your health or life is on the line, the loss of jewelry or a piercing is a comparatively minor consideration.

Circumstances are quite different when you undergo scheduled medical or dental procedures or get treated for a non-life-threatening health problem. Since it can be tough to reinsert jewelry once you remove it, take precautions to preserve your piercing. You might need to educate your care provider, but the effort will be worthwhile to avoid leaving a hole empty, risking shrinkage or closure.

Many health care workers insist that you remove body jewelry for all procedures or tests, especially when the area in question is adjacent to a piercing. This sometimes reflects thoughtless adherence to policy rather than genuine medical necessity. Having a piercing-friendly medical or dental professional can be quite advantageous. Your piercer may be able to recommend practitioners who are knowledgeable about piercing or help you to educate your own.

Discuss your piercing with your doctor or dentist, preferably before scheduling an appointment in which the presence of your jewelry may be an issue. Inquire about the feasibility of wearing a nonmetallic replacement when you are asked to remove metal from your body. Obtain one before your appointment and arrange for an insertion if you will require help. If you cannot get a retainer in advance, certain substitutes can function as a temporary retainer to keep the channel open until jewelry can be reinserted. A sterile floss threader (available in a dental office), or sterile tubing from a catheter needle or thick suture material (available in a hospital), are suitable options.

Studies have shown that removing piercing jewelry is generally not necessary for magnetic resonance imaging (MRI), X-rays, and many other procedures unless the piercing is directly in the area of examination or treatment.[1] High-quality metal body jewelry is *nonferromagnetic* (not magnetic), so it won't react to the MRI equipment. Beware, however, of cheap body jewelry, which may indeed be dangerous due to the high-powered magnets. I had a cranial MRI with no issues while wearing thirty-nine pieces of quality body jewelry!

If you wear metal, it will be visible on the test results, but this is only a problem when the ornament obscures the area of concern. CT or PET scan images are affected by metal in the region of the examination, so you will need to remove regular body jewelry for this type of analysis.

Dentists, orthodontists, periodontists, and hygienists are often especially disapproving of tongue and other oral piercings. Sometimes they are downright hostile, which can make dental procedures even more challenging for piercees than they usually are for most people. You may be subjected to poor treatment, lectures on the dangers of piercings, or even the refusal of urgent procedures unless you remove your jewelry. Dentists are justified in having negative attitudes: poorly fitted jewelry and excessive play do cause substantial damage to teeth and oral structures. But there is never an excuse for a health care professional to mistreat you.

Many dentists don't know about the crucial measures that can be followed to diminish the risks. Explain to yours that you wear jewelry of the proper size and avoid playing with it to preserve your oral health. Once they know that you are conscious of piercing safety and care about your teeth, you might earn their respect. Show your dentist chapter 12 of this book, or bring them a copy of the APP brochure "Oral Piercing Risks and Safety Measures."[2] Sharing the information will educate them, and they can pass along their newfound knowledge to colleagues and other pierced patients who have not been informed about the vital facts. Your health is the priority, always. Do your best to plan proactively, but never sacrifice medical or dental treatment to avoid a reprimand or the risk of losing a piercing.

BODY JEWELRY AND CT SCANS

I once had a radiology tech who was as curious as I was to find out what would happen if we attempted to do my cranial CT scan without removing the jewelry from my twenty-five above-the-neck piercings. The results resembled a modern art piece with lots of small geometric lines extending from every ring and bar in my head. It looked interesting, but it was not at all useful for analysis or diagnosis of anything. I was convinced: I had to remove all of my oral and facial ornaments for this radiology exam, which was no quick or easy task—even for a trained professional.

RETAINERS

Retainers are worn for two primary purposes: to obscure piercings from view, or to keep them open when ordinary jewelry must be removed, such as for sports or medical care. Most studios offer a selection, and many options are available online. Some are specific to a particular type of piercing, while others are more multi-purpose.

The possibilities for safe and effective concealment of most piercings increase considerably after you have healed. You can disguise many above-the-neck piercings using jewelry so tiny that it is barely visible. You can wear a transparent piece or one that looks like a freckle. There are flesh-colored retainers or ends for barbells or labrets that blend in with the surrounding tissue. Replacing an ornamental end is more straightforward than changing out an entire piece of jewelry. For example, if you wear a labret stud, you can swap a fancy adornment for a small concealment disc as needed.

Glass retainers in a nose-bone style or that fasten with an O-ring can be worn to conceal ear and nostril piercings. Silicone plugs in skin tones can help to camouflage large-gauge piercings. Hook-shaped eyebrow retainers and other designs held in by gravity or jewelry shape are much less secure and could come out during sleep or physical activity. Nonmetallic PTFE barbells are excellent for body piercings because they stay in much more securely than those with an O-ring closure, and the material is inert.

Acrylic retainers are common, but not recommended due to safety concerns with the material. For short-term wear to avoid accidental closure of a healed piercing, they may be worth the risk if no other option is available. Never wear acrylic in fresh or inflamed piercings, and quickly remove it from a healed piercing if you experience any irritation.

If you can't locate a retainer in your current jewelry gauge, it is preferable to put in a thinner one instead of leaving the channel empty. It may be necessary to stretch back up later, but the piercing won't completely close, which can happen when nothing occupies the hole.

DIY RETAINERS

You can create your own retainers to avoid wearing metal jewelry or for concealment. If the smallest, flattest body jewelry available for your piercing still isn't discreet enough, coat the visible portion of it with nail polish that matches your skin tone. Use a product that is free of formaldehyde, toluene, and phthalates, and make sure the painted surface doesn't rest against your skin. To minimize the shine, tap it with your finger while the lacquer is still a little tacky. You can wear the piece once it is completely dry. Examine your concealment coating regularly and maintain it by repeating the process as needed.

You can also make a custom-fit retainer yourself from an inert polymer. Some piercers sell suitable materials that are generally quite inexpensive. For thinner gauges, small, transparent snips of medical monofilament (like thick sutures) may work. Use scissors to trim a length to fit your piercing and burn one end into a small knob with a lighter so that the retainer doesn't slip through. You can tap the heated end against a glass surface to flatten it. Remove your jewelry and insert the polymer piece into the hole. These are very discreet, but they aren't useful for regular wear because the unsecured retainer is held in place by gravity or the tightness of your tissue; it can easily fall out if moved or bumped. Nipples, navels, and ear cartilage tend to have snug channels and may keep in an unsecured retainer reasonably well, but earlobes are generally loose, and the piece may slip out.

Piercees in the military and others who are under close inspection can use this type of retainer trimmed just shy of the full length of a piercing. Once inserted, the polymer keeps the interior of the hole open, and the ends shrink down. This is as invisible as a retainer can get, but you should wear it *only* if your piercing is well healed, and you are familiar enough with it to be confident that you can retrieve the plastic at will. To prevent embedding, this type of internal retainer should be used only for short periods. An insertion taper can be helpful to push it out and reinsert jewelry.

A plastic piece that is a little longer than the piercing can be fastened with small, clear silicone O-rings. This will be a bit more stable, but also more apparent. It may take some experimentation to find the retainer that works best for you. Healed piercings can be disguised for many situations; but if you must endure harsh scrutiny and piercing is forbidden, you will have to go without jewelry or a retainer.

TRAVELING WITH PIERCINGS

Travel can be taxing under any circumstances, but being away from home with piercings can present additional challenges. Eating different foods, riding in crowded buses, changing time zones, and having jet lag all add to the strain on your body. Even old piercings can flare up from differences in temperature, humidity, water quality, and the stress of being on the road. They may become red or irritated, or secrete fluid, even after a long dry spell. Don't panic; simply resume your aftercare routine. Your piercing will usually settle down when your body accommodates to the new location, or you return to your familiar environment.

Anyone who has suffered from Montezuma's revenge knows that foreign fauna and flora can make traveling quite disagreeable, with or without piercings. Exposing your system to unfamiliar microorganisms can lead to illness or infection. It is an excellent idea to boost your immune system before and during a trip by following the health-promoting behaviors explained in "Healthy Habits for Rapid Healing," page 229. Take precautions against disease and wash your hands frequently. If you are planning to visit a part of the world that might prove risky, bring along waterproof bandages to cover your piercing. Going on a jungle safari, trekking across glaciers, and surfing untried waters are perilous journeys when you have a new piercing. Recreational endeavors like these can also aggravate a healed one. Plan your piercings and vacations accordingly, as certain activities are inadvisable or prohibited when you have an open wound.

Especially if you are still healing, be prepared to maintain your aftercare regimen during your trip by bringing supplies with you. Ready-to-use products such as saline spray are especially convenient when you're camping or staying in environments that make it hard to bathe as usual. You might need to use bottled water for rinsing, depending on the quality of the local supply on tap. If you're advised not to drink the water or brush your teeth with it, that's a sure sign that you should also avoid getting it on an open wound, including a healing piercing.

METAL DETECTORS AND SECURITY
Piercees are often concerned that their piercing(s) will set off a metal detector in an airport or other venue. Security personnel will react differently to the presence of piercings, and so will the machinery. Many heavily pierced people travel extensively without so much as a single beep. Yet stories circulate regarding piercees enduring strip searches or having to remove body jewelry to board a plane.

If your travel companions are unaware of your penchant for piercing, you may be concerned about an unplanned disclosure during a security screening. Clothing might help to mask or confuse the issue: wear a metal zipper you can blame for a beep instead of a genital piercing, or perhaps an underwire bra to take responsibility for your nipple piercings. If revealing a piercing while traveling is unacceptable, wear nonmetallic jewelry. Quality metal body jewelry is nonferromagnetic and will not set off the walk-through metal detectors. However, the handheld wands are often more sensitive and sometimes do sound an alarm when scanning directly over metal body jewelry. According to the TSA, if your metal body jewelry happens to cause a machine to beep, a pat-down may be required. Or you may be asked to remove your body piercing in private as an alternative to the hands-on screening.[3]

Depending on the location of your piercing, you may be examined in a private room by a security officer of your gender. If you wish to take your trip, it is best to be calm and cooperative. Don't wear or carry long spike-style jewelry during travel, as these could be construed as weapons and confiscated. Spikes aside, you should not be compelled to remove body jewelry, since it isn't a security threat.

DEPILATING
Removing hair around piercings can be tricky. Here are some things to keep in mind:
- ○ Hygiene is of paramount concern when shaving around a healing piercing. Rinse your razor thoroughly and change the blade frequently. Finish by

washing the area with soap and water to guard against infection. Store your razor carefully and keep it well away from your toilet to avoid the bacterial plume emitted upon flushing.

o Even if your piercing is fully healed, always rinse the area well after shaving. Hair particles can cause irritation and infection if they get into the channel.

o Although somewhat painful, plucking can remove the last stubborn whiskers that are closest to your jewelry and cannot be shaved off. Use clean tweezers.

o Wait several weeks before waxing near a piercing, and have it done only by a skilled professional. The tiny goggles used for tanning are perfect for protecting your jewelry.

o Don't use cream depilatories near a healing piercing. These contain strong chemicals that can irritate or inflame the delicate tissue.

o Depending on placement, it might be easier to remove jewelry during shaving once a piercing is healed.

MENSTRUATION

The menstrual cycle causes a complex set of physical changes in the body that can affect piercings. During menstruation and just prior to its onset, breasts and genitals may swell and become tender. Even established piercings in these areas may flare up during this time of the month. Therefore, if you are planning to get a nipple or genital piercing, it is generally best to schedule it shortly after your period ends so you will have some time to heal before your cycle starts again.

Your menstrual fluid will not adversely affect a healing genital piercing, but your hands must be clean before you touch the area when using sanitary products. Make sure that the string of a tampon is not looped around genital jewelry before you pull it. If you wear pads, change them often.

PIERCING AND PREGNANCY

It is highly inappropriate to get a new piercing while you are pregnant.[4] Beyond the fact that no reputable professional will perform a piercing if they know you are expecting, your body is already occupied with a momentous and complex task: creating and nurturing your baby. Getting pierced during pregnancy also unnecessarily exposes your unborn child to risks, including infection (because of the expected changes to your immune system), allergic reaction, bloodborne disease, and medication used to treat complications.

If you anticipate becoming pregnant in the next year or so, postpone getting a piercing with an extended healing time, especially the nipple or navel. If a navel piercing is not yet healed, as your abdomen grows and the area changes, further healing cannot occur. After you confirm that you are expecting, remove your jewelry if you have a fresh or unhealed nipple or navel piercing. Bolster your system to optimize your pregnancy instead of depleting it by trying to heal a piercing.

ESTABLISHED PIERCINGS

Other than navel, nipple, or genital piercings, most healed piercings do not experience particular problems due to pregnancy. However, any piercing can be affected by the extensive changes taking place in your body. Even old ear piercings can have flare-ups due to the hormone fluctuations that routinely occur during pregnancy.

GENITAL JEWELRY

Babies are sometimes delivered with genital jewelry in place, and no obstetric complications have been reported in the medical literature.[5] However, it is prudent to remove all metal jewelry from genital piercings before vaginal childbirth to avoid the possibility of tearing the piercing or causing trauma to the infant. It is improbable that piercings of the hood (HCH, VCH, or triangle) would cause problems. Labia piercings are more apt to get in the way, and the jewelry in a fourchette should be taken out. Talk to your doctor or midwife about their policy on piercings so that you can be prepared when delivery day arrives. If you intend to wear a genital piercing during childbirth, the jewelry or retainer should be small enough to avoid catching or interfering during delivery, but large enough to accommodate engorgement and local swelling. Depending on hospital policy, you may be able to leave genital piercings in place if a cesarean section is planned.

NAVEL PIERCINGS AND PREGNANCY

If you experience no issues with a healed navel piercing, simply leave the jewelry in place. However, dramatic alterations to the size and shape of the belly are typical; your innie can become an outie. Once the tissue begins to stretch, you could experience discomfort, inflammation, and sometimes migration. Switching to a flexible polymer maternity retainer usually resolves these problems. If the piercing still doesn't feel comfortable, you should abandon it until after delivery.

NIPPLE PIERCING AND BREASTFEEDING

Pregnant piercees may worry about breastfeeding with pierced nipples, but piercings do not seem to interfere with lactation in most cases. An average nipple has up to twenty pore-like milk ducts, rather than a single spout. Therefore, a nipple piercing in a standard gauge size with uneventful healing won't block them all.

The ability to nurse could be impaired if a troubled nipple piercing causes excess scarring or damages nerves. If you remove the jewelry from a well-healed nipple piercing, some milk might seep or flow from the empty channel, which could produce a faster supply than your baby needs.[6]

Leaving out your nipple jewelry during breastfeeding is safest for your infant. Jewelry removal eliminates the most serious risk of your baby choking on a ring or bar that becomes unfastened. You also diminish the potential for other nursing problems, such as difficulty latching on or damage to the soft tissue of your infant's mouth. Another consideration is the risk of bacteria entering the baby's system from the jewelry. Some piercees have successfully nursed while wearing flexible retainers instead of metal. *Do not* wear the style that has an O-ring closure, because it is not secure enough to stay on during nursing.

If you decide to remove your jewelry and leave it out until you are done nursing, the piercing may shrink or close by the time your baby is weaned. If your piercing was fully healed, there is a chance the hole could remain open. It may be possible to encourage a well-established channel to stay viable by regularly passing a small, clean insertion taper through it. If the piercing has sealed shut and you wish to be repierced, it is best to wait at least three months after you stop nursing to allow the tissue to normalize.

THE POINT

Even if you don't plan to keep a piercing "through sickness and in health, for as long as you both shall live," coexisting with it can take some effort and patience. You and your piercings are likely to have some good times, and some tough ones—just like a marriage. It can be difficult to anticipate all the ways a piercing can impact you over the years. For better or worse, you will likely need to make decisions and perhaps even compromises in the ongoing relationship between your piercing and your daily life.

20

SEX!

The act of piercing is exotic and primal, perhaps because penetrating the body with a needle is a metaphor for intercourse itself. While sexual enhancement is a primary impetus for certain piercings, it is not a universal motivation. The assumption that all piercees wear tongue, nipple, and genital piercings for erotic reasons is erroneous. On the other hand, piercings can be erotically charged even when they are in areas that are not inherently erogenous. Piercees have described experiencing sensual pleasure from ear, navel, and neck surface piercings, and improbable spots including the septum and eyebrow. Virtually any piercing has the potential to arouse and excite.

CAN PIERCINGS ENHANCE YOUR SEX LIFE?

"I absolutely love my piercings—being 'vajazzled' makes me feel sexy, sexually confident, and at an age (fifty-six) that most wouldn't think you could revamp things in the sex department, trust me, you can!" —Z.

Many people get genital piercings to enrich their sexual experiences, whether they want to call attention to a particular spot or augment their own sensation or a partner's. Because sex is such a dynamic and individual activity, only you can determine whether your piercing is an utter delight, or if it gets in the way. A period of accommodation is to be expected while you figure out how a new piercing performs in conjunction with your inclinations and erogenous zones. You may need to change your jewelry size or style for optimal pleasure. Once healed, give yourself some time to learn and adapt. The vast majority of my clients enjoy their piercings tremendously; many describe heightened sensation and satisfaction that is sometimes described as "life-changing." On occasion, someone will find that a specific piercing is incompatible with their proclivities. The good news is that it is easy to be rid of a piercing if you decide it isn't serving you.

Though piercings can improve your love life, they are not a panacea for problems, including unskilled or incompatible partners. Intimate piercings can also help—or hurt—the genital size match of a couple. If you and your lover have a snug fit already, adding an ampallang or apadravya could be unhelpful because these increase width at the head of the penis. However, if you have more ease between you, the added jewelry could be just the thing to make you more compatible, resulting in increased gratification for both parties.

SAFER SEX

A new genital piercing can only benefit from resting and avoiding friction and trauma. Still, I do not set a particular period of abstinence from sexual activities while healing; I've found that telling people not to have sex doesn't always work. Instead, I issue two non-negotiable rules:

1. **Be gentle.** Pay attention to your body. If your piercing feels the slightest bit sore, you must stop or modify what you're doing. As you begin to heal and the piercing feels less tender, you must still be vigilant to avoid injuring fragile new cells. Being too rough during healing can result in migration, excess scar tissue formation, and other complications.

2. **Be clean and hygienic.** You *must* use protective barriers to prevent infection via the sharing of bodily fluids. For oral sexual contact, use a *dental dam* (sheet of latex or polyurethane) to shield the vulva for cunnilingus and a flavored or unlubricated condom during fellatio. Before contact near a healing piercing, thoroughly wash hands and sex toys, and use condoms for intercourse and on insertables like dildos and bullet-type vibrators. If other barriers aren't suitable, apply a waterproof dressing such as Tegaderm before sexual activities to keep your partner's body fluids from getting on your piercing. All of these precautions are mandatory to prevent infection during the *entire initial healing period*, even if you and your partner are monogamous and healthy. If you can't effectively protect your piercing, then you must abstain.

3. Appropriate body jewelry is smooth, so high-quality condoms that fit correctly should perform well. Water-based lubricant helps reduce excess friction to protect the integrity of the material. The sensitivity of your healing piercing can make up for the addition of an unfamiliar barrier. Pleasure Plus condoms have some extra room that can accommodate frenum and Prince Albert jewelry. Avoid prophylactics and lubricants with the spermicide nonoxynol-9 (N-9); the harsh chemical detergent can burn, sting, and harm the delicate cells of a fresh piercing (as well as vaginal or rectal tissue).[1]

> ## TIP OF THE DAY
> Using a regular condom and a pair of sharp scissors, you can make a dam to shield vulva piercings during cunnilingus. Make a single cut through the rolled edge to the center, and the prophylactic will unroll into a rectangular shape that you can use over the genitals as a barrier in place of a dental dam. Condoms are more readily available than dental dams, and they are thinner and come in more colors and flavors, too!

POTENTIAL DOWNSIDES

There are some possible drawbacks to genital piercings: they might cause damage from accidents or rough sex. During the healing period, this risk is virtually eliminated because you and your partner must always be gentle and use barrier protection. If you will not be using barriers after healing, you'll need to wear body jewelry that is compatible to avoid catching during sexual activities. When one partner wears a circular barbell and the other a closed ring, there is a chance of mishaps. Consider adding a captive bead to close off the center gap of the circular barbell.

An accidental entanglement can result in disaster:

> "My circular barbell got caught in my wife's captive bead ring that was in her VCH . . . she pushed me back. I screamed, 'No!' but it was too late. In pushing me back, my PA ripped away her ring and took her entire clitoral hood, or at least a good 80 percent of it, with it. If you get caught, don't try to rip apart, and don't panic. Stop and work the problem [out]. Move easily and gently, and unhook yourself."—B.

Genital piercings might physically get in the way, depending on your preferred activities, specific placement, and jewelry. Some wearers find that vibrators make excessive noise from contact with metal. Fellatio could be problematic with ampallang, apadravya, and large Prince Albert piercings. Jewelry can chip or crack teeth. Consider your personal inclinations when deciding on a piercing. Functional and practical aspects are relevant for sexually active piercees.

PIERCINGS AND PARTNERS

If intimacy with a new sweetheart is imminent, it is probably a good idea to talk about your genital piercing, or at least give a hint before your clothes come off. In a way, being pierced can both attract and limit possible mates:

> "I've been approached by women because of them. At the same time, I've been shunned by others. To me, it's balanced out . . . but at least I have a sense of contentment."—R.

Piercings can be a source of conflict when you are involved with somebody who does not appreciate your taste in body modification. You may have to decide whether your partner or your piercings are a bigger priority, and who ultimately controls your body. Relationships have ended over such discrepancies.

> "My girlfriend left me when I got my first eyebrow piercings. . . . Now I have a girlfriend that loves my piercings and wants to get some with me!"—F.

OVERSTIMULATION, SENSATION, AND DESENSITIZATION

There is often a period of localized hypersensitivity when a piercing is new. The overstimulated nerve endings calm as healing begins, and the body grows accustomed to the constant presence of jewelry, usually within the first week. For better or worse, genital piercings are not permanently stimulating. Regardless of piercing placement, there is no concern—or hope—of becoming a continuous human orgasm machine. That said, increased pleasurable sensations are a common consequence when nipple or genital piercings are touched or caressed, whether new or healed. Many piercees report spectacular enhancements, including experiencing orgasm from activities that had never produced the result before. Some describe having an improved libido, at least for a while.

When piercings are appropriately placed and handled according to accepted practice, there is no physiological basis for a permanent reduction in sensitivity from any standard piercing placement. Piercings (including those of the nipples and genitals) have been rumored to result in eventual desensitization of the area. I was even asked by an anxious, uninformed young man, "Two years after my nipple piercing, will I lose all feeling there like my friend told me I would?" Urban myths abound, but there is no empirical evidence that the continued presence of jewelry will diminish any of the sensation with which a person is naturally blessed.[2]

Occasionally, diminished feeling in the localized area is described after a vulva piercing has healed. This can usually be attributed to the typical spike in sensitivity following a piercing and normalizing of sensation once it has settled and the wearer has become accustomed to it. Rather than a decrease in original feeling, this is usually a matter of getting used to a piercing that was highly responsive when it was new.[3] This is seldom an issue with penis piercings because the nerve endings are distributed over a much larger area.

> ## JUST ONCE
> I've performed thousands of genital piercings since the 1980s. In that time, I can recall only one case in which a woman complained of decreased sensitivity, about a year after getting a vertical hood piercing. She removed her jewelry, and everything soon returned to normal.

WHICH PIERCINGS ARE BEST?

Innumerable variables in anatomy and motivation make that a question without a universal answer. Whether to appeal to your aesthetic sense, increase your own sensitivity, or stimulate your partner, there is a piercing to suit your preferences, and hopefully, your build too.

Placement and jewelry selection can affect function. For example, I usually position the VCH for maximum stimulation. But if you are hypersensitive, there might be a way to situate the piercing for ornamentation. If your clitoris is recessed and your hood is long, the piercing could be placed a little lower, so it doesn't touch the glans. Smaller jewelry might minimize the sensation. See chapter 14 for details on a wide range of genital piercing options.

WHICH VULVA PIERCING IS BEST?

First you have to pose the relevant question: best for what?
- Fastest healing: VCH, inner labia, or Princess Albertina
- Jewelry a partner feels during penetration: Outer or inner labia, Princess Albertina, or fourchette
- Highest visibility: Christina, high outer labia, or a high HCH
- Most clitoral stimulation: VCH, HCH, triangle, or clitoris, depending on anatomy

WHICH PENIS REGION PIERCING IS BEST?

- Fastest healing: Prince Albert
- Jewelry a partner feels during penetration, and potential G-spot stimulation: Ampallang, apadravya, or reverse Prince Albert
- Most clitoral stimulation: Pubic piercing (with a ring that has a large or textured bead)
- Highest visibility: Upper frenum, pubic, or hafada piercing
- Jewelry that is not inserted during penetration: Pubic, lorum, scrotum, or guiche
- For your own sensation and delight: Personal preferences vary, so try the piercing(s) to which you are attracted

Even sound can enhance the effects:

> "The jingling of the scrotals and frenums as I walk around turn her on as well, and the jingling that occurs during sex I think heightens her pleasure . . . kind of like 'copulation music.'"—S.

KISSING AND ORAL SEX

In general, the enjoyment of kissing relates to compatibility. If your lover is fond of wet, sloppy kisses but you favor a drier variety, it won't matter whether jewelry is present; your pleasure will fall short. Oral piercings can add a distinct focus to the act of kissing, but they aren't intrusive, as some might imagine.

Similarly, there are differences of opinion about receiving oral sex from someone wearing tongue or lip jewelry. Some will say nothing is better, yet others don't feel anything different. Multiple factors affect the experience, including the technique and enthusiasm of the giver; jewelry size, type, and placement; and the receiver's sensitivity. When a vulva is on the receiving end, jewelry seems to make more of an impact, but there is no unanimous accord as to whether it feels good or is "too much."

INFIBULATION

In prior eras, infibulation was a means of imposing abstinence (see page 9); today, however, it is usually part of a BDSM relationship with a trusted partner. If you have a desire for enforced chastity, certain piercings and body jewelry can be used to prohibit physical stimulation, erections, or penetration. It may be hard for the uninitiated to understand, but infibulation itself can be a form of erotic interaction through the consensual exchange of power and control.

Piercings must be fully healed and settled before attempting any form of infibulation. The fine, malleable nature of genital tissue makes it difficult to achieve long-term chastity using piercings. Continuous pressure and heavy weight nearly always cause soreness or migration eventually. An ordinary padlock is sometimes used to connect the rings in multiple piercings, but should never be put through your tissue. Proper body jewelry locks are made that are safe for wear in the body. A variety of other devices and closures are available to control the genitals via piercings.

Vulva options: The inner labia are generally too stretchy for preventing sexual access unless your piercings are placed at the base of the tissue near the body, and tightly fastened. If you have elongated inner labia that are pierced near the edge, penetration may still be possible, even if you wear a single ring through both sides. Affixing multiple piercings on the upper portion of the outer labia might prevent clitoral stimulation (or, depending on jewelry, could augment it). Connecting outer labia piercings adjacent to the vaginal opening is most effective for infibulation. Jewelry may need to be changed to wear tampons for monthly periods; otherwise, you will need to use pads.

Penis region options: The most common infibulation techniques are to connect a pair of foreskin piercings, or to fasten a Prince Albert (or frenum) to guiche or scrotum jewelry. Piercings are sometimes used to affix cages or other custom-made chastity devices.

> "Physically I pretty much look the same, but I definitely smile more when I look in the mirror. My confidence makes everything better, including the bedroom."—C.

THE POINT

A piercing is sometimes what you make of it; if you want yours to be an aphrodisiac, then it can function as one. If you just like the way it looks, that's valid, too. Piercings can boost your self-esteem, inflame passions, and bring your sensuality into focus. Joining your lover for a visit to a studio to get intimate piercings may deepen your connection and even inspire new forms of love play. If you feel attracted to a genital piercing, find a qualified professional, and give it a go!

PART 7

PIERCING IN MODERN CULTURE

PIERCEES AND THE
ESTABLISHMENT 320

A CAREER IN PROFESSIONAL
PIERCING 324

THE FUTURE OF PIERCING 329

21

PIERCEES AND THE ESTABLISHMENT

Most people who get piercings derive great enjoyment from them, but body modification sometimes causes problems when dealing with society. Despite increased acceptance, authority figures in Western culture are not always sympathetic to the practice of piercing. The devout sometimes cite sacred scriptures prohibiting body art; medical professionals may see only the threat of disease; psychologists have been known to decry piercing as self-mutilation, and lawmakers view it as a problem to be regulated. Though piercing has become far more widespread and is considered mainstream in certain areas, some people with visible body art still experience discrimination and prejudice.

DOCTOR/PATIENT HOSTILITY

At the most fundamental level, piercings can seem wrong to doctors. They are trained to close wounds, not keep them open. Furthermore, many physicians still have no specific training in dealing with piercings. They frequently used to assume that whatever was wrong with you was due to a piercing. For example, a doctor blamed a woman's healed cartilage piercings for her ear infection, even though she'd intermittently experienced the same ailment since childhood. Fortunately, this seems to happen less frequently nowadays.

Though piercing has become pervasive, psychologists and mental health professionals still sometimes associate it with pathologies like depression or self-harm. Additionally, piercing uses instruments familiar to doctors, such as needles and forceps, so many in the health care field find the procedure uncomfortably close to practicing medicine.

Medical professionals with negative attitudes toward body art may be judgmental or believe that all piercees are uncaring about their health or ignorant about piercing's risks. They may disapprove of piercings because of skewed experiences: body modification generally comes to their attention only when complications arise. By reading this book, you probably have more education about piercing than most medical personnel have had in their curricula.

YOUR PIERCING OR YOUR JOB

Stereotyping of modified people has declined, but you might still run into obstacles with employers who have negative attitudes about pierced individuals. It is entirely permissible to be refused employment because you wear body art; there is no federal protection for it in the workplace. This is not discrimination in the legal sense, because appearance is always a key component of getting and keeping a job. When interviewing, try to downplay noticeable piercings by wearing small jewelry or concealment pieces, if you believe there might be an issue. The standard aspects remain essential for every job applicant: punctuality, preparedness, and proper grooming.

Even in professions outside the white-collar realm, wearing body jewelry may be limited or prohibited. Practical matters, such as health and safety issues, can also affect piercings in the workplace. Employees who wear earphones, stethoscopes, or other audio equipment can end up with irritated ear piercings. Masks may interfere with septum or nostril piercings. Cooks, landscapers, mechanics, construction workers, and others who toil in dirty or sweaty environments often find that their piercings do not fare well.

The organization Support Tattoos and Piercings at Work (STAPAW) lists mainstream companies that hire people with piercings, and petitions businesses and corporations to revise dress-code policies to permit body art.[1] To find work opportunities, you can also ask modified friends for job leads and watch for pierced employees in action.

DIRTY BUSINESS

I had a client who experienced endless problems trying to heal her ear and facial piercings, though she assured me that she followed all aftercare instructions without fail. It finally came to light that she worked in a waste treatment plant, and the environment was simply prohibitive to healing.

DRESS CODES

Whether at school or work, you may have to contend with a dress code that restricts or bans piercings. Trying to combat this type of imposed conformity can be frustrating. One problem is that dress codes often contain ambiguous standards: jewelry must be "in good taste" or "not distracting." That is subjective and difficult to define, leaving room for interpretation by whoever is in charge.

If you run into trouble, determine whether there is a written policy and, if so, read it. If the guidelines are vague or do not specifically refer to piercing, or if there is no printed policy at all, you should be in a better position to negotiate. Fortunately, many dress codes have evolved and eased in response to the ongoing and growing popularity of body art. To her delight, a registered nurse discovered that her employer had loosened restrictions against visible piercings:

> "This means that I can finally get my nose repierced after all these years . . . I'm glad to see that employers in health care are realizing that people with piercings are capable of being professional and hard workers. I've had many elderly patients and their families notice my tongue, and all they said is, 'I don't understand why you kids do that.' When asked if their opinion of me as a nurse changed, all have quickly replied no, they still think I am professional."—E.

PIERCED CELEBRITIES

It is more common than ever to see famous people being open about (and acting proud of) their body art. Celebrities sporting multiple ear piercings, navel, nostril, septum, and even nipple piercings are often spotted.

THE HALLS OF LEARNING

Private and religious educational institutions have almost unlimited power to formulate rules about student conduct, including dress codes. Dealing with school authorities can be a challenge at the best of times, but if you are brazen enough to attempt to defy your school bureaucracy, it helps if you are well behaved and earning good grades. Arguably, wearing piercings in school is not nearly as distracting to students as puberty, and no one can ban that—although many wish they could.

THE MILITARY

Despite a long history of tattooing among military personnel, the armed forces rigidly require conformity of appearance. Though tattoo regulations have loosened substantially, piercing is still banned by all United States military service branches. They have issued edicts like US Army Regulation 670-1, which states, "Attaching, affixing or displaying objects, articles, jewelry, or ornamentation to, through, or under their skin, tongue, or any other body part is prohibited. This applies to all Soldiers on or off duty."[2] A single pair of small, simple stud earrings is acceptable for earlobe piercings on servicewomen. Trying to fight against their strict standards is a losing proposition; if you can't obey the rules, don't join.

PIERCING REGULATIONS

Tattooing has a long history of regulation, but legal systems scrambled to catch up when piercing exploded in popularity. Nearly every state now has legislation addressing some aspect of piercing, with the majority prohibiting piercing of minors without parental permission. Laws establishing minimum standards for preventing the spread of disease are beneficial, but the statutes in some states do not address specifics. Many do require registration or licensure by the governing body (which varies by location), but relatively few have a certification process for piercers. Even in states with the most comprehensive and stringent regulations, enforcement is not always up to par. The point is, even if a studio or piercer is licensed by their state, this does not guarantee that they are competent or safe. Ask a reputable piercer, use the internet, or contact your local health authorities to find out about laws in your area.[3]

ONE OF THE LUCKY ONES: A PIERCED PROFESSOR

"I often get questions, especially when I travel, as people try to find context for who I am, because in their professional lives they are not accustomed to seeing an adult male with a septum piercing, in addition to my eyebrow, earlobes, and other piercings. . . . In fact, I am a tenured full professor in health education, and had my first piercing (earlobe) twenty-five years ago. I'm in my eighteenth year in my current faculty position. My septum piercing—no, I do not remove it when I work—has been a part of who I am for more than a decade. Am I treated differently because I have piercings? Yes. Do I have colleagues who think my piercings are unprofessional? Yes. Why do I have piercings? Why not? . . . I am who I am and I have no desire to be like anyone else. I desire only to be the best and most unique me that I can be. That's what should be truly important in life. I am past president of a national professional association. I have published in scholarly journals in my field and fortunately continue to excel in my profession. I am sure that there are times when I am overlooked because of my appearance, my race, and/or my sexual orientation. Therefore, everyone, particularly a new professional or a student in secondary school or in college, should think very carefully before getting body art. There will be those who will treat us differently because of the decisions we have made to tattoo or pierce our bodies. However, if I were to do it over again, would I obtain body art? Yes!"—Reginald Fennell, PhD

FREEDOM'S JUST ANOTHER WORD

Ultimately, as a pierced person, you must consider your priorities when interacting with the powers that be in our society. You may have to sacrifice some of your piercings to land a job or feed yourself or your family; there is no disgrace in that. On the other hand, a young man who once dreamed of being a firefighter told me, "I wanted to be a firefighter for a while, but to be honest . . . I loved my mods more. Sometimes you've got to make a choice."

22

A CAREER IN PROFESSIONAL PIERCING

Most piercers regularly receive enthusiastic inquiries such as, "How can I become a piercer?" and, "Hey, will you teach me to pierce?"

Piercing seems like a totally awesome career: you don't have to go to college for a degree, you can have your own style, including all the body modifications you want, and you get to be in a cool studio where it's probably more like a party than drudgery.

Unfortunately, if that's what you think, you are in for a rude awakening. Professional piercing is a real job—and it isn't about you; it's about your clients. An extended period of training is followed by years of demanding work and the certainty that you won't become a millionaire. Unless a piercer is exceptionally talented, businesslike, and skilled in self-promotion, this line of work is apt to be closer to a subsistence-level job. See details on piercer income levels, employment benefits, and more in the survey summary, Appendix C, page 334.

To be a good piercer, you need specific qualities and capabilities. It also takes extensive education, even though you will find no courses in piercing offered at your local university, community college, or vocational school. Obtaining worthwhile training is difficult, because there are limited opportunities for instruction.

ATTRIBUTES

Perhaps surprisingly, a piercer's primary concern isn't with jewelry and needles—it's with people. If you are considering becoming a piercer, first ask yourself if you have the personal traits required in this service-oriented profession. Are you tolerant and able to interact closely with all types of people? Can you summon the patience and empathy necessary to deal with nervous clients? Do you have strong verbal skills to communicate effectively with them?

Piercing is a profession that also demands particular physical and practical attributes. A quality practitioner must have the natural artistic aptitude to place piercings and jewelry aesthetically. You also need sharp vision, excellent hand-eye coordination, and superior manual dexterity. You must have the stamina to perform your last procedure of the day with the same energy and concentration as your first. If you get sick easily or have allergy-prone skin, think twice about becoming a piercer. While few piercings are gory, if you faint at the sight of blood, this is clearly not a job for you.

RISKS

When you pierce, you assume a real risk: a disease could be transmitted to you via a needlestick accident. Extensive training and consistent focus are indispensable to avoid the health hazards of working with "sharps," because hepatitis and other bloodborne pathogens are widespread. You also run the risk of developing illnesses, sensitivities, or allergies from harsh chemical disinfectants or medical gloves. Less obvious is the emotional toll. Working with clients who get pierced to reclaim their bodies after being assaulted is just one of the many intense and draining (yet rewarding) experiences piercers deal with regularly.

FORMAL EDUCATION

At a minimum, all piercers should undergo training in CPR and first aid, and study bloodborne pathogens. Some regulations require a piercer to pass courses on these subjects to receive a license. If you are seriously interested in pursuing a career in professional piercing, classes in biology, chemistry, anatomy, medical terminology and ethics, phlebotomy, and patient relations are recommended. These are available in nursing, emergency medical technician (EMT), and medical assistant programs at most community colleges, and some can be taken online.

Even if you never intend to manage or own a studio, general business classes in accounting, computers, customer relations, marketing, photography, and entrepreneurship can only benefit you. If you're unable to locate a piercer willing to take you on, you will have some familiarity with alternate fields you may want to pursue instead.

PIERCER TRAINING

There is no recognized program for obtaining a certificate or diploma in piercing, so don't be fooled into thinking you could get one, hang out your shingle, and start poking holes in people for a profit. There are a variety of ways piercers learn, but only one—apprenticeship—is recommended.

Some receive all of their so-called training by watching videos. This method provides a bare minimum of information and is highly inadvisable. Videos are a poor substitute for in-person practical tutelage, and some of them contain techniques that are harmful or even criminally negligent. A beginner cannot distinguish piercing facts from fabrications. The best videos offer valid tips, but they should never be used as a sole form of instruction. Some of them provide excellent training—for what *not* to do. I've actually used them for this purpose while teaching my staff to pierce. An online course, even a long one, can't provide sufficient education to make you a safe, capable piercer.

Other piercers learn using the trial-and-error method: they practice on friends and/or the paying public. Obviously, this is not recommended either.

Some trainees will attend a workshop or seminar to learn. These courses usually last a few days to a week, and the participants ordinarily do piercings on friends, volunteers, or each other under the supervision of an instructor. The top programs provide an abundance of vital information about hygiene, sterilization, cross-contamination control, piercing techniques, appropriate jewelry, aftercare, and more. Unfortunately, even the best short course is not a substitute for comprehensive hands-on instruction under a mentor's guidance. There's just no way to impart a thorough enough education to make someone a competent piercer in such a brief period. Even the most adept pupil will still require additional one-on-one training to pierce skillfully, or their clients will suffer through numerous trials and errors. In vetting workshops, ask: "Will this course make me a piercer?" The most ethical ones will honestly inform you that it will not.

A piercer who posts a handsome "Certificate of Training" on their wall may have received it in the mail with a video and "piercing kit"; they may have had a week or so of solid instruction—or they may have taken a substandard class from someone who was out to make a fast buck.

APPRENTICESHIPS

An apprenticeship is an extended training period in a studio under a capable mentor. In the best case, the instructor will be an accomplished expert and will teach the apprentice everything they know. Unqualified mentors can only turn out inferior piercers, bringing down the overall level of competency in the entire industry. Even a respected and experienced piercer is not necessarily blessed with the ability to impart their knowledge to others.

Be very suspicious of anyone who claims they can teach you to pierce in a brief period—especially if you must pay a substantial fee. Many a piercer has forked over thousands of dollars for a three-month program only to find that it was dangerously incomplete and unprofessional. Most ethical piercers will not take you as a trainee unless they intend to keep you on staff. There is little point in devoting intensive time and energy to your instruction if you will leave to set up a competing studio or have to seek a job in a glutted market.

Studios rarely advertise openings for legitimate apprenticeships because piercers can pick from a flock of hopefuls they already know. Networking and persistence are needed to land a position. Talk to piercers and develop a rapport with any you trust and admire. Have piercings done on yourself and make it clear to your piercer how interested and resolute you are about pursuing piercing as a career. Consider volunteering to help out around the studio so you can get to know one another better; be persistent but not pesky.

Once you land an apprenticeship, you may be asked to sign a confidentiality agreement, a noncompete clause, or other legal forms. Even if you are walking on air, don't sign anything you don't feel comfortable with or don't understand. If it is not written in plain language, have an attorney look it over. It is imperative to work out the precise terms before starting. Who is paying whom, and how much? What exactly will your duties include? How long is the anticipated duration of your training? When will you actually start to pierce?

APPRENTICESHIP COSTS

A quarter of piercers surveyed (see page 334) earned income as an apprentice, but the rest paid for their educations; for most of them, it cost $1,000 or less.

EVALUATING AN APPRENTICESHIP

Thanks to the Association of Professional Piercers' "Suggested Apprentice Body Piercer Guidelines and Curriculum," there are now standardized criteria for specific apprenticeship terms and curricula, and for the credentials of a piercer who is eligible to teach.[1]

In addition to plenty of supervised hands-on instruction in piercing procedures, a comprehensive apprenticeship should provide education on anatomy, cross-contamination prevention, needlestick protocol, autoclave use and maintenance, bloodborne pathogens, jewelry quality and selection, aftercare, troubleshooting, bedside manner, customer service, client paperwork, and much more. The APP's guidelines include the following as a minimum standard:

- 1,200 hours working with a mentor piercer: This training (documented daily, cosigned by both apprentice and mentor) involves observing the mentor performing piercings, maintaining paperwork, processing tools (if applicable), and doing client consultations as well as other piercing studio–related responsibilities.
- 100 hours of documented procedure observation. This should include no fewer than a hundred piercing procedures. Those hundred piercing procedures should feature a variety of piercing locations and techniques.
- 100 piercings performed under mentor supervision. The apprentice should never attempt a piercing they haven't done before without mentor supervision.

Before taking on an apprentice, the mentor(s) should meet the following minimum criteria:

- Five years of professional piercing experience
- Up-to-date CPR, first aid, and bloodborne pathogens training

A number of other suggested prerequisites are encouraged but optional, including APP membership and two letters of recommendation (of the mentor) by piercers from other studios.

THE APP'S "PIERCING APPRENTICE'S BILL OF RIGHTS"
Every piercing apprentice has the right:

- To a clean, safe work environment, with Personal Protective Equipment (PPE) provided at no cost to them
- To appropriate bloodborne pathogens training, paid for by the shop they are training at
- To a workplace free of hazing
- To a professional work relationship with their mentor. This relationship must be devoid of sexual, verbal, or any other type of illegal harassment
- To an apprenticeship compliant with local labor laws
- To observation and instruction by their mentor for every piercing they are attempting for the first time
- To decline to perform piercings they are not properly trained to do
- To a reasonable work schedule, in compliance with local labor laws
- To a knowledgeable mentor with enough experience to train a new piercer
- To pursue employment in another field or with another body art studio

CONTINUING EDUCATION
Experienced industry leaders (myself included) sometimes offer webinars, workshops, or seminars. These can be an excellent way to supplement your knowledge, particularly in technical or advanced topics. The APP provides a wide range of continuing education classes to piercers during its annual conference. It is a unique and inspiring educational event for beginning and experienced piercers alike. You need not be a member of the organization to attend conference classes, though you must be one to join in the annual APP members' retreat.

THE POINT
Some of this industry's pioneers learned by piercing themselves and their friends, but there were no other alternatives when they began. Better options should be available now. If you are determined to become a piercer, spend a few years getting pierced and studying related subjects. Make an honest evaluation of your character and capabilities to decide if a career in professional piercing is right for you.

23

THE FUTURE OF PIERCING

Piercing has undergone a genuinely explosive revolution in recent decades. After an extended history among indigenous peoples followed by years of obscurity at the fringes of Western society, piercing has achieved massive worldwide popularity in contemporary culture. Regardless of individual motivations, modern piercing has touched the lives of countless people. Even if you don't have piercings of your own, you surely know someone who does (though you may be unaware of it). There is something special about piercing and other forms of modification that stirs the innate human desire to adorn the body. This deep-seated drive is an essential element that will help to sustain the popularity piercing has achieved.

While body art still is not universally accepted or considered entirely mainstream, time and repeated exposure have helped to lift piercing from the dark realm of subversive practices. It continues to develop into a more "normal" activity, and ongoing familiarity is leading to ever greater acceptance.

GROWTH OF THE INDUSTRY
In addition to the original population that engaged in piercing, other diverse subcultures have embraced the practice. Factions of belly dancers, bikers, steampunks, goths, Wiccans, sorority sisters, rappers, naturists, the LGBTQ+ community, and other groups have shared piercing as a common pursuit. None of them mandate piercing, but it can strengthen connections between people who share other mutual interests. In some cases, piercing functions as a formal or informal ritual or rite of passage. This can have great significance for those who participate, and it may serve to deepen their bonds.

The internet and mobile apps have also contributed enormously to the escalation of piercing. Millions of people around the world share information and photos on social media. These virtual experiences help to connect piercing fans, inspire trends, and form an essential backbone for piercing in today's world.

Openly pierced celebrities continue to inspire fads and fashions when they are shown flaunting their latest adornments. They continuously generate cycles of trends as fans emulate piercings and jewelry styles worn by their favorite influencers and stars.

EXTREME BODY ART: STEREOTYPES AND NEGATIVE PERSPECTIVES

Though piercing is widespread, limits remain on how much is considered acceptable, and negative stereotypes about heavily modified people persist. Unfortunately, we sometimes perpetuate disapproving perceptions ourselves. To gain respect, we must demonstrate to the people around us—families, neighbors, and strangers—that we are like everyone else (though extra fancy and full of holes).

When you show off extreme body art, you become a liaison between worlds, whether you want to or not. Try to be tolerant with strangers. It does require patience when you are asked, "Didn't that hurt?" for the thousandth time, but through an understanding attitude, you can foster acceptance wherever you go.

When you are heavily adorned, it is unreasonable to expect that people will not look—or even gawk—at you, depending on the extent of your modifications. Handle the attention with tact and maturity; don't react with a "What are you looking at?" sneer. You know what inspires their stares. Instead of fulfilling negative expectations with an angry, aggressive response, surprise oglers by being personable instead. Do your best to be informative and articulate. When you consistently behave in this manner, you will dispel biased beliefs toward the abundantly adorned, one person at a time.

A LIFESTYLE OPTION: HERE TO STAY

One great advantage of our modern society is the remarkable array of acceptable ways to customize yourself and your life. You can live off the grid, or in a city, suburb, tiny house, or commune. You can opt for a BDSM, vegan, minimalist, or rave lifestyle—or another alternative of your choice. You can hire a stylist to update your look or a doctor to alter your appearance. If having your fat surgically sucked out and injecting botulism toxin into your face have become standard practices for beautification, it is not a big stretch to understand how a ring or gem in a nose, eyebrow, or navel piercing could gain prevalence.

Piercing has been a part of our world for millennia, and now that it has earned a place in the grand buffet of personal options, there is no taking it off the table. You can choose for yourself: to pierce or not to pierce. The decision is yours.

THE POINT

Years ago, I read a brief passage written by Jim Ward about a "piercing urge," a passionate yearning for piercing that cannot be sated by any other means. This book provides the information necessary to help you fulfill that impulse as safely as possible—or perhaps to accept and comprehend piercing as a personal preference if you never understood the attraction. There are numerous variables to consider: piercers and studios, hygiene and sterility, piercing placements and techniques, jewelry styles and quality, aftercare regimens, and more. The details and options can seem endless. But now that you are knowledgeable, you can make educated choices and deal with your piercing responsibly. You have an excellent chance of getting a piercing that heals well and will give you years (or a lifetime) of enjoyment.

Appendix A: Gauge Conversion Chart

	16g
	14g
	12g
	10g
	8g
	6g
	4g
	2g
	0g
	00g
	7/16"
	1/2"
	9/16"
	5/8"
	11/16"
	3/4"

Brown & Sharpe Gauge	Inches	Decimal Inches	Millimeters (Rounded)	Millimeters
20	1/32	.032	.8	.81
18	5/127	.040	1.0	1.02
16	3/64	.051	1.2	1.29
14	1/16	.064	1.6	1.63
12	5/64	.081	2	2.05
10	3/32	.102	2.5	2.59
8	1/8	.128	3.2	3.26
6	5/32	.162	4	4.12
—	3/16	.178	—	4.76
4	13/64	.204	5	5.19
2	1/4	.258	6	6.54
0	5/16	.325	8	8.25
00	—	.365	9	9.27
—	3/8	.375	10	9.50
000	—	.410	—	10.41
—	7/16	.438	11	11.11
0000	1/2	.460	12	11.86
—	9/16	.563	14	14.29
—	5/8	.625	16	15.90
—	11/16	.688	18	17.46
—	3/4	.750	19	19.00
—	13/16	.813	20	20.64
—	7/8	.875	22	22.20
	15/16	.938	24	23.81
	1	1.000	25	25.40

Appendix B: Minimum Healing Times Chart

Ampallang: 6–9 months

Apadravya: 6–9 months

Bridge, vertical: 4–6 months

Bridge: 4–6 months

Christina: 6–9 months

Clitoral hood, horizontal (HCH): 6–8 weeks

Clitoral hood, vertical (VCH): 4–8 weeks

Clitoris: 4–8 weeks

Dydoe: 3–4 months

Ear cartilage/antitragus: 6–9 months

Ear cartilage/conch: 6–9 months

Ear cartilage/ faux rook or daith: 6–9 months

Ear cartilage/forward helix: 6–9 months

Ear cartilage/helix: 6–9 months

Ear cartilage/rook: 6–9 months

Ear cartilage/snug: 6–9 months

Ear cartilage/tragus: 6–9 months

Earlobe: 4–8 weeks

Eyebrow: 6–8 weeks

Foreskin: 2–3 months

Fourchette: 6–8 weeks

Frenum: 3–4 months

Guiche: 3–4 months

Labia, inner: 4–8 weeks

Labia, outer: 3–4 months

Labret: 6–8 weeks

Lingual frenulum: 4–8 weeks

Lip, side: 6–8 weeks

Lip, upper: 2–3 months

Lorum: 3–4 months

Navel: 6–9 months

Nipple, large: 6–9 months

Nipple, small: 3–4 months

Nostril: 4–6 months

Prince Albert: 4–8 weeks

Princess Albertina: 4–6 weeks

Princess Diana/Duke: 4–8 weeks

Pubic: 4–6 months

Reverse Prince Albert: 4–6 months

Scrotum: 3–4 months

Septum: 4–8 weeks

Surface: 6–9 months

Teardrop: 3–4 months

Tongue/tongue tip: 4–8 weeks

Triangle: 3–4 months

Appendix C: The Piercer Survey

My joint venture with the APP marked the first time *any* substantive statistical data about piercers has been collected by the industry. We asked 940 professionals working in the United States sixty-four questions about apprenticeships and training, studio practices and policies, income and employment benefits, and much more. Below is a summary of some of the information we gathered. (All figures are pre-COVID-19.)

THE BASICS

Based on zip code zones, respondents work in all regions throughout the United States. One-third are APP members. The bulk of participants are full-time piercers, nearly 20 percent are part-timers, and fewer than 10 percent work less than twenty hours per week. More than a quarter are business owners as well as piercers.

A young population staffs the industry. More than 36 percent of piercers surveyed are 18–29 years of age, over a quarter are 30–35 years old, and another 20 percent are in the 36–41 age group. Approximately 10 percent are 42–47, and there are just a few of us old-timers (about 5 percent) in the 50-and-up range.

The vast majority—90 percent—learned through an apprenticeship, but a third of them had training that lasted only six months. A mere 20 percent studied under a mentor for two years or longer, which is the usual amount of time I took to train my staff. A quarter earned income as an apprentice, but the rest paid for their educations; for most of them, it cost $1,000 or less.

Studios are primarily small businesses; almost half have just a single full-time piercer, another quarter have two full-time piercers on staff, and the rest have three or more. Plenty of shops also have part-time piercers, with almost half having one, 14 percent having two, and surprisingly, nearly 16 percent having five part-time piercers.

Over 40 percent of piercers work as independent contractors. Less than one-third pierce as employees, with one-quarter paid an hourly wage, and less than 20 percent receiving a salary. Most piercers (two-thirds) receive a commission on piercings, and close to half also get a percentage on jewelry or other merchandise. Credit-card tips appear to make up a substantial portion of piercer income, with about half earning in this manner as well.

Close to 20 percent of piercers surveyed earned under $20,000 annually, and even fewer took in between $30,000 and $40,000; fewer still made between $40,000 and $50,000. Less than 10 percent made more than $80,000 per year.

Your personal annual income specifically from being a body piercer in 2019?

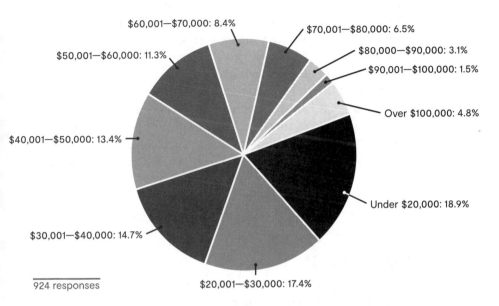

$60,001–$70,000: 8.4%
$70,001–$80,000: 6.5%
$80,000–$90,000: 3.1%
$50,001–$60,000: 11.3%
$90,001–$100,000: 1.5%
Over $100,000: 4.8%
$40,001–$50,000: 13.4%
Under $20,000: 18.9%
$30,001–$40,000: 14.7%
$20,001–$30,000: 17.4%

924 responses

A significant number of piercers are relative neophytes, as one-third of respondents have been piercing for less than five years. Still, there are plenty of seasoned professionals out there (see below).

How long have you been piercing professionally (outside of an apprenticeship)?

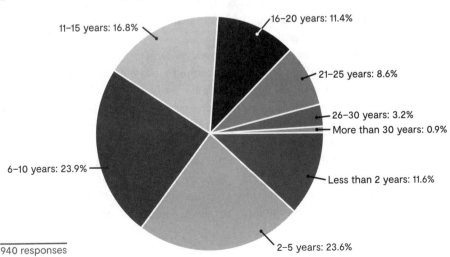

16–20 years: 11.4%
11–15 years: 16.8%
21–25 years: 8.6%
26–30 years: 3.2%
More than 30 years: 0.9%
6–10 years: 23.9%
Less than 2 years: 11.6%
2–5 years: 23.6%

940 responses

335

THE SURPRISES

Nearly all of the piercers surveyed perform most of the common above-the-waist piercings, but the numbers are far more variable regarding genital work. While 80 percent offer VCH piercings, only a third do triangles. Though two-thirds of piercers offer Prince Albert and frenum piercings, less than half do ampallangs, apadravyas, and pubic piercings. I hadn't realized that there was such a difference in the particular piercings offered by individual practitioners.

The industry lacks diversity to an embarrassing extent: over 80 percent of piercers surveyed are white! About 4 percent are Native American, less than 3 percent are Black, and 13 percent are Hispanic/Latinx. Just 1.5 percent are Asian or Asian Indian, and the remainder made up less than a full percent. This formerly male-dominated field is now composed of 55 percent women, 39 percent men, and close to 7 percent who identify as genderqueer or nonbinary. Given the gay origins of body piercing, we're a fairly heterosexual group too, with over half claiming that identity, and only 4 percent gay/lesbian. However, another 43 percent are bisexual, pansexual, or queer.

THE CONCERNS

Nearly one-fourth of respondents purchase presterilized equipment. This is somewhat worrying because sterility can be guaranteed only if the manufacturers adhere to the medical industry's stringent requirements, and not all of them do.

I was disheartened to find that 37 percent use a bulk-dispensed skin prep product, because individually packaged products are considerably safer. Also disturbing, over 15 percent used their skin prep (soap or surgical scrub) as a lubricant. These products are *not* intended for that purpose. Soap generally isn't even suggested for the exterior during healing, and this practice deposits it right inside the fresh channel! Even more piercers (16 percent) don't apply any lube at all. Over half use a water-based lubricant (the type I advocate), and nearly 10 percent use an ointment, which is also not advisable.

Beware: A small number of piercers surveyed (2 percent) use dry heat, which is not an acceptable sterilization practice for the industry. About 60 percent use a cassette-type sterilizer, and nearly three-quarters have a front-loading, standard autoclave. Some shops have more than one type. Only a tiny fraction of studios (.32 percent) are fully disposable, though I anticipate that number will rise substantially in the coming years.

It was dismaying to see how poorly piercers are preparing for the future. Under ⁓ercent have a 401(k) savings plan through work, and 36 percent had less than ⁓ings at the time of the survey. Less than one-third of piercers surveyed ⁓⁓h is about half of the average US homeownership rate.[1]

Two-thirds of piercers receive no traditional employment benefits whatsoever. Under 20 percent receive paid vacations, and slightly less than that accrue sick pay. Even fewer are compensated for overtime (14 percent). Over one-third of respondents have no medical insurance at all. Only 12.5 percent have health insurance through their work as piercers, and about the same quantity have state Medicaid. Some are insured through a family member (17.5 percent), and more than 20 percent pay out of pocket for coverage.

Many other topics were covered, and more of the findings will be available from the Association of Professional Piercers at www.safepiercing.org.

Notes

INTRODUCTION

1. *Webster's Revised Unabridged Dictionary*, s.v. "thrill (*v.*)," accessed July 11, 2020, http://www .dictionary.net/thrill.

CHAPTER 1

1. Beth Wilkinson, *Coping with the Dangers of Tattooing, Body Piercing, and Branding* (New York: Rosen Publishing Group, 1998), 77.

CHAPTER 2

1. Rufus C. Camphausen, *Return of the Tribal: A Celebration of Body Adornment* (Rochester, VT: Park Street Press, 1997), 42; and Wilkinson, *Coping with the Dangers*, 25.

2. Alice Klein, "Kangaroo-Bone Nose Piercing Is Oldest Bone Jewellery Ever Found," *New Scientist*, November 2016, https://www.newscientist.com/article/2113247-kangaroo-bone-nose-piercing- is-oldest-bone-jewellery-ever-found.

3. Hannah Osborne, "Earliest Evidence of Facial Piercing in Africa Discovered in 12,000-Year-Old Skeleton," *Newsweek*, January 2020, https://www.newsweek.com/earliest-facial-piercing-africa- ancient-skeleton-1484600.

4. Camphausen, *Return of the Tribal*, 6, 13.

5. Kristin Baird Rattini, "Who Was Tutankhamun?" *National Geographic*, April 2019, https://www .nationalgeographic.com/culture/people/reference/tutankhamun.

6. Metropolitan Museum of Art, relief panel ca. 883–859 BCE, Assyrian, accessed July 11, 2020, https://www.metmuseum.org/art/collection/search/322611.

7. "Fashion and Beauty Secrets of 2,500 Year Old Siberian 'Princess' from Her Permafrost Burial Chamber," *Siberian Times*, August 2012, https://siberiantimes.com/culture/others/features /fashion-and-beauty-secrets-of-a-2500-year-old-siberian-princess-from-her-permafrost-burial- chamber.

8. George M. Gould and Walter L. Pyle, "Anomalies and Curiosities of Medicine: Being an encyclo- pedic collection of rare and extraordinary cases, and of the most striking instances of abnormality in all branches of medicine and surgery, derived from an exhaustive research of medical literature from its origin to the present day" (Philadelphia: W. B. Saunders, 1897), 752, http://resource.nlm.nih.gov/57221200R.

9. Jody P. Rubin, "Celsus's Decircumcision Operation: Medical and Historical Implications," *Urology* 16, no. 1 (1980): 121–24, The Circumcision Reference Library, www.cirp.org/library /restoration/rubin.

10. Cornelius Celsus, *De Medicina (On Medicine)*, trans. W. G. Spencer, Loeb Classical Library Edition, vol. 3, bk. 7 (Cambridge, MA: Harvard University Press, 1938), 425, http://penelope .uchicago.edu/Thayer/E/Roman/Texts/Celsus/7*.html.

11. Donald E. Brown, James W. Edwards, and Ruth P. Moore, "The Penis Inserts of Southeast Asia: An Annotated Bibliography with an Overview and Comparative Perspectives" (occasional paper Center for South and Southeast Asia Studies, University of California, Berkeley, 1988), 16.

and Moore, "The Penis Inserts of Southeast Asia," 6, 13.

Brief History of the Evolution of Body Adornment in Western Culture: ugene, OR: Tribalife Publications, 2003), 96.

14. "Discover Indonesia Online," accessed July 13, 2020, http://indahnesia.com/indonesia /KALDEC/decoration.php.

15. Joseph Campbell, *The Masks of God*, vol. 1, *Primitive Mythology* (New York: Penguin Group, 1998), 254–55.

16. Brown, Edwards, and Moore, "The Penis Inserts of Southeast Asia," 14.

17. Jon Reidel, "War of 1812 Dig Yields Surprises for UVM Archaeologists," *The View,* June 29, 2005, University of Vermont, http://www.uvm.edu/theview/pdfs/062905.pdf.

18. Bernhardt J. Harwood, *The Golden Age of Erotica* (Los Angeles: Sherbourne Press, 1965), 305–6.

19. "Earrings," updated July 2020, https://www.encyclopedia.com/fashion/encyclopedias-almanacs-transcripts-and-maps/earrings.

20. Perlingieri, *A Brief History of the Evolution of Body Adornment*, 19.

21. Slim Price, "The Great Omi," *Sideshow World,* accessed July 13, 2020, http://www.sideshowworld .com/13-TGOD/SP-C/4-Omi/tgodgreatomi.html.

22. Lois Bibbings and Peter Alldridge, "Sexual Expression, Body Alteration, and the Defence of Consent," *Journal of Law and Society* 20, no. 3 (Autumn 1993): 356–70.

23. Carol Caliendo, Myrna L. Armstrong, and Alden E. Roberts, "Self-Reported Characteristics of Women and Men with Intimate Body Piercings," *Journal of Advanced Nursing* 49, no. 5 (2005): 474–84.

CHAPTER 3

1. William E. Keene, Amy C. Markum, and Mansour Samadpour, "Outbreak of *Pseudomonas aeruginosa* Infections Caused by Commercial Piercing of Upper Ear Cartilage," *Journal of the American Medical Association* 291, no. 8 (February 2004): 981–85, https://pubmed.ncbi.nlm .nih.gov/14982914.

2. Ahmed Messahel and Brian Musgrove, "Infective Complications of Tattooing and Skin Piercing," *Journal of Infection and Public Health* 2 (2009): 7–13, https://www.sciencedirect.com /science/article/pii/S1876034109000070.

3. Donna I. Meltzer, "Complications of Body Piercing," *American Family Physician* 72, no. 10 (November 2005), www.aafp.org/afp/20051115/2029.html.

4. "HIV Transmission," Centers for Disease Control and Prevention (CDC), accessed July 13, 2020, https://www.cdc.gov/hiv/basics/transmission.html.

5. "Hepatitis B Questions and Answers for the Public," Centers for Disease Control and Prevention (CDC), accessed July 13, 2020, https://www.cdc.gov/hepatitis/hbv/bfaq.htm#bFAQc09.

6. Rania A. Tohme and Scott D. Holmberg, "Transmission of Hepatitis C Virus Infection through Tattooing and Piercing: A Critical Review," *Clinical Infectious Diseases* 54, no. 8 (2012): 1167–78, https://pubmed.ncbi.nlm.nih.gov/22291098.

7. Dayton Preslar and Judith Borger, "Body Piercing Infections," *Stat Pearls,* National Institutes of Health, National Library of Medicine, updated April 2020, https://www.ncbi.nlm.nih.gov /books/NBK537336.

8. Junaid Hanif et al., "'High' Ear Piercing and the Rising Incidence of Perichondritis of the Pinna," *British Medical Journal* 322 (April 2001): 906–7, https://www.ncbi.nlm.nih.gov/pmc /articles/PMC1120071/pdf/906.pdf.

9. "Ear Piercing and Acupuncture Points," 2016, https://www.acupuncture.org.uk/public-content /public-ask-an-expert/ask-an-expert-about-acupuncture/ask-an-expert-about-acupuncture-pressure-points/3231-ear-piercing-and-acupuncture-points.html.

CHAPTER 4

1. Dennis Watkins, "Painful Expectations," *Scientific American Mind* 290, no. 1 (January 2004), www.sciam.com/article.cfm?id=painful-expectations.

2. Tetsuo Koyama et al., "The Subjective Experience of Pain: Where Expectations Become Reality," *Proceedings of the National Academy of Sciences of the United States of America* 102, no. 36 (September 2005): 12950–55, www.pnas.org/content/102/36/12950.full.

3. Jerry Emanuelson, "Some Preliminary Information: The Prevalence of Needle Phobia," The Needle Phobia Page, accessed July 14, 2020, https://www.needlephobia.com/prevalence.html.

CHAPTER 5

1. Marilda H. T. Brandão et al., "Ear Piercing as a Risk Factor for Contact Allergy to Nickel," *Jornal de Pediatria* [*Journal of Pediatrics*, Brazil] 2, no. 86 (2010): 149–154, http://www.jped.com.br/conteudo/10-86-02-149/port.pdf.

CHAPTER 6

1. Brad Kelechava, "ISO Health Care Product Sterilization Standards Adopted by Association for the Advancement of Medical Instrumentation (AAMI)," *American National Standards Institute*, April 2018, https://blog.ansi.org/2018/04/iso-aami-health-sterilization-standard-adopt/#gref.

CHAPTER 8

1. Christophe André, "Proper Breathing Brings Better Health," *Scientific American*, January 2019, https://www.scientificamerican.com/article/proper-breathing-brings-better-health.

2. Kristin Anderson and Rose L. Hamm, "Factors That Impair Wound Healing," *Journal of the American College of Clinical Wound Specialists* 4 (2014): 84–91, https://www.ncbi.nlm.nih.gov/pmc/articles/PMC4495737.

3. "Find Green-e Certified Carbon Offsets," Green-e, 2020, https://www.green-e.org/certified-resources/carbon-offsets.

CHAPTER 9

1. Adam R. Puchalski and Inder J. Chopra, "Radioiodine Treatment of Differentiated Thyroid Cancer despite History of 'Iodine Allergy,'" *Endocrinology, Diabetes & Metabolism* (March 2014), https://www.ncbi.nlm.nih.gov/pmc/articles/PMC3965283.

2. "Facts about Iodine and Iodophors," 3M, 2016, https://multimedia.3m.com/mws/media/716284O/3m-skin-and-nasal-antiseptic-facts-about-iodine-and-iodophors.pdf.

CHAPTER 10

1. "About Gold Jewellery," World Gold Council, accessed July 14, 2020, https://www.gold.org/about-gold/about-gold-jewellery.

2. "Measuring Layer Thickness on Gold Plated Surfaces," Artisan Plating, accessed July 14, 2020, https://artisanplating.com/measuring-layer-thickness-on-gold-plated-surfaces.

CHAPTER 11

1. L. Kirkeby et al., "Immunoglobulins in Nasal Secretions of Healthy Humans: Structural Integrity of Secretory Immunoglobulin A1 (IgA1) and Occurrence of Neutralizing Antibodies to IgA1 Proteases of Nasal Bacteria," *Clinical and Diagnostic Laboratory Immunology* 7, no. 1 (January 2000): 31–39, https://www.ncbi.nlm.nih.gov/pmc/articles/PMC95818.

2. "Osteonecrosis," Medline Plus, National Institutes of Health, National Library of Medicine, updated July 8, 2020, https://medlineplus.gov/osteonecrosis.html.

CHAPTER 12

1. Francesco Covello et al., "Piercing and Oral Health: A Study on the Knowledge of Risks and Complications," *International Journal of Environmental Research and Public Health* 17, no. 2 (January 2020): 613, https://www.ncbi.nlm.nih.gov/pmc/articles/PMC7013412.

2. Dayton Preslar and Judith Borger, "Body Piercing Infections," *Stat Pearls*, National Institutes of Health, National Library of Medicine, updated April 23, 2020, https://www.ncbi.nlm.nih.gov/books/NBK537336.

3. Patricia A. Frese, "Oral Piercings: Implications for Dental Professionals," *Dental Continuing Education Course No. 423*, accessed July 15, 2020, https://www.dentalcare.com/en-us/professional-education/ce-courses/ce423/aftercare-for-piercings.

4. Tarwinder Rai, "Oral Piercings Can Cause Serious Dental Problems, Warns Dentist," *Medical Xpress*, July 2015, https://medicalxpress.com/news/2015-07-oral-piercings-dental-problems-dentist.html.

5. "Lip Piercing Can Lead to Receding Gums," *Science Daily*, March 2005, https://www.sciencedaily.com/releases/2005/03/050326010029.htm.

6. "Tongue Piercings Damage the Gums and Teeth," *Dentistry Today*, June 2018, https://dentistrytoday.com/news/industrynews/item/3467-tongue-piercings-damage-the-gums-and-teeth.

CHAPTER 13

1. David Schlossberg, *Infections of Leisure* (Herndon, VA: ASM Press, 2004), 409.

2. Samantha Lindsay, "Important: Read This before Getting a Belly Button Piercing," *PrepScholar*, July 2016, https://blog.prepscholar.com/belly-button-piercing.

3. "Umbilical Hernia," Mayo Clinic, May 2020, https://www.mayoclinic.org/diseases-conditions/umbilical-hernia/symptoms-causes/syc-20378685.

4. John-Paul Regan and Jesse T. Casaubon, "Abdominoplasty (Tummy Tuck)," *Stat Pearls*, National Institutes of Health, National Library of Medicine, updated May 2020, https://www.ncbi.nlm.nih.gov/books/NBK431058.

5. Katie Warchol, "How Your Blood Flow Helps Heal Wounds," *ProMedica HealthConnect*, updated March 2017, https://promedicahealthconnect.org/body-and-conditions/how-your-blood-flow-helps-heal-wounds.

6. Richard P. Schaedel, "The Karankawa of the Texas Gulf Coast," *Southwestern Journal of Anthropology* 5, no. 2 (Summer 1949): 117–37.

7. Kelly Shanahan, "10 Common Breast Cancer Myths Dispelled," *Breast Cancer Now*, September 2019, https://breastcancernow.org/information-support/have-i-got-breast-cancer/breast-cancer-causes/10-common-breast-cancer-myths-dispelled#piercing.

CHAPTER 14

1. H. A. Ramesh et al., "Wound Healing Activity of Human Urine in Rats," *Research Journal of Pharmaceutical, Biological and Chemical Sciences* 1, no. 3 (June 2010): 750–58, https://www.researchgate.net/publication/286888210_Wound_healing_activity_of_human_urine_in_rats.

2. J. Kenig, P. Richter, and Ł. Sikora, "Menstruation—Still a Contraindication to Elective Surgery?" *Polski przeglad chirurgiczny* [Polish Surgical Review] 86 (2014): 57–59, https://www.researchgate.net/publication/260431579.

3. Kayla McDonell, "7 Symptoms of Candida Overgrowth (Plus How to Get Rid of It)," Healthline, August 2017, https://www.healthline.com/nutrition/candida-symptoms-treatment.

4. Vaughn S. Millner et al., "First Glimpse of the Functional Benefits of Clitoral Hood Piercings," *American Journal of Obstetrics and Gynecology* 193, no. 3 (September 2005): 675–76.

5. Dictionary.com, s.v. "Labium (*n.*)," accessed July 15, 2020, https://www.dictionary.com/browse /labium.

6. Rebecca Chalker, *The Clitoral Truth: The Secret World at Your Fingertips* (New York: Seven Stories Press, 2002).

7. Simon LeVay, Janice Baldwin, and John Baldwin, *Discovering Human Sexuality*, 3rd ed. (New York: Sinauer Associates, Oxford University Press, 2015).

8. Kreklau et al., "Measurements of a 'Normal Vulva' in Women Aged 15–84: A Cross-Sectional Prospective Single-Centre Study," *British Journal of Obstetrics and Gynecology* (June 2018), https://obgyn.onlinelibrary.wiley.com/doi/10.1111/1471-0528.15387.

9. Ann E. Stapleton, "Systematic Review with Meta-Analysis of Cranberry-Containing Products Are Associated with a Protective Effect against Urinary Tract Infections," *Evidence Based Medicine* 18, no. 3 (June 2013): 110–11, https://www.ncbi.nlm.nih.gov/pmc/articles/PMC4091907.

10. Alvaro E. Donaire and Magda D. Mendez, "Hypospadias," *Stat Pearls*, National Institutes of Health, National Library of Medicine, May 2020, https://www.ncbi.nlm.nih.gov/books /NBK482122.

11. "A Glossary of Terms Relating to Circumcision, the Genitals & Urinary Organs," International Circumcision Forum, updated January 2020, http://www.circinfo.com/glossary/got-en-w.pdf.

12. Dr. B. Hagen, Deutsche Gesellschaft für Völkerkunde, "Die künstlichen Verunstaltungen des Körpers bei den Batta" [The Artificial Defacements of the Body in the Batta], *Zeitschrift für Ethnologie* 16 (1884): 217–25.

13. Brown, Edwards, and Moore, "The Penis Inserts of Southeast Asia," 4, 33.

14. "Foreskin Restoration for Circumcised Men," Circumcision Information and Resource Pages, August 2013, www.cirp.org/pages/restore.html.

CHAPTER 15

1. Miller-Keane and Marie O'Toole, "Wound Care," *Encyclopedia and Dictionary of Medicine, Nursing, & Allied Health*, 7th ed. (2003), https://medical-dictionary.thefreedictionary.com /wound+care.

2. Michael Mercandetti, "Wound Healing and Repair," Medscape, April 2, 2019, https:// emedicine.medscape.com/article/1298129-overview.

3. *The Free Dictionary*, accessed July 16, 2020, http://medical-dictionary.thefreedictionary.com /Sebum.

4. Philip Youderian, "Bacterial Motility: Secretory Secrets of Gliding Bacteria," *Current Biology* 8, no. 12 (June 1998), https://www.cell.com/current-biology/comments/S0960-9822(98)70264-7.

5. P. P. Hegde, A. T. Andrade, and K. Bhat, "Microbial Contamination of 'in Use' Bar Soap in Dental Clinics," *Indian Journal of Dental Research* 17, no. 2 (2006): 70–73, http://www.ijdr.in /article.asp?issn=0970-9290;year=2006;volume=17;issue=2;spage=70;epage=3;aulast=Hegde.

6. Paper Towel Drying with Warm Air Drying," *Infection Control and Hospital Epidemiology* 26, no. 3 (February 2005): 316–20, https://www.researchgate.net/publication/7940259_Efficiency_ of_Hand_Drying_for_Removing_Bacteria_from_Washed_Hands_Comparison_of_Paper_ Towel_Drying_with_Warm_Air_Drying.

7. Marla Raineri, "Help Injuries Heal Faster by Taking a Whole Body Health Approach," The BetterPT Blog, 2019, https://www.betterpt.com/post/help-injuries-heal-faster-by-taking-a-whole-body-health-approach.

8. S. A. Divya et al., "Role of Diet in Dermatological Conditions," *Journal of Nutrition & Food Sciences* 5, no. 5 (2015), https://www.longdom.org/open-access/role-of-diet-in-dermatological-conditions-2155-9600-1000400.pdf.

9. Nathaniel F. Watson et al., "Recommended Amount of Sleep for a Healthy Adult: A Joint Consensus Statement of the American Academy of Sleep Medicine and Sleep Research Society," *Sleep* 38, no. 6 (June 2015), https://www.ncbi.nlm.nih.gov/pmc/articles/PMC4434546.

10. Tracey J. Smith et al., "Impact of Sleep Restriction on Local Immune Response and Skin Barrier Restoration with and without 'Multinutrient' Nutrition Intervention," *Journal of Applied Physiology* (September 2017), https://pubmed.ncbi.nlm.nih.gov/28912361.

11. K. Ousey et al., "The Importance of Hydration in Wound Healing: Reinvigorating the Clinical Perspective," *Journal of Wound Care* 25, no. 3 (March 2016): 122–30, https://pubmed.ncbi.nlm.nih.gov/26947692.

12. Jean-Philippe Gouin and Janice K. Kiecolt-Glaser, "The Impact of Psychological Stress on Wound Healing: Methods and Mechanisms," *Immunology and Allergy Clinics of North America* 31, no. 1 (February 2011), https://www.sciencedirect.com/science/article/abs/pii/S0889856110000810.

13. Wayne Jonas, "Use Exercise to Increase Your Body's Ability to Heal," *Psychology Today*, December 2019, https://www.psychologytoday.com/us/blog/how-healing-works/201912/use-exercise-increase-your-body-s-ability-heal.

14. S. Chatterjee, A. Basu, and T. K. Choudhury, "A Comparative Study of Conventional Wound Irrigants and Their Effectiveness in Wound Healing," *Journal of Surgical Academia* 2, no. 2 (2012): 2–6, https://jsurgacad.com/sites/default/files/article/2012/02-MS1058%20(2-6).pdf.

15. R. Fernandez and R. Griffiths, "The Effects of Water Compared with Other Solutions for Wound Cleansing," *Cochrane Database of Systematic Reviews* 2 (2012), https://www.cochranelibrary.com/cdsr/doi/10.1002/14651858.CD003861.pub3/pdf/CDSR/CD003861/CD003861_abstract.pdf.

16. William C. Shiel Jr., "Medical Definition of Debridement," MedicineNet, December 2018, https://www.medicinenet.com/script/main/art.asp?articlekey=40481.

17. Jose Tarun et al., "Evaluation of pH of Bathing Soaps and Shampoos for Skin and Hair Care," *Indian Journal of Dermatology* 59, no. 5 (September–October 2014): 442–44, https://www.ncbi.nlm.nih.gov/pmc/articles/PMC4171909.

18. John Ross, "The Bacterial Horror of Hot Air Hand Dryers," Harvard Health Blog, May 2018, https://www.health.harvard.edu/blog/the-bacterial-horror-of-the-hot-air-hand-dryer-2018051113823.

19. U.S. Food & Drug Administration, "Antibacterial Soap? You Can Skip It, Use Plain Soap and Water," U.S. FDA Consumer Updates, May 2019, https://www.fda.gov/consumers/consumer-updates/antibacterial-soap-you-can-skip-it-use-plain-soap-and-water.

20. Gabriel W. Rangel, "Say Goodbye to Antibacterial Soaps: Why the FDA Is Banning a Household Item," Harvard University Science in the News, January 2017, http://sitn.hms.harvard.edu/flash/2017/say-goodbye-antibacterial-soaps-fda-banning-household-item.

21. Serhan Sakarya et al., "Hypochlorous Acid: An Ideal Wound Care Agent With Powerful Microbicidal, Antibiofilm, and Wound Healing Potency," *Wounds: A Compendium of Clinical Research and Practice* 226, no. 12 (November 2014): 342–50, https://www.researchgate.net/publication/272677446_Hypochlorous_Acid_An_Ideal_Wound_Care_Agent_With_Powerful_Microbicidal_Antibiofilm_and_Wound_Healing_Potency.

22. Michael H. Gold et al., "Topical Stabilized Hypochlorous Acid: The Future Gold Standard for Wound Care and Scar Management in Dermatologic and Plastic Surgery Procedures," *Journal of Cosmetic Dermatology* 19, no. 2 (February 2020): 270–77.

23. "Warm Compress or Soak," Drugs.com, February 2020, https://www.drugs.com/cg/warm-compress-or-soak.html.

24. Johan P. E. Junker et al., "Clinical Impact upon Wound Healing and Inflammation in Moist, Wet, and Dry Environments," *Advances in Wound Care* 2, no. 7 (September 2013): 346–358, https://www.liebertpub.com/doi/abs/10.1089/wound.2012.0412.

25. Kapil S. Agrawal et al., "Acetic Acid Dressings: Finding the Holy Grail for Infected Wound Management," *Indian Journal of Plastic Surgery* 50, no. 3 (September–December 2017): 273–80, https://www.ncbi.nlm.nih.gov/pmc/articles/PMC5868106.

26. Tamsyn Sa Thring, Pauline Hili, and Declan P. Naughton, "Antioxidant and Potential Anti-inflammatory Activity of Extracts and Formulations of White Tea, Rose, and Witch Hazel on Primary Human Dermal Fibroblast Cells," *Journal of Inflammation* 8, no 1 (October 2011): 27, https://pubmed.ncbi.nlm.nih.gov/21995704.

27. Allen Gabriel, "Wound Irrigation," Medscape, December 2017, https://emedicine.medscape.com/article/1895071-overview.

28. Junker et al., "Clinical Impact Upon Wound Healing," 346–358.

29. "Body Piercings: Cleaning and Healing," University Health Services, University of California, Berkeley, accessed July 16, 2020, https://uhs.berkeley.edu/health-topics/body-piercings.

30. "Body Piercings," UC Berkeley.

31. "Bactine Frequently Asked Questions: Usage," Bactine.com, accessed July 16, 2020, https://bactine.com.

32. "Body Piercings," UC Berkeley.

33. H. Schreier et al., "Molecular Effects of Povidone-Iodine on Relevant Microorganisms: An Electron-Microscopic and Biochemical Study," *Dermatology* (1997), https://www.karger.com/Article/Abstract/246043.

34. David J. Weber, William A. Rutala, and Emily E. Sickbert-Bennett, "Outbreaks Associated with Contaminated Antiseptics and Disinfectants," *Antimicrobial Agents and Chemotherapy* 51, no. 12 (December 2007): 4217–24; American Society for Microbiology, https://aac.asm.org/content/51/12/4217.

35. Pamela A. Brown and Julie Phelps Maloy, *Quick Reference to Wound Care*, 2nd ed. (Sudbury, MA: Jones and Bartlett Publishers, 2005), 33–39.

36. Hiroko-Miyuki Mori et al., "Wound Healing Potential of Lavender Oil by Acceleration of Granulation and Wound Contraction through Induction of TGF-β in a Rat Model," *BMC Complementary Alternative Medicine* 16 (2016): 144, https://www.ncbi.nlm.nih.gov/pmc/articles/PMC4880962.

37. Christiane Staiger, "Comfrey: A Clinical Overview," *Phytotherapy Research* 26, no. 10 (October 2012): 1441–48, https://www.ncbi.nlm.nih.gov/pmc/articles/PMC3491633.

38. C. F. Carson, K. A. Hammer, and T. V. Riley, "*Melaleuca alternifolia* (Tea Tree) Oil: A Review of Antimicrobial and Other Medicinal Properties," *Clinical Microbiology Reviews* 19, no. 1 (January 2006): 50–62, https://pubmed.ncbi.nlm.nih.gov/16418522.

39. Enrico de Lazaro, "Bioactive Compound in Essential Oils Enhances Wound Healing: Study," *Sci News*, December 31, 2019, http://www.sci-news.com/medicine/beta-carophyllene-essential-oils-wound-healing-07971.html.

40. Xiaoqing Guo and Nan Mei, "Aloe Vera: A Review of Toxicity and Adverse Clinical Effects," *Journal of Environmental Science and Health, Part C* 34, no. 2 (April 2, 2016): 77–96, https://www.ncbi.nlm.nih.gov/pmc/articles/PMC6349368.

41. Wilson Sim et al., "Antimicrobial Silver in Medicinal and Consumer Applications: A Patent Review of the Past Decade (2007–2017)," *Antibiotics* 7, no. 4 (December 2018): 93, https://www.ncbi.nlm.nih.gov/pmc/articles/PMC6315945.

42. Ananda A. Dorai, "Wound Care with Traditional, Complementary and Alternative Medicine," *Indian Journal of Plastic Surgery* 45, no. 2 (May–August 2012): 418–24, https://www.ncbi.nlm.nih.gov/pmc/articles/PMC3495394.

43. Charles P. Gerba, Craig Walis, and Joseph L. Melnick, "Microbiological Hazards of Household Toilets: Droplet Production and the Fate of Residual Organism," *Applied Microbiology* 30, no. 2 (August 1975): 229–37, http://aem.asm.org/cgi/content/ abstract/30/2/229.

44. David L. Johnson et al., "Lifting the Lid on Toilet Plume Aerosol: A Literature Review with Suggestions for Future Research," *American Journal of Infection Control* 41, no. 3 (2013): 254–58, https://www.ncbi.nlm.nih.gov/pmc/articles/PMC4692156.

45. Adam D. Munday et al., "Neutrophil-Derived Oxidants Induce a Gain-of-Function Phenotype in GPIbα," *Blood* 122, no. 21 (November 15, 2013): 3510, https://ashpublications.org/blood/article/122/21/3510/15312/Neutrophil-Derived-Oxidants-Induce-a-Gain-Of.

46. Zofia M. Prokopowicz et al., "Hypochlorous Acid: A Natural Adjuvant That Facilitates Antigen Processing, Cross-Priming, and the Induction of Adaptive Immunity," *Journal of Immunology* 184, no. 2 (January 2010): 824–35, https://www.jimmunol.org/content/jimmunol/184/2/824.full.pdf.

47. Sakarya et al., "Hypochlorous Acid," 342–50.

48. Gold et al., "Topical Stabilized Hypochlorous Acid," 270–77.

CHAPTER 16

1. Becky Ham, "Pre-Surgery Stress Linked to Signs of Slow Wound Healing," Health Behavior News Service, October 23, 2003, https://www.newswise.com/articles/pre-surgery-stress-linked-to-signs-of-slow-wound-healing; and Jean-Philippe Gouin, "The Impact of Psychological Stress on Wound Healing: Methods and Mechanisms," *Immunology and Allergy Clinics of North America* 31, no. 1 (February 2011), https://www.sciencedirect.com/science/article/abs/pii/S0889856110000810

2. Tracey Quail Davidoff, "Tattoos and Piercings: What the Urgent Care Provider Needs to Know," *The Journal of Urgent Care Medicine* (April 2018), https://www.jucm.com/tattoos-and-piercings-what-the-urgent-care-provider-needs-to-know.

3. Cindy M. Schorzman, "Common Complications Involved in Body Piercing," *Wounds International* 1, no. 5 (November 2010): 19–21, https://www.woundsinternational.com/journals/issue/482/article-details/common-complications-involved-in-body-piercing.

4. "Daniel Hindle Lip Piercing Death Prompts Advice Pack," *BBC News*, March 2011, https://www.bbc.com/news/uk-england-south-yorkshire-12743471.

5. Lippincott, *Lippincott's Nursing Procedures*, 6th ed. (Ambler, PA: Wolters Kluwer, Lippincott Williams & Wilkins, 2013).

6. Silvina B. Pugliese and Sharon E. Jacob, "A Review of Neomycin," *The Dermatologist* 23, no. 7 (July 2015), https://www.the-dermatologist.com/content/review-neomycin.

7. Donna Meltzer, "Complications of Body Piercing," *American Family Physician* 72, no. 10 (November 2005): 2029–34, https://www.aafp.org/afp/2005/1115/p2029.html.

8. V. Jacobs et al., "Mastitis Nonpuerperalis after Nipple Piercing: Time to Act," *International Journal of Fertility and Women's Medicine* 48, no. 5 (September/October 2003): 226–31, www.medscape.com/medline/abstract/14626379.

9. "Antibiotics Not Necessary to Treat Most Abscesses, Even in the Presence of MRSA," Infection Control Today, April 2007, https://www.infectioncontroltoday.com/view/antibiotics-not-necessary-treat-most-abscesses-even-presence-mrsa.

10. "Pyogenic Granuloma," Dermatologic Disease Database, accessed July 17, 2020, https://www.aocd.org/page/PyogenicGranuloma.

11. Elena Conde, "Overgranulation: When the Wound Bed Is Over-Activated," When a Wound in the Skin Won't Heal, January 2019, https://www.elenaconde.com/en/overgranulation-when-the-wound-bed-is-over-activated.

12. Bruno de Assis Quelemente, Ana Beatriz Pinto da Silva Morita, and Angelo Teixeira Balbi, "Use of Hypertonic Solutions of Sodium Chloride in Hypergranulating Wounds," *Revista de Enfermagem UFPE [Journal of Nursing, Brazil]* 3, no. 2 (March 2009), https://www.researchgate.net/publication/49594064_Use_of_hypertonic_solutions_of_sodium_chloride_in_hypergranulating_wounds.

13. "Folliculitis," Mayo Clinic, March 2018, https://www.mayoclinic.org/diseases-conditions/folliculitis/symptoms-causes/syc-20361634.

14. "Folliculitis," https://www.mayoclinic.org/diseases-conditions/folliculitis/diagnosis-treatment/drc-20361662.

15. Nancy Larson, "When You Should See a Doctor for a Cut or Scrape," Very Well Health, July 2020, https://www.verywellhealth.com/should-i-see-a-doctor-about-my-cut-or-scrape-1298587.

16. *Encyclopedia Britannica*, s.v. "Scar," accessed July 17, 2020, https://www.britannica.com/science/scar.

17. Rei Ogawa and Satoshi Akaishi, "Endothelial Dysfunction May Play a Key Role in Keloid and Hypertrophic Scar Pathogenesis—Keloids and Hypertrophic Scars May Be Vascular Disorders, *Medical Hypotheses* 96 (November 2016): 51–60, https://www.sciencedirect.com/science/article/pii/S0306987716302766.

18. David Jansen, "Keloids," Medscape, updated June 2020, https://emedicine.medscape.com/article/1298013-overview#a2.

19. Sarah Jane Commander et al., "Update on Postsurgical Scar Management," *Seminars in Plastic Surgery* 3, no. 3 (2016): 122–28, https://www.ncbi.nlm.nih.gov/pmc/articles/PMC4961501/pdf/10-1055-s-0036-1584824.pdf.

20. Jo-An M. Atkinson et al., "A Randomized, Controlled Trial to Determine the Efficacy of Paper Tape in Preventing Hypertrophic Scar Formation in Surgical Incisions That Traverse Langer's Skin Tension Lines," *Plastic and Reconstructive Surgery* 116, no. 6 (November 2005): 1648–56, https://pubmed.ncbi.nlm.nih.gov/16267427.

21. Anna I. Arno et al., "Up-to-Date Approach to Manage Keloids and Hypertrophic Scars: A Useful Guide," *Burns* 40, no. 7 (November 2014): 1255–66, https://www.sciencedirect.com/science/article/abs/pii/S0305417914000710.

22. Erica C. Davis and Valerie D. Callender, "Postinflammatory Hyperpigmentation: A Review of the Epidemiology, Clinical Features, and Treatment Options in Skin of Color," *The Journal of Clinical and Aesthetic Dermatology* 3, no. 7 (July 2010): 20–31, https://www.ncbi.nlm.nih.gov/pmc/articles/PMC2921758.

23. "Top Ten Contact Dermatitis Allergens Identified in Mayo Clinic Study," Science Daily, March 2006, https://www.sciencedaily.com/releases/2006/03/060303204044.htm.

24. "Nickel Allergy," Mayo Clinic, May 2019, https://www.mayoclinic.org/diseases-conditions/nickel-allergy/symptoms-causes/syc-20351529.

25. Maureen Choi, "Itchy Eyes? Why Your Manicure Is the Most Likely Culprit," *Living Healthy*, August 2017, https://www.livinghealthy.com/articles/itchy-eyes-why-your-manicure-is-the-most-likely-culprit.

26. "Nickel Allergy," https://www.mayoclinic.org/diseases-conditions/nickel-allergy/diagnosis-treatment/drc-20351534.

27. Michael Mercandetti, "Wound Healing and Repair," Medscape, April 2, 2019, https://emedicine.medscape.com/article/1298129-overview

28. Peter Ambe et al., "Swallowed Foreign Bodies in Adults," *Deutsches Arzteblatt International* 109, no. 50 (December 2012): 869–75, https://www.ncbi.nlm.nih.gov/pmc/articles/PMC3536040.

29. Scott DeBoer, Michelle McNeil, and Troy Amundson, "Body Piercing and Airway Management: Photo Guide to Tongue Jewelry Removal Techniques," *Journal of the American Association of Nurse Anesthetists* 76, no. 1 (February 2008): 19–23, https://www.ncbi.nlm.nih.gov/pubmed/18323315.

CHAPTER 17

1. Jung Hwa Park et al., "Effect of Cleaning and Sterilization on Titanium Implant Surface Properties and Cellular Response," *Acta Biomater* 8 no. 5 (May 2012): 1966–1975, https://pubmed.ncbi.nlm.nih.gov/22154860; Dayane de Melo Costa et al., "Reprocessing Safety Issues Associated with Complex-Design Orthopaedic Loaned Surgical Instruments and Implants," *Injury* 49, no. 11 (November 2018): 2005–12, https://pubmed.ncbi.nlm.nih.gov/30236794.

CHAPTER 18

1. Erica Skadsen, "General and Material Information," Organic Natural Body Jewelry, accessed July 18, 2020, www.organicjewelry.com/generalinfo.html.

2. R. V. Dietrich, "Horn," Central Michigan University College of Science and Technology, accessed July 18, 2020, http://stoneplus.cst.cmich.edu/zoogems/horn.html.

3. R. V. Dietrich, "Ivory," Central Michigan University College of Science and Technology, accessed July 18, 2020, http://stoneplus.cst.cmich.edu/zoogems/ivory.html.

4. "States Banning the Sale of Fossil Ivory and Proposed Legislation," *Journal of Paleontological Sciences* no. 14 (May 2020), https://aaps-journal.org/Fossil-Ivory-Legislation.html.

5. Wei Song et al., "Comparison of In Vitro Biocompatibility of Silicone and Polymethyl Methacrylate during the Curing Phase of Polymerization," *Journal of Biomedical Materials Research* 106 no. 7 (October 2018): 2693–99, https://pubmed.ncbi.nlm.nih.gov/29480542.

6. Mark Pellman, "PVD Coatings for Medical Device Applications (Physical Vapor Deposition)," *Products Finishing*, July 2000, https://www.pfonline.com/articles/pvd-coatings-for-medical-device-applications.

7. Sydney Whalen, "Subdermal Implants: Understanding the Risks of This Controversial Body Modification Trend," Zwivel, June 2017, https://www.zwivel.com/blog/subdermal-implants-body-modification.

8. Thomas Steffen et al., "Safety and Reliability of Radio Frequency Identification Devices in Magnetic Resonance Imaging and Computed Tomography," *Patient Safety in Surgery* 4, no. 1 (February 2010): 2, https://www.ncbi.nlm.nih.gov/pmc/articles/PMC2825188.

9. "Transdermal Implant," BMEzine.com Encyclopedia, accessed July 18, 2020, https://web.archive.org/web/20080829185756/http://wiki.bmezine.com/index.php/Transdermal_implant.

10. Deborah Addington, *Play Piercing* (Emeryville, CA: Greenery Press, 2011).

CHAPTER 19

1. Scott DeBoer et al., "Body Piercing/Tattooing and Trauma Diagnostic Imaging: Medical Myths vs. Realities," *Journal of Trauma Nursing* 14, no. 1 (January–March 2007): 35–38.

2. "Oral Piercing Risks & Safety Measures," Association of Professional Piercers, accessed March 9, 2021, https://safepiercing.org/oral-piercing-risks-safety-measures.

3. "Frequently Asked Questions: Should I Remove My Body Piercing?," Transportation Security Administration, accessed July 18, 2020, https://www.tsa.gov/travel/frequently-asked-questions.

4. Amos Grunebaum, "Body Piercings during Pregnancy: Are They Safe," BabyMed, June 2020, https://www.babymed.com/body-piercings-during-your-pregnancy-are-they-safe.

5. Brigette Lee et al., "Complications Associated with Intimate Body Piercings," *Dermatology Online Journal* 24, no. 7 (July 2018): 2, https://escholarship.org/content/qt5gp333zr/qt5gp333zr.pdf.

6. "Nipple Piercing," National Institutes of Health, Drugs and Lactation Database, National Library of Medicine, December 2018, https://www.ncbi.nlm.nih.gov/books/NBK500564/pdf /Bookshelf_NBK500564.pdf.

CHAPTER 20

1. Jen Gunter, "Condoms with Extras? No Thanks," *The New York Times*, February 2020, https://www.nytimes.com/2020/02/07/well/condoms-with-extras-no-thanks.html.

2. "Pierced Clit," Columbia University Health Services, Go Ask Alice!, March 2017, https://goaskalice.columbia.edu/answered-questions/pierced-clit.

3. "Desensitization," BMEzine Encyclopedia, accessed July 19, 2020, https://wiki.bme.com/index .php?title=Desensitization.

CHAPTER 21

1. Support Tattoos and Piercings at Work, accessed July 19, 2020, https://www.stapaw.com.

2. "Guide to the Wear and Appearance of Army Uniforms and Insignia, Army Regulation 670-1," Department of the Army, May 2017, https://armypubs.army.mil/epubs/DR_pubs/DR_a/pdf /web/ARN6028_DAPam670-1_Web_FINAL.pdf.

3. "Tattooing and Body Piercing State Laws Statutes and Regulations," The National Conference of State Legislature, March 2019, https://www.ncsl.org/research/health/tattooing-and-body-piercing.aspx.

CHAPTER 22

1. "APP Suggested Apprentice Body Piercer Guidelines and Curriculum (2019 ed.)," Association of Professional Piercers, https://safepiercing.org/become-a-piercer.

APPENDIX C

1. Jennifer Rudden, "Homeownership Rates in the United States from 1990 to 2019," Statista, March 2020, https://www.statista.com/statistics/184902/homeownership-rate-in-the-us-since-2003/.

Glossary

A

abdominoplasty: Cosmetic surgery of the abdomen; *also* tummy tuck

abscess: Pus-filled pocket of infection trapped under the skin

acrylic: General term for many varieties of plastic, including those sold under the brand names Plexiglass and Lucite

adipose: Containing fat; found in the tissue just below the dermis

adjuvant: Substance that enhances the immune system's response to the presence of a toxin or foreign invader

aerosolize: To become airborne in microscopic particles

aesthetics: Physical appearance, especially when considered pleasing

aftercare: Wound care; the treatment given healing piercings

alar cartilage: Cartilage on the sides of the nose that is commonly pierced in a nostril piercing

allicin: Onion or garlic extract, used in scar-reduction products

alloy: A mixture of metals and elements combined to create different properties than the materials have individually

American ampallang: Horizontal glans penis piercing that does not pass through the urethra

American Society for Testing and Materials (ASTM): Now ASTM International; organization that provides technical standards for materials, products, and systems

American Wire Gauge (AWG): Standard of measurement for wire thickness used for sizing American body jewelry and piercing needles; *also* Brown & Sharpe

ampallang: Genital piercing that passes horizontally through the head of the penis; *see also* American ampallang and European ampallang

anaphylaxis: Life-threatening allergic reaction

anatomy: Physical structure; one of the factors in piercing placement

anchor: *See* surface anchor

ankyloglossia: Greek for "crooked tongue." *See* tongue-tied

anneal: To heat and cool a metal, alloy, or glass to specific temperatures at certain time intervals to change its properties

anodize: Process of altering the way a metal surface refracts light (which appears to change its color) by creating an oxide film

anti-care: *See* dry wound care

anti-eyebrow piercing: *See* teardrop piercing

antihelix: Curved elevation of cartilage in front of the helix that runs parallel to it; the mid-antihelix is the site of the snug piercing

antimicrobial: Chemical substance that inhibits or destroys microbes such as bacteria, viruses, and fungi

antitragus: Small vertical ridge of cartilage above the earlobe (next to the intertragus notch)

apadravya: Genital piercing that passes vertically through the head of the penis; comprising a Prince Albert piercing on the bottom and a reverse Prince Albert piercing on the top

apex: Highest point; in piercing, the deepest anatomical point, such as under the clitoral hood or inside the navel

APP: *See* Association of Professional Piercers

arterioles: Tiny arteries that transport oxygenated blood from the heart to the capillaries

aseptic: Free of disease-causing microorganisms

Ashley: Piercing in the center of the lower lip

aspirate: To inhale into your lungs

Association of Professional Piercers (APP): International nonprofit membership organization dedicated to the dissemination of vital health and safety information related to body piercing to piercees, piercers, health care providers, legislators, and the general public

atrophic scar: Pit or depression below the surface of the skin, caused by a wound

Austin bar: Horizontal surface piercing at the tip of the nose

autoclave: Machine used for sterilizing equipment or materials

avascular: Not well supplied with fluid and ducts, especially blood circulation of veins, arteries, and capillaries

AWG: *See* American Wire Gauge

B

bacterial endocarditis: *See* infective endocarditis

bacteriostatic: Restricts growth and activity of microorganisms

Bactroban: Prescription-only antibiotic effective for topical treatment of localized infections; *also* mupirocin

barbell: Basic body jewelry style; a bar post and two ends that are often spherical in shape

bar-style jewelry: Body jewelry with a post portion that functions like a barbell

basal cells: Base layer of skin cells; the first layer of cells formed in wound healing

BCR: Ball closure ring. *See* captive bead ring

BDSM: Combined acronym referring to bondage and discipline (BD), domination and submission (DS), and sadomasochism (SM); consensual forms of human sexual behavior

belly button: *See* navel

benign: Not a threat to life or long-term health; noncancerous

bent bar: *See* curved barbell

Betadine: Iodine-based surgical scrub commonly used to clean the skin before piercing

biocompatible: Suited for wear in the body without causing irritation, allergy, or infection

biofilm: Thin, slimy adherent layer of microbes that can cause wound infection

biohazard can: Waste receptacle used for disposables (other than needles) that may contain blood or blood products

biohazard room: *See* sterilization room

biological indicator: *See* spore test

biopsy punch: *See* dermal punch

bloodborne disease: Illness caused by exposure to bloodborne pathogens such as HIV or hepatitis B or C

bloodborne pathogen: Microorganism that can cause disease when present in blood

blood poisoning: *See* septicemia

blowout: Complication from overstretching; skin pushes out from inside the piercing

body modification: Practices that change the body, including piercing, tattooing, branding, and scarification

borosilicate: Type of glass used for body jewelry, laboratory beakers

bottom: Submissive partner in a BDSM scene or relationship

bridge piercing: Horizontal piercing through the tissue between the eyes or a little lower, on the bridge of the nose; *also* Erl, nasion, or mid-brow

Brown & Sharpe: Standard of measurement for wire gauge (thickness); *also* American Wire Gauge

bull ring: *See* circular barbell

C

caliper: Instrument used to measure internal or external dimensions of jewelry and other objects

candidiasis: Overgrowth of a fungus, *Candida albicans*; called a yeast infection

cannula: Needle covered with a flexible sleeve, commonly used for piercing in Europe; *also* catheter needle

captive: Captive bead ring; *also* the captive bead or other captive piece or ornament

captive bead: Closure that fits in the gap of a captive bead ring to secure the jewelry; *also* captive

captive bead ring: Ring with a captive bead or captive piece that can be changed or replaced

captive circular barbell: Circular barbell with a captive bead added to the center

captive piece: An alternate ornament or design that is worn in a captive bead ring and functions the same way as a captive bead

captive tube: Cylindrical captive piece suited to healed piercings

cartilage: Dense, avascular tissue that is commonly pierced in the upper ear and nostril

catheter needle: *See* cannula

CBR: *See* captive bead ring

cellulitis: Inflammation of the cells; spreading infection of tissues beneath the skin

chamfer needle: *See* O-needle

cheese-cutter effect: Cutting of tissue caused by jewelry that is too thin in gauge

Christina: Vertical surface piercing at the top of the cleft of Venus, extending up the pubic mound; *also* Venus

circular barbell: Ring-style jewelry that operates like a barbell: the ends screw off and on; *also* bull ring or horseshoe

cleft of Venus: Furrow at the base of the pubic mound where it divides to form the labia majora; *also* pudendal cleft

clicker: Hinged jewelry style commonly worn in septum and daith piercings

clitoral glans: External portion of the clitoris usually covered by the clitoral hood; *also* clitoral head

clitoral head: *See* clitoral glans

clitoral hood: Protective fold of tissue that covers the clitoral glans; *also* prepuce

clitoris: Highly sensitive erectile organ at the front of the vulva

cold abscess: Infection of *Mycobacterium abscessus* (lacks tenderness and inflammation)

cold sterilant: Hospital-strength liquid disinfectants that reduce the number of microorganisms; not accepted as a sole sterilization method for piercing equipment or jewelry

collagen: Fibrous protein that provides strength and resilience to skin

compression technique: Application of firm pressure following cartilage piercing to reattach surface tissue to the cartilage underneath to prevent bumps during healing

compression therapy: Continuous mechanical pressure used to flatten scars

concave taper: An insertion taper shaped at the back end to fit with a convex jewelry end

conch: Deep bowl-shaped central shell of the ear; *also* concha

concha: *See* conch

conch piercing: Piercing of the conch

contact dermatitis: Skin rash from contact with an allergen or irritant substance

contaminate: Make unclean, especially as a result of contact with something harmful such as disease-causing microorganisms

contraction: Step in the second phase of the healing process in which the edges of the wound pull together

coronal ridge: Flared rim of tissue on the glans

C-ring: Circular barbell widened to conform to anatomy; same as a U-ring, but less open

crus helix: *Also* crus of helix; *see* helix crus

crusties: Nonmedical term for the normal dried discharge around healing piercings

cryotherapy: Treatment using cold or ice

CSR wrap: Moisture-repellent, autoclavable material used as a sterile protective drape around the area being pierced

curette: A medical tool with a small loop on the end that can be used to support tissue for certain piercings

curve: *See* curved barbell

curved barbell: Barbell variation that forms approximately one-fourth of a circle; *also* bent bar and curve

cytotoxic: Poisonous or harmful to cells

D

Dahlia: Set of piercings near the corners of the mouth; *also* Dahlia bites or Joker bites

Dahlia bites: *See* Dahlia

daith: Piercing of the innermost ridge of cartilage just above the ear canal at the root of the helix crus

dead stretching: Expansion of a piercing simply by pushing in a larger object

debridement: Removal of dead, contaminated, or adherent tissue or foreign material from a wound

deep Prince Albert piercing: Prince Albert piercing placed further down the penis shaft

dental dam: Sheet of latex or polyurethane used in dental procedures; can shield the vulva to prevent sharing of bodily fluids during oral sexual contact

depilation: Removal of hair via shaving, waxing, depilatory cream, laser, or other means

dermal anchor: *See* surface anchor

dermal elevator: Tool used to lift the tissue to create cavities for insertion of subdermal or transdermal implants; *also* dermal separator

dermal punch: Medical tool for tissue biopsies; can be used to create a piercing; *also* biopsy punch

dermal separator: *See* dermal elevator

dermis: Thick layer beneath the epidermis containing connective tissue, hair follicles, blood and lymph vessels, sweat and oil glands, and nerves

development: Lasting change in the shape, dimensions, and texture of localized tissue following piercing

deviated septum: A displacement from the midline of the tissue that divides the nostrils

Diana piercing: *See* Princess Diana piercing

disinfection: Process of reducing the number of microorganisms from a surface or object by applying antimicrobial chemical agents

divot: Small depression in the skin left by piercing; also refers to the infranasal depression between mouth and nose

dolphin piercing: Deep Prince Albert piercing connected by a single piece of jewelry to a traditional Prince Albert piercing

D-ring: Variation of the captive ring; the flat part of the D is worn through a piercing

dry wound care: No wetting or washing of the area for weeks or months and all care or cleaning products are avoided; *also* anti-care

dydoe piercing: Genital piercing through the coronal rim of the glans penis

E

ear cartilage piercing: General term for an ear piercing that is not through the soft tissue of the earlobe; also traditional placement through the helix (or through the scapha near the helix)

earlet: *See* eyelet

ear-piercing gun: Device used to insert a pointed earring (not used by professional piercers)

edema: Swelling caused by a buildup of excess fluid in the tissues

energy pull: *See* pull

epidermis: Thin outermost layer of skin; protects the dermis just beneath it

episiotomy: Incision made to enlarge the vaginal opening to facilitate childbirth

epithelial cells: Skin cells; cells forming the protective covering on most external and internal surfaces of the body and its organs

epithelialization: Process in the growth phase of wound healing involving the formation of skin to completely cover a wound as epithelial cells grow together and thicken

Erl piercing: *See* bridge piercing

essential oils: Concentrated liquid plant compounds

European ampallang: Horizontal glans penis piercing that passes through the urethra

externally threaded jewelry: Style in which the threads are on the part of the jewelry that passes through the body

eyelet: Hollow tube-style jewelry worn through the body, usually in stretched piercings; also earlet or grommet

F

female circumcision: *See* female genital cutting (FGC)

female genital cutting (FGC): Alteration or partial or entire removal of external genitalia of a girl for cultural or religious reasons; *also* female genital mutilation (FGM) and female circumcision

female genital mutilation (FGM): *See* female genital cutting (FGC)

female guiche: *See* fourchette piercing

ferromagnetic: Magnetic; attracted by a magnet

fibula: Fastening device historically used for infibulation (to ensure chastity)

fifth cranial nerve: *See* trigeminal nerve

fistula: Flesh tunnel; the channel that forms when a piercing heals (epithelializes) with jewelry inside it

flare-up: Regression in healing as a piercing secretes and becomes inflamed and/or tender

flash-cycle cassette sterilizer: *See* StatIM

flatback barbell: *See* labret stud

flora: Microorganisms (primarily bacteria) that normally inhabit a part of the body

Foerster sponge forceps: A medical clamp with an oval head commonly used to support and secure tissue, especially for tongue piercings

folliculitis: Inflammation and infection in or around a hair follicle

forceps: Medical grasping tool used by some piercers to secure and support tissue for piercing

foreskin piercing: Piercing of the skin covering the glans of the penis

forward helix piercing: Placed at the root of the helix, the juncture of the ear cartilage and the face

fourchette: "Little fork" in French; *See* fourchette piercing

fourchette piercing: Vertical piercing at the rear border of the vaginal opening

fraenum: *See* frenulum

freehand: Piercing method in which the only tool used is a piercing needle (no forceps or needle receiving tubes)

frenulum: Fibrous cord of connecting tissue

frenulum labiorum pudenda: Anatomical term for location of the fourchette piercing

frenum ladder: Multiple frenum piercings placed in a row

frenum loop: Band worn around the penis shaft secured by a barbell through a healed frenum piercing

frenum piercing: Genital piercing through the pliable tissue on the penis shaft

frowny: Piercing of the lower lip frenulum

fungi: Microorganisms, including mold and yeast, that feed off other organisms to survive; can cause infection; *sing.* fungus

G

gauge: Numerical standard of measurement for thickness of metal wire; sometimes used as a verb to mean stretching a piercing, or as a noun referring to a stretched hole or the jewelry worn in one

gauging: Colloquial term for stretching

gauging up: *See* gauging

genital beading: Implant in which beads are placed within genital tissue to add sensation and/or alter appearance

genital ribs: Variation of genital beading in which rod-shaped pieces are used

gentian violet: Purple water-based fungicide used as ink in surgical markers and other methods of marking piercing placement

germicidal: Kills microorganisms that cause disease

glabella: Anatomical term for tissue between the brows; location of the bridge piercing

glans: Head of the penis or tip of the clitoris

Golden Rule of Piercing Hygiene: Do not touch healing piercings with unwashed hands

gold-filled: *See* gold-plated

gold-overlay: *See* gold-plated

gold-plated: Base metal coated with a thin layer of gold to create affordable jewelry with the look of gold; *also* gold-filled, gold-overlay, rolled gold, and vermeil

Gräfenberg spot: *See* G-spot

granulation: Phase in the second stage of the healing process; body produces cells, including collagen and elastin

granulation tissue: Small, grainy tissue particles that grow to cover healing wounds

grommet: *See* eyelet

growth phase: Second stage of the wound healing process that includes granulation and contraction; *also* proliferative phase

G-spot: Sexually sensitive area on the front wall of the vagina; *also* Gräfenberg spot

guiche: A piercing located in the perineum, behind the scrotum and across the perineal raphe

H

hafada piercing: Scrotum piercing, especially when placed on one or both sides in the upper portion of the natural fold

half gauges: Odd-numbered gauge sizes in between the usual even-numbered sizes used for body jewelry and equipment

Heimlich maneuver: Upward abdominal thrusts to dislodge an obstruction stuck in the windpipe

helix: Curled outer rim of the external ear; location for the traditional ear cartilage piercing

helix crus: Anatomical term for daith piercing placement at the innermost ridge of cartilage just above the ear canal; *also* crus helix and crus of helix

helix root: Where the curl of the helix originates at the top of the ear nearest the head; location of the forward helix piercing

hemostasis: Stoppage of bleeding; part of the first stage of early wound healing

hill: In contrast to *valley*, an anatomical rise or ridge; genitals in which the clitoral hood is pronounced and higher than the outer labia

HOCl: *See* hypochlorous acid

horseshoe: *See* circular barbell

hyperextend: Go beyond the normal range of movement for the body or a joint

hypergranulation tissue: Excessive growth of granulation tissue

hypertonic: Containing more salt than human fluids (as opposed to *isotonic*)

hypertrophic scar: Thick, lumpy scar that sits above the surface of the skin

hypochlorous acid: Broad-spectrum antimicrobial and anti-inflammatory used topically for wound care; *also* HOCl

hypospadias: Congenital anomaly in which the urinary meatus is not located at the tip of the penis

I

implant: Extreme body modification in which a foreign object is placed beneath the skin; includes subdermal and transdermal implants

implant designation: Numbered codes that represent a precise standard for a material from the American (now International) Society for Testing and Materials (ASTM) and/or the International Standards Organization (ISO)

implant grade: An implant designation for material with biocompatibility levels accepted for medical implant usage

induration: Localized hardening of normally soft tissue, often seen in wounds or infections

industrial: *See* industrial piercing

industrial piercing: Single barbell through two or more piercings, usually across the top of the ear cartilage; *also* industrial, industrial project, or scaffold piercing

industrial project: *See* industrial piercing; also can indicate a more elaborate combination or uncommon placement

infection: Invasion and multiplication of disease-causing microorganisms, producing an injurious effect

infective endocarditis: Potentially deadly infection of the inner lining of the heart or heart valves (previously referred to as bacterial endocarditis)

inferior crus of the antihelix: Small ridge of cartilage that originates near the face in the upper part of the ear; anatomical term for the location of the rook piercing

infibulation: Restriction of sexual activity through mechanical means

inflammation: Normal, localized protective response to injury that protects the body from infection but is problematic if it becomes chronic

inflammatory phase: First stage in the process of wound healing; includes hemostasis and the laying down of basal cells

infranasal depression: Natural midline dip between mouth and the nose; site of philtrum piercing; *also* divot

infused herbal oil: Essential oil mixed into an oil base

infusion: Tea from flowers, leaves, or roots steeped longer than usual to extract their properties

inner conch: True conch piercing in the concha of the ear

inner labia: Delicate hairless folds of flesh situated between the outer labia; *also* labia minora

innie: Concave navel configuration

insertion: To put jewelry into an existing piercing; *also* jewelry insertion and reinsertion

insertion pin: *See* insertion taper

insertion taper: Tool used to facilitate jewelry insertion or reinsertion and for stretching piercings to a thicker gauge; *also* insertion pin, or taper

intact: An uncircumcised penis

interdigital spaces: Between the fingers or toes

internally threaded: Jewelry with the threads on the ball or end; the portion that passes through the body is tapped with a hole to receive the threads

interstitial fluid: Liquid between cells of the body; a component of crusties

intertragus notch: Groove at the bottom of the opening to the ear canal above the earlobe and below the tragus

inverse vertical labret: Vermillion piercing in the center of the lip that exits inside the mouth

iron cross: Combination of a horizontal and vertical piercing, usually in a nipple or penis head; also magic cross

irrigation: *See* wound irrigation

isotonic: Matches the salinity of human fluids (as in normal saline, 0.9 percent sodium chloride solution)

ivory: Dentine portion of a mammal's tooth

J

J-bar: *See* J-curve

J-curve: J-shaped barbell variation suited to VCH and navel piercings

jewelry insertion: *See* insertion

Joker bites: *See* Dahlia

K

karat: Measure of gold purity; 24 karat is pure gold, 18 karat is 18 parts gold out of 24 parts metal in an alloy

keloid: Large, dense growth of excessive scar tissue much bigger than the original wound

keratin: Fibrous protein that is not water soluble; one of the components of sebum

keratinocyte: Primary type of cells in the epidermis

L

labia: "Lip" in Latin; external skin folds of the vulva; *sing.* labium

labia majora: *See* outer labia

labia minora: *See* inner labia

labret piercing: Lip piercing; from the Latin *labrum*

labret stud: Short barbell with a disc on one end and an ornament (ball, gem, etc.) on the other; *also* flatback barbell

ladder: Rows of piercings, commonly of frenum, labia, or other genital placement

laparoscopy: Medical procedure in which instruments are inserted through small incisions; frequently done in the navel

L-bend: L-shaped jewelry worn in a nostril piercing

lingual frenulum: Thin web of tissue connecting the tongue to the floor of the mouth

LITHA: Minimal aftercare consisting of regular hygiene; acronym for Leave It the Heck Alone

lobule: Fleshy portion of the earlobe; the lobe

localized argyria: Permanent dark discoloration of skin caused by exposure to silver or silver salts; *also* tarnish tattoo

lorum piercing: Horizontal piercing where the penis meets the scrotum

lumen: Space inside a tubular structure, such as the hollow interior of a needle or receiving tube

lymph: Pale fluid of the lymphatic vessels; chiefly plasma and white blood cells

M

magic cross: *See* iron cross

mandible: Lower jawbone or vertical piercing under the tongue, through the floor of the mouth to the underside of the jaw; *also* sprung

Master Piercer: Honorary title earned for expertise, dedication, and contributions to professional piercing bestowed by another Master Piercer

maturation: Final stage in the wound healing process in which the collagen becomes more organized and strengthens; *also* remodeling

Medusa: *See* philtrum piercing

microbe: Microscopic organism such as a bacterium or fungus, especially one that can transmit disease

microbicide: A substance that kills microbes

microdermal: *See* surface anchor

mid-brow: Location and alternate name of the bridge piercing

midline: In the center; structure or imaginary line that divides the body into left and right halves

migration: When a piercing moves from its original position; either settles and heals, or continues to move and rejects

mill certificates: Documents to provide evidence of a particular grade of metal; *also* mill certs or mill test certificates

mill certs: *See* mill certificates

mill test certificates: *See* mill certificates

mini barbell: Barbells in small gauges suited to above-the-neck piercings

mirror finish: High-shine, super-smooth surface

mons pubis: *See* pubic mound

mons veneris: *See* pubic mound

motility: Ability to move independently (exhibited by some bacteria)

mupirocin: *See* Bactroban

Mycobacterium abscessus: *See* cold abscess

N

nasallang: Industrial piercing of the nose through both nostrils and septum

nasion: Area between the eyes; location for bridge piercing

nasolabial folds: Smile lines around the mouth extending roughly from the corners of the nose to the corners of the mouth

natural materials: Horn, bone, wood, amber, stone, and other materials that are worn in healed piercings; *also* organics

navel: Scar left where the umbilical cord was attached; *also* umbilicus and belly button

necrosis: Death of tissue or cells caused by injury or disease

needle blade: Type of needle used in the United States for piercing; *also* piercing needle

needle blanks: Metal tubes in a range of sizes that can be used as disposable transfer pins, insertion tapers, and receiving tubes

needle receiving tube: Hollow tube used in piercing procedures; *also* receiving tube and NRT

negative space: Area between or around; unpierced skin left between holes for aesthetics and safety

nesting: Normal tendency of oral jewelry to indent a millimeter or so into the soft tissue

nipple development: *See* development

noncytotoxic: Doesn't kill cells

nonferromagnetic: Not magnetic; not affected by a magnet

noniodized: Without iodine

normal saline: Isotonic sodium chloride solution, having the same salt concentration (0.9 percent) as body fluids

nose bone: Short post worn in a nostril piercing with a tiny ball that is passed through the tissue to keep the jewelry in place

nostril piercing: Cartilage piercing on the side of the nose

nostril screw: Post-style jewelry with a curved tail that rests inside the nostril or behind the ear; does not require a backing like a traditional stud earring

NRT: *See* needle receiving tube

O

Occupational Safety and Health Administration (OSHA): US government agency that regulates workplace safety

O-needle: Piercing needle with a sharp circular bevel instead of a pointed tip, that may be used for cartilage and surface piercings; *also* chamfer needle

Orbital: Two piercings joined together with a ring

organics: *See* natural materials

orofacial piercing: Piercing from the exterior facial surface through to the interior of the mouth; includes piercings of the upper and lower lips

OSHA: *See* Occupational Safety and Health Administration

outer conch: Piercing in the scapha or anti-helix nearer the concha area than the helix

outer labia: Thick fleshy folds of the vulva where hair grows; *also* labia majora

outie: Protruding navel configuration

P

PA: *See* Prince Albert piercing

palang: Term used by the Dyaks in Borneo for piercing of the penis head and the object ("crossbar") worn in it; apparent origin of the word *ampallang*

palladium: Inert elemental metal sometimes alloyed with gold or platinum for jewelry

PA piercing: *See* Prince Albert piercing

parotid duct: Conduit for saliva from the parotid gland

parotid gland: Largest of the salivary glands

pathogenic: Able to cause disease

pathogens: Germs such as bacteria or viruses that can cause disease

Pennington forceps: A medical clamp with a triangular jaw commonly used to support and secure tissue for piercing

perineal raphe: Faint ridge of tissue that runs from scrotum to anus; location of guiche piercing

perineum: Area between the anus and the rear part of the external genitalia; location of guiche and fourchette piercings

peritoneum: Membrane that lines and protects the abdominal cavity

philtrum piercing: In the natural indentation between mouth and nose (the infranasal depression); *also* Medusa, divot, and upret

phlebotomy: *See* venipuncture

physical vapor deposition: *See* PVD

pierce and stretch: Technique of making a piercing, then immediately stretching it larger using an insertion taper (not recommended)

Piercee's Bill of Rights: List of piercees' rights by the Association of Professional Piercers

piercing needle: Super-sharp beveled needle made specifically for performing piercings; *also* needle blade

pin-coupling taper: Insertion taper style; the back end is a pin shaped to fit inside internally threaded or threadless jewelry

plasma: Liquid part of blood composed of serum, water, salt, enzymes, antibodies, proteins, and clotting factors

platinum: Inert, expensive, precious, elemental metal suited for piercing jewelry

play piercing: Temporary piercings; insertion of a needle or needles (and occasionally jewelry) for a performance, ritual, or BDSM or erotic scene

pneumothorax: Collapsed lung caused by air in the space between the lung and chest wall

polymer: In piercing, inert synthetic plastics such as PTFE that are commonly used for retainers

Polytetrafluoroethylene: *See* PTFE

povidone iodine: *See* Betadine

preauricular pit: Tiny natural hole in the skin that is sometimes present where a forward helix piercing is placed

prepuce: Fold of tissue that covers the glans; the clitoral hood or foreskin

Prince Albert piercing: Genital piercing on the underside of the penis at the juncture of the head and shaft; jewelry rests inside the urethra and is worn out the tip of the urinary meatus

Princess Albertina: Piercing of the female urinary meatus

Princess Diana piercing: Genital piercing placed under the clitoral hood like a VCH piercing, but off to the side(s)

proliferative phase: *See* growth phase

prophylaxis: Preventive treatment

PTFE: Inert, flexible, autoclavable form of Teflon used as a nonmetallic jewelry alternative; *also* Polytetrafluoroethylene

pubic mound: Soft pad of rounded flesh on the pubic bone present in all genders; *also* pubis, mons pubis, and mons veneris (when above the vulva)

pubis: *See* pubic mound

pudendal cleft: *See* cleft of Venus

pull: Temporary piercing(s) are tethered and pulled in a controlled manner to achieve certain mental or physical states; *also* energy pull

pus: Thick, opaque fluid consisting of white blood cells, dead cells, and bacteria; produced by inflammation and infection

pustule: Small round area of inflamed skin with a visible collection of pus; a pimple

PVD: High-tech version of electroplating deposits a durable film of black, copper, and other colors; used on body jewelry and in other industries; *also* physical vapor deposition

pyogenic granuloma: *See* hypergranulation tissue

Q

Q-tip test: Placing a lubricated swab beneath the clitoral hood to check anatomical suitability (sufficient depth) for a VCH piercing

R

receiving tube: *See* needle receiving tube

reinsertion: Inserting jewelry in a piercing that has been left empty

rejection: Piercing migration in which jewelry is pushed completely out of the body

relaxing: *See* resting

remodeling: *See* maturation

resorption: Erosion of bone, cartilage, gum, or other tissue, which is absorbed by the body

resting: Practice of removing large-gauge jewelry for a time to relieve tissue of weight and pressure; *also* relaxing

retainer: Alternative worn in a piercing for concealment, or to keep it open when ordinary jewelry must be removed, such as for sports or medical care

retiring: Removing jewelry to abandon a piercing

reverse PA: *See* reverse Prince Albert piercing

reverse Prince Albert piercing: Vertical midline piercing from the urethra to the top of the penis glans, the upper part of an apadravya piercing; *also* reverse PA

reverse vertical labret: *See* inverse vertical labret

ring expanding pliers: *See* ring opening pliers

ring opening pliers: Jewelry tool used to widen a ring, usually for inserting a captive bead or to spread the gap of a circular barbell into a C-ring or U-ring; *also* ROP, snap-ring pliers, ring expanding pliers, or RXP

ring-style jewelry: Jewelry style that functions like a ring, including the circular barbell

rolled gold: *See* gold-plated

rook piercing: Placement through the small ridge of cartilage that originates near the face in the upper part of the ear (the inferior crus of the antihelix)

ROP: *See* ring opening pliers

RXP: *See* ring opening pliers

S

sadhu piercing: Lower conch piercing, especially in a large gauge

scaffold piercing: *See* industrial piercing

scalpelling: Using the cutting instrument to create or enlarge a piercing

scapha: Elongated depression of the ear that separates the helix and antihelix

scar: Mark left in the skin by the healing of a wound

screw threads: *See* threads

scrumper: *See* smiley

seam ring: Jewelry style that must be bent for insertion and removal

sebum: Naturally occurring product of the body that collects in healed piercing channels; contains fat, keratin, and cellular material from oil glands

septicemia: Severe total body infection caused by harmful microorganisms throughout the bloodstream; *also* blood poisoning

septril: Midline piercing between the nostrils into a stretched septum piercing

septum forceps: Specialized clamp with a short piece of needle receiving tube soldered onto each end; sometimes used for septum, conch, and triangle piercings

septum piercing: Piercing in the tissue dividing the nostrils

septum retainer: Open-ended U-shaped or modified staple-shaped jewelry that conceals a septum piercing by flipping up and hiding inside the nostrils

septum spike: Straight jewelry with tapered ends worn in a healed septum piercing

septum stench: The pungent, rotten odor of sebum in a septum piercing

serous: Relating to serum

serum: Clear liquid part of blood; essentially plasma, without the clotting factor

serous exudate: Lymph, dead cells, and interstitial fluid; forms crusties in piercings

sharps disposal: Special container for safely discarding used piercing needles

side lip piercing with ring: Self-descriptive type of orofacial piercing

single-point piercing: Alternate name for a surface anchor or the procedure to insert one

slotted forceps: Clamp that has a segment of the jaws removed so the tool can be taken off easily, even after jewelry is in place

SM: Sadomasochism; *see* BDSM

smiley: Piercing of the upper web that attaches the center of the lip to the gums; *also* scrumper

snake bites: Piercing placement on either side of the lips or tongue; *also* venoms, vipers, or viper bites

snake eyes: Horizontal scoop piercing across the tip of the tongue, *also* transverse tongue tip piercing

snap-ring pliers: *See* ring opening pliers

snug piercing: Horizontal ear cartilage piercing framing the antihelix, a protrusion between the conch and the helix

soda-lime glass: Common type used in art glass, most windows, and kitchen glassware

spore: Form of certain microbes (including pathogenic bacteria and fungi) that often survive harsh environments in a dormant stage; when conditions improve, they can germinate and resume their life cycle

spore test: Validation of autoclave function to determine if all spores were destroyed using strips of heat-resistant spores run through a sterilization cycle then evaluated by a testing laboratory; *also* biological indicators

sprung: *See* mandible

Standard Precautions: Infection control practices for dealing with blood or other potentially infectious body fluids; formerly Universal Precautions

StatIM: Cassette autoclave with a fast sterilization cycle; *also* flash-cycle cassette sterilizer

step-down threading: Externally threaded jewelry with screw-threads that are smaller

than the post, so they can fit inside a piercing needle or insertion taper

sterile: Free of all microorganisms; an object that has passed through the process of sterilization

sterilization: Destruction of all microorganisms, including fungi, bacteria, viruses, and spores

sterilization room: Separate room for processing contaminated items; *also* biohazard room

stretching: Practice of gradually enlarging a piercing to a thicker gauge size

stretching crescent: Curved or circular insertion taper worn like jewelry; not suggested for use in stretching

stretch mark: Form of scarring; narrow band of discoloration caused by expanding and weakening of the skin

subdermal implant: Form of body modification in which an implant is placed under the skin through an incision and the object is enclosed under the surface

sublingual: Under the tongue

supine: Lying on the back

supra-alar crease: Natural niche on the side of the nose where it flares; common location for nostril piercing

surface anchor: Tiny specialized jewelry worn in a single L-shaped opening formed in the tissue (term for jewelry and procedure); *also* anchor, dermal anchor, and microdermal

surface bar: Barbell variation for surface piercings shaped like an open staple, with a longer straight bar post between two shorter upright legs

surface piercing: Piercing of a flat area of the body that lacks a defined fold, flap, or protrusion of tissue

suspension: Temporary piercing in which sterile hooks are inserted through the flesh and used to suspend a piercee by special rigging

sweet spot: Anatomical location optimal for piercing placement

T

tandem piercing: Pair of piercings simultaneously performed by two piercers

taper: *See* insertion taper

tapping: Drilled-out hole in threaded jewelry that fits the screw threads

tarnish tattoo: *See* localized argyria

teardrop piercing: Facial surface piercing atop the crest of the cheekbone; *also* anti-eyebrow

thermoplastic: Material that can be shaped somewhat after heating and that will retain its new form once cooled

thermotherapy: Treatment using heat

threaded: Having screw threads for securing removable ends on body jewelry

threaded end: Ball, gem, or other ornament that has the threads (rather than the tapping)

threaded-pin taper: Insertion taper style in which the larger end screws into the tapping on the jewelry

threadless jewelry: Alternate jewelry closure instead of threads; the removable end has a pin that presses into a hole in the post where it is secured by tension

threadlocker: Product applied to threads to help prevent the jewelry from unscrewing

threads: Spiral thread pattern cut into threaded jewelry that screws into a hole in the tapped portion

thrush: Oral yeast infection; candidiasis

tissue manipulation: Localized massage of the skin to prepare it for piercing

tongue-tied: Having restricted tongue movement due to a tight lingual frenulum; *also* ankyloglossia

tongue-tip piercing: Piercing within the first half-inch of the tongue

tragus: Small protrusion of cartilage that juts out from the face over the center of the ear canal

transdermal implant: Implant placed under the skin through an incision with an opening made to allow an ornament to show above the surface

transfer pin: A small needle blank used to connect a needle and internally threaded jewelry for the transfer into a new piercing

transverse: Horizontal or crosswise

transverse tongue tip piercing: *See* snake eyes

triangle piercing: Genital piercing at the base of the hood just beneath the clitoral shaft

trigeminal nerve: Main sensory nerve on each side of the head and face and the motor nerve of muscles used for chewing; *also* fifth cranial nerve

true navel piercing: When the protrusion of an outie navel is pierced (not recommended)

tummy tuck: *See* abdominoplasty

Tygon: Flexible autoclavable silicone medical tubing sometimes used as a nonmetallic jewelry alternative

U

ultrasonic unit: Machine that removes debris using agitation from sonic waves in liquid

umbilicus: *See* navel

underdeveloped: Anatomy that is small or has not grown to its full extent

Universal Precautions: *See* Standard Precautions

upret: *See* philtrum piercing

urethra: Tube that delivers urine from the bladder out of the body

urinary meatus: External urethral opening where Prince Albert and Princess Albertina piercing jewelry is worn

U-ring: Custom-bent circular barbell widened out to a U-shape to conform to anatomy; same style as a C-ring, but opened even wider

V

valley: In contrast to *hill*, an anatomical groove or crevice; genitals in a very vertical configuration with outer labia higher than the hood

vascularity: Supply of fluid and ducts, especially blood circulation of veins, arteries, and capillaries

vasoconstriction: Narrowing of blood vessels

VCH: *See* VCH piercing

VCH piercing: Genital piercing through the clitoral hood, placed so the jewelry rests in contact with the clitoral glans; *also* vertical clitoral hood piercing

venipuncture: Drawing blood or inserting an intravenous line; *also* phlebotomy

venoms: *See* snake bites

venules: Tiny veins that transport deoxygenated blood from the capillaries

venus: *See* Christina

vermeil: *See* gold-plated

vermillion border: Juncture where the facial surface meets the pigmented area of the lips

vermillion: Pigmented area of the lips where lipstick or lip balm is applied

vermillion piercing: A piercing through the pigmented portion of the lip; most commonly inverse vertical labret or Ashley

vertical bridge piercing: Vertical facial surface piercing between the eyebrows or slightly above them

vertical clitoral hood piercing: *See* VCH piercing

vertical lip piercing: Vertical surface piercing through the pigmented part of the lip

viper bites: *See* snake bites

vipers: *See* snake bites

vulva: External genitalia including labia majora and minora, clitoral hood, and clitoris

W

wound care: Promotion of wound healing by minimizing factors that inhibit healing, enhancing the healing process, and reducing risk of infection; aftercare

wound debridement: *See* debridement

wound healing: Series of stages in the process of the body regenerating dermal and epidermal tissue following injury

wound irrigation: The steady flow of a solution across a wound surface

wound shaping: Technique used to form the piercing channel in the shape of the jewelry or alter the way jewelry sits

wrecking ball fractures: Cracks in teeth caused by jewelry in an oral piercing

Y

yeast infection: *See* candidiasis

Select Bibliography

Armitage, Cecil Hamilton. *The Tribal Markings and Marks of Adornment of the Natives of the Northern Territories of the Gold Coast Colony.* Royal Anthropological Institute of Great Britain and Ireland. London: Harrison and Sons, 1924.

Association of Professional Piercers. *APP Manual,* US Edition. Association of Professional Piercers, 2013.

Brown, Donald E., James W. Edwards, and Ruth P. Moore. "The Penis Inserts of Southeast Asia: An Annotated Bibliography with an Overview and Comparative Perspectives." Occasional Paper No. 15, University of California, Berkeley, 1988.

Califia, Pat. *Public Sex: The Culture of Radical Sex.* 2nd ed. San Francisco: Cleis Press, 2000.

Camphausen, Rufus C. *Return of the Tribal: A Celebration of Body Adornment.* Rochester, VT: Park Street Press, 1997.

Curry-McGhee, Leanne K. *Tattoos and Body Piercing Overview Series.* San Diego, CA: Lucent Books, 2005.

De la Haye, Amy, and Cathie Dingwal. *Surfers, Soulies, Skinheads & Skaters: Subcultural Style from the Forties to the Nineties.* Woodstock, NY: Overlook Press, 1996.

Dunbar, Andrew, and Dean Lahn. *Body Piercing.* New York: St. Martin's Press, 1998.

Featherstone, Mike, ed. *Body Modification.* London: Sage Publications, 2005.

Gay, Kathlyn, and Christine Whittington. *Body Marks: Tattooing, Piercing, and Scarification.* Brookfield, CT: Millbrook Press, 2002.

Hewitt, Kim. *Mutilating the Body: Identity in Blood and Ink.* Bowling Green, OH: Bowling Green State University Popular Press, 1997.

Lloyd, J. D., ed. *Body Piercing and Tattoos: Examining Pop Culture.* Farmington Hills, MI: Greenhaven Press, 2003.

McNab, Nan. *Body Bizarre, Body Beautiful.* Darby, PA: Diane, 1999.

Mercury, Maureen. *Pagan Fleshworks: The Alchemy of Body Modification.* Rochester, VT: Park Street Press, 2000.

Miller, Jean-Chris. *The Body Art Book: A Complete, Illustrated Guide to Tattoos, Piercings, and Other Body Modifications.* New York: Berkeley Books, 2004.

Musafar, Fakir and Mark Thompson. *Spirit + Flesh.* Santa Fe, NM: Arena Editions, 2015.

Perlingieri, Blake Andrew. *A Brief History of the Evolution of Body Adornment in Western Culture: Ancient Origins and Today.* Eugene, OR: Tribalife Publications, 2003.

Pimsler, Ari and Shawn Porter. *Better Safe than Ari: The Collected Sacred Debris Interviews Vol. 1 & 2.* San Francisco: Blurb, Incorporated, 2018.

Pitts, Victoria L. *In the Flesh: The Cultural Politics of Body Modification.* New York: Palgrave Macmillan, 2003.

Polhemus, Ted. *Streetstyle: From Sidewalk to Catwalk.* London: Thames and Hudson, 1994.

Robinson, Julian. *The Quest for Human Beauty: An Illustrated History.* New York: W.W. Norton & Company, 1998.

Rubin, Arnold, ed. *Marks of Civilization: Artistic Transformations of the Human Body.* Los Angeles: Museum of Cultural History, University of California, 1988.

Steele, Valerie. *Fetish: Fashion, Sex, and Power.* New York: Oxford University Press, 1997.

Vale, V., and Andrea Juno. *Modern Primitives: An Investigation of Contemporary Adornment & Ritual.* San Francisco: Re/Search Publications, 1999.

Ward, Jim. *Running the Gauntlet: An Intimate History of the Modern Body Piercing Movement.* Berkeley, CA: Re:Ward, Inc., 2013.

Wilkinson, Beth. *Coping with the Dangers of Tattooing, Body Piercing, and Branding.* New York: Rosen Publishing Group, 1998.

Wruck, Charlotte. *Jewels for Their Ears: Why Earrings Are as Popular Today as They Were 10,000 Years Ago.* New York: Vantage Press, 1980.

About the Author and Contributor

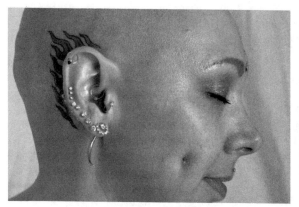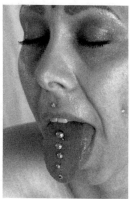

TODD FRIEDMAN

Elayne Angel has been a professional piercer for more than thirty years, and was honored with the President's Lifetime Achievement Award by the Association of Professional Piercers in 2006. A contributing writer for *PAIN Magazine,* she has served multiple terms on the Board of Directors for the Association of Professional Piercers, including as president. She lives in Mérida, Mexico, guest pierces at fine studios around the United States, performs online anatomy and piercing problem consultations, and provides customized continuing education for professional piercers.

Jef Saunders has been piercing since the late nineties. He too is a former APP president, and recipient of the APP President's Award. He lives in Ann Arbor, Michigan, and owns Gamma Piercing with his wife, Laura Jane. Jef is a piercing instructor at the Fakir Intensives and provides piercing education in multiple formats for piercers around the world.

Visit www.piercingbible.com.

Index

A

abdominoplasty, 154
abscesses, 250–51
acrylic jewelry, 96, 289
acupuncture, 29
Addington, Deborah, 300
A+D Original Ointment, 239
Aerosmith, 15
aesthetics, 55
aftercare
  alternative, 240–42
  avoiding trauma, 230–32
  cleaning, 232–35
  components of, 222, 226–27
  dry wound care, 238
  evolution of, 222–23
  guidelines on, from piercers, 223, 240
  healthy habits, 229–30
  hygiene, 227–29
  hypochlorous acid (HOCl), 235–36, 245
  ice packs and compresses, 236–38
  jewelry rotation, 234
  "Leave It the Heck Alone" (LITHA) method, 238
  for oral piercings, 243–44
  products not recommended for, 238–40
  wound debridement, 233, 238
  wound irrigation, 232–33
  See also healing
alcohol, 239, 243, 244
allergies, 23–24
alloys, 92
aloe vera gel, 242
amber jewelry, 288
American ampallang piercing, 209, 210
American Wire Gauge (AWG), 81, 280
ampallang piercing, 209–11
anesthetics, 65
angle-related bumps, 318–19
annealing, 83, 97
anti-care, 238
anti-eyebrow piercing, 130

antitragus piercing, 114
antler jewelry, 288
anxiety, 33–34, 56, 57–58, 65, 246–47
apadravya piercing, 209, 211–13
apprenticeships, 326–28
Aranda, 11
argyria, localized, 260
Ashley piercing, 147
Association of Professional Piercers (APP), 49, 91, 327–28, 334, 337
athletics, 32, 230–31, 302
Austin bar, 127
autoclaves, 44–45
Aztec culture, 10

B

bacitracin, 239
Bactine, 239
ball closure rings. See captive bead rings
bamboo jewelry, 287
bandages, 231
bar-style jewelry
  barbells, 88–89
  circular barbells, 86–87
  curved barbells, 89
  J-curve (J-bar), 89, 90
  jeweled navel curves, 89
  surface bars, 90
  threadless, 90–91
beauty mark, 145
belly piercing. See navel piercing
bent bars, 89
benzalkonium chloride (BZK), 239
benzethonium chloride (BZT), 239
Betadine, 239
biocompatibility, 91
biological indicators, 44–45
biopsy punches, 295–97
bleeding, 27, 66, 225
blood thinners, 57
blowouts, 24, 282
body jewelry. See jewelry
body modification, forms of, x

bone jewelry, 287
breastfeeding, 309–10
breast piercings, 11
breathing techniques, 65
bridge piercing, 130
Brown & Sharpe, 81
bumps
  angle-related, 318–19
  irritation, 107, 113, 252

C

calipers, 81
candida, 171
cannulas, 70
captive bead rings (CBRs), 83–84
captive circular barbells, 87
careers
  piercing prohibitions and, 32, 321–22
  in professional piercing, 324–28, 334–37
castile soap, 234
"catching the tube," 262
catheter needles, 70
cellulitis, 251–52
Celsus, 10
cheek piercing, 148, 150
cheese-cutter effect, 25
children, piercings for, 36–39, 61
choking, 264
Christina piercing, 187–89
circular barbells, 86–87
cleansers, 233–34, 235, 239
clitoral hood piercings
  horizontal, 170, 176–78
  Princess Diana/Duke, 175–76
  triangle, 170, 178–81
  vertical, 170, 171–75
clitoris piercing, 170, 189–91
cock rings, 194
complications, 247–65
compresses, warm, 236–38
compression technique, 74
conch piercing, 106, 110–11
constellation piercings, 105
consultations, 56

contact dermatitis, 232, 260–61
continuing education, 328
corks, 70
corset piercing, 301
C-rings, 87
"crusties," 224–25
CT scans, 304
curated ear, 105
curved barbells, 89
curves, 89
customized circular barbells, 87
Cyprian Society, 215

D

Dahlia piercings, 147
daith piercing, 112, 113
Dakota, Erik, 111
dead stretching, 280
debridement, 233, 238
deep Prince Albert, 198
dental emergencies/
    appointments, 303–4
depilating, 307–8
dermal anchor, 294–95
dermal punches, 295–97
dermatitis, 232, 260–61
diabetes, 23
dimple piercing, 148, 150
discoloration, 259
discrimination, 320
divot piercing. See philtrum
    piercing
DIY (do-it-yourself) piercings,
    20–21
doctors
    attitudes of, toward
        piercings, 320
    as piercers, 48, 50
dolphin piercing, 199
dress codes, 321–22
dry wound care, 238
Duff, Lou, 178, 179
Duke piercings, 175–76
Dyak tribe, 209
dydoe piercing, 212, 215–16

E

ear piercings
    antitragus, 114
    body piercings vs., 31
    cartilage (helix or scapha),
        10, 106–9, 112

conch, 106, 110–11
curated (constellation), 105
daith, 112, 113
forward helix, 106, 113–14
guns, 21–22
    for infants and children,
        37–38
    lobe, 11, 102–5, 106
    rook, 111–12
    sexual orientation and, 6
    snug, 112, 115
    tragus, 106, 110
edema, 65, 230
Elizabeth II, Queen, 11
employment
    piercings and, 32, 321–22
    in professional piercing,
        324–28, 334–37
endocarditis, infective, 23
energy pulls, 300
environmental impact, 67
essential oils, 242
ethical issues
    in apprenticeships, 328
    for piercers, 42–43
European ampallang piercing,
    209, 210
exercise, 230–31, 302
eyebrow piercing, 127–29

F

facial piercings
    eyebrow, 127–29
    other, 129–31
    risky, 26
    See also ear piercings; nose
        piercings; oral piercings
faux rook piercing, 112
faux snug piercing, 115
fistulas, 27
fixed bead rings, 84–85
Foerster sponge forceps, 71
forceps, 70–72
foreskin piercing, 217–19
forward helix piercing, 106,
    113–14
fourchette piercing, 170,
    185–87, 205
freehand piercings, 73
frenulum labiorum
    pudenda, 186

frenum piercing, 199–202
frowny, 148
Fulani, 10

G

gauge measurements, 69, 81,
    278, 332
gauging up. See stretching;
    individual piercings
Gauntlet, 13–14, 80, 98, 178, 202
gemstone jewelry, 288
genital beading, 298–99
genital piercings
    bleeding and, 168
    cost of, 60
    hygiene and, 168
    pain and, 167
    selecting piercer for, 166–67
    sex and, 5, 311–17
    shaving and waxing and, 169
    transgender considerations
        for, 169
    underwear and, 168
    urinating and, 168–69
    See also penis region
        piercings; vulva piercings
genital ribs, 299
glass jewelry, 96, 289–90
gold jewelry, 94–95
gold-plated jewelry, 96–97
Granger, Ethel and Will, 11
granuloma, 253
Great Omi, 12
group identification, 3–4
guiche piercing, 195, 205–7

H

hafada piercing, 217
half-gauges, 69
hand washing, 228
healing
    determining complete, 226
    factors affecting, 224
    healthy habits and, 31,
        229–30
    minimum times for,
        226, 333
    problems with, 247–65
    process of, 224–26
    secretions and, 224–25
    symbolic, 4

workplace environment
and, 321
See also aftercare; *individual piercings*
health history, 23, 31
heart disorders, 23
helix piercing, 106–9, 112
hemostats, 274
hepatitis, 22
herbs, 241–42
HIV, 22, 23
honey, 242
horizontal clitoral hood (HCH)
piercing, 170, 176–78
horn jewelry, 287
hydrogen peroxide, 239
hygiene
aftercare and, 227–29
jewelry and, 273
piercers and, 43–47, 61, 62,
68, 273
hypergranulation tissue, 156,
253–54
hyperpigmentation, 259
hypochlorous acid (HOCl),
235–36, 245
hypospadias, 197

I
Iban Dayaks, 10
ice packs, 236
immune system disorders, 23
implant designations, 92, 93
implants, 297–98, 299
industrial piercings, 292–93
infant ear piercing, 37–38
infections
abscesses, 250–51
localized, 249–50
risk of, 22–23
yeast, 171, 240
infibulation, 9–10, 217, 316–17
infranasal depression, 146
insertion tapers, 76–77, 270–71
interstitial fluid, 225
intertragus notch, 110
iodine, 239
iron cross, 162, 209
irritation bumps, 107, 113, 252
ivory jewelry, 287–88

J
J-curves (J-bars), 89, 90
jeweled navel curves (JNCs), 89
jewelry
adjusting, 67
aspirated, 265
bar-style, 88–90
changing, 270–73
choking on, 264
choosing, 63, 78–79, 97–98,
272
cleaning, 268
embedded, 261–62
finish of, 97
for healed and stretched
piercings, 285
hygiene and, 273
for initial piercings, 91–95
losing, 275
materials for, 91–97, 285–90
new, 275–76
novelty, 79, 97, 98
primitive origins of, 79
quality of, 98
reinserting, 105, 284
removing, 248
replacement parts for, 67
ring-style, 82–85, 87
rotating, 234
shapes of, 80
sizes and measurements of,
67, 81–82
sterilizing, 61, 62
swallowed, 264–65
tapered, 281
tarnished, 268
threaded, 85–88
threadless, 90–91
tightness and, 226
tools for, 273–74
See also individual piercings
Joker piercings, 147

K
Kama Sutra, 10
Karankawa tribe, 158
karats, 94
keloids, 25, 256, 258–59
keratin, 225
King, Paul, 15
kissing, 316

Kopka, Dan, 202
Kravitz, Lenny, 207

L
labia piercings
inner, 170, 184–85
outer, 170, 182–84
labret piercing, 10, 140–44
ladders, 170, 182, 199, 200
Lakshmi, 9
laparoscopy, 154
latex sensitivity/allergy, 68
L-bends, 118
"Leave It the Heck Alone"
(LITHA) method, 238
legal regulations, 322–23
lifestyle considerations, 31–32
lingual frenulum piercing, 148
lip piercings, 10, 140–47
Listerine, 239–40
Loomis, Roland, 12
lorum piercing, 199, 202–3
lowbret piercing, 149
lubrication, 241
lupus, 23

M
Maasai, 10
Madonna, 145
magic cross, 209
maintenance, 268–70, 281–82
Malloy, Doug, 8, 13, 14–15,
205, 215
mandible piercing, 148
mantis, 120
massage, 281–82
Mayan culture, 10
medical emergencies/
appointments, 303–4
medical treatments, piercings
as, 28
Medusa piercing. *See* philtrum
piercing
menstruation, 171, 308
metal detectors, 307
microdermal piercing, 294–95
mid-brow piercing, 130
migration, 24, 262–63
military personnel, 322
mill certificates, 92–93
Millner, Vaughn, 172
Modern Primitives, 12, 14

Monroe, 145
moral support, 59
motivations, 2–7
MRIs, 303–4
Musafar, Fakir, 12, 13, 111
myths, 27–28

N

nasallang, 127, 293
natural materials, 96, 285–88
navel piercing, 15–16, 151–57, 309
needle blanks, 72–73
needle phobia, 35
needle receiving tubes (NRTs),
    72, 74
Neosporin, 239
niobium jewelry, 93–94
nipple piercing, 158–65, 309–10
nose bones, 118
nose piercings
    care of, 115–16
    nostril, 10, 116, 117–22
    other, 127
    preparation for, 115
    septum, 10, 116, 122–26, 323
nostril screws, 91, 118

O

obsidian jewelry, 290
Olmec culture, 10
O-needle surface piercing, 292
Operation Spanner, 14
oral piercings
    aftercare for, 243–44
    Ashley, 147
    beauty mark, 145
    cheek, 148, 150
    Dahlia, 147
    dimple, 148, 150
    frowny, 148
    Joker, 147
    kissing and, 316
    labret, 10, 140–44
    lingual frenulum, 148
    lip, 10, 140–47
    lowbret, 149
    Madonna, 145
    maintenance of, 269–70
    mandible, 148
    Monroe, 145
    philtrum, 146–47

preparation for, 57
questionable, 147–49
risks of, 26, 132, 149
scrumper, 148
smiley, 148
sprung, 148
tongue, 11, 17, 133–40, 149
vermillion, 147
oral sex, 316
orbitals, 292, 293–94
organics. See natural materials
ornamented clicker and seam
    rings, 91
Ötzi the Iceman, 9
Oversby, Alan, 14

P

pain, 34–35, 66
parents
    advice for, 37
    attitudes of, 36
    consent of, 36, 37
parotid ducts, 148, 150
patches, protective, 231
penis region piercings
    ampallang, 209–11
    apadravya, 209, 211–13
    bleeding and, 193
    cock rings and, 194
    deep Prince Albert, 198
    dolphin, 199
    dydoe, 212, 215–16
    erections and, 194
    foreskin, 217–19
    frenum, 199–202
    guiche, 195, 205–7
    hafada, 203, 217
    history of, 11, 200
    infibulation and, 317
    lorum, 199, 202–3
    Prince Albert, 15, 194–99, 212
    pubic, 207–9, 217
    reverse Prince Albert, 212,
        213–15
    risky, 26
    scrotum, 199, 203–5, 217
    sensation and, 193
    sex and, 10, 315
    urinating and, 193
    See also genital piercings
Pennington forceps, 71

philtrum piercing, 146–47
piercees
    age and, 3, 33, 36–39
    appropriate behavior for,
        59–60
    moral support for, 59
    motivations of, 2–7
    societal attitudes toward, 27,
        32, 320–23, 329–30
piercers
    apprenticeships for, 326–28
    attitude of, 42
    career as, 324–28, 334–37
    consultations with, 56
    education and training for,
        325–26, 328
    ethics of, 42–43
    finding, 47–50
    hygiene and, 43–47, 61, 62,
        68, 273
    income of, 334–35
    legal regulations for, x–xi,
        322–23
    licenses for, 40
    medical professionals as,
        40, 48, 50
    personal attributes of,
        324–25
    professional organization
        for, 49
    risks for, 325
    skills of, 40–42
    studio standards for, 43–44
    survey of, 334–37
    tipping, 61
    watching, 47–48
    websites of, 47
Piercing Fans International
    Quarterly (PFIQ), 13–14
piercing needles, 69–70
piercing procedures
    anesthetics and, 65
    caution about, 76
    pain during, 34–35, 66
    setup for, 68
    steps in, 74–76
    techniques for, 73–74
    tools and equipment for,
        44–46, 69–73, 76–77
    See also individual piercings

piercings
  advanced, 291–95
  aftermath of, 66
  anticipation before, 33–34, 56
  athletics and, 32, 302
  concealing, 32, 305–6
  cost of, 60–61
  depilating and, 307–8
  DIY (do-it-yourself), 20–21
  environmental impact of, 67
  experimental, 299
  future of, 329–31
  history of, 8–17, 102, 158
  lifestyle considerations and,
    31–32
  maintenance of, 268–70,
    281–82
  as medical treatments, 28
  menstruation and, 308
  minimizing trauma to,
    230–32
  motivations for, 2–7, 54
  number of, 55–56
  obstacles to, 33, 35
  picking, 54–55
  placement of, 25–26, 54–55,
    64–65
  play, 299–300
  popularity of, x, 15–17, 329–30
  pregnancy and, 308–10
  preparing for, 56–58, 64–65
  re-, 263–64
  responsibility and, 30
  retiring, 283–84
  risks of, xii, 20–27, 29
  as rituals, 4–5, 61–62
  secretions and, 224–25
  self-expression and, 6, 7, 14
  sex and, 311–17
  tandem, 161
  traveling with, 306–7
  troubleshooting, 246–65
  urge for, 330–31
  waivers and release forms
    for, 63
  weight loss/gain and, 302–3
  See also aftercare; healing;
    jewelry; stretching;
    individual piercings
pimples, piercing, 254–55
plastic jewelry, 95, 289

platinum jewelry, 95
play piercing, 299–300
pliers
  ring closing (RCPs), 273, 274
  ring opening (ROPs), 273, 274
PMMA (polymethyl-
    methacrylate), 289
porcupine quills, 287
pregnancy, 308–10
prejudice, 320
preparation
  mental, 57–58
  physical, 56–57
  supplies, 56
Prince Albert piercing, 15, 194–
    99, 212
Princess Albertina piercing,
    191–92
Princess Diana piercings,
    175–76
PTFE (polytetrafluoroethylene),
    95
pubic piercing, 207–9, 217
pulls, 300
punks, 13
pus, 225
PVD (physical vapor
    deposition) coatings, 290
pyogenic granuloma, 253

R
reinsertions, 105, 284
rejection, 24, 262–63
relaxation techniques, 65
relaxing, 281
release forms, 63
repiercing, 263–64
resorption, 298–99
resting, 281
retainers, 248, 303, 305–6
reverse Prince Albert piercing,
    212, 213–15
rhino piercing, 127
Ridler, Horace, 12
risks, 20–27, 29
rituals, 4–5, 61–62
rock jewelry, 288
rook piercing, 111–12

S
sadhus, 111
sailors, 11

saline, 232–33
scaffold piercings, 292–93
scalpelling, 297
scapha piercing, 106–9
scarring, 25, 256–59
schools, piercings in, 321–22, 323
scrotum piercing, 199, 203–5, 217
scrumper, 148
seam rings, 84
Sebastian, Mr., 14
sebum, 225
secretions, 224–25
security screenings, 307
self-expression, 6, 7, 14
septicemia, 251
septril, 127
septum piercing, 10, 116,
    122–26, 323
serous exudate, 205
sex, 5, 311–17
sexual orientation, 6
sharps disposal, 46
shaving, 307–8
sideburn piercing, 131
silicone jewelry, 289
silver
  colloidal, 242
  jewelry, 96
Silverstone, Alicia, 15
Simonton, Richard. See Malloy,
    Doug
single-point piercing, 295
skin
  dermatitis, 232, 260–61
  dry, 259
  sensitive, 232
smiley, 148
smoking, 229
snake bites, 136
snake eyes, 149
SnapPlugs, 280
snug piercing, 112, 115
soaps, 233–34, 235, 239
spore tests, 44–45
sports, 32, 230–31, 302
sprung piercing, 148
StatIM, 45, 62
steel jewelry, 93
stereotypes, 330
sterilizers, 44–46
stone jewelry, 288

stretching
  crescents or rings, 281
  dead, 280
  gauge measurements, 69,
    81, 332
  history of, 276, 277
  in-between sizes for, 280
  maintenance of, 281–82
  over-, 276, 282
  popularity of, 276
  speed of, 277
  techniques for, 277–78, 280
  tips for, 278–79
  trouble with, 24, 282
  weights and, 279–80
stretch marks, 155
students, 321–22
subdermal implants, 297
Support Tattoos and Piercings
    at Work (STAPAW), 321
supra-alar crease, 117
surface anchor, 294–95
surface bars, 90, 291
surface piercings, 291–92
suspension, 300
swimming, 231

T
tandem piercings, 161
tanning, 231–32
tapers. See insertion tapers
"tarnish tattoo," 260
tattoos, x, xii
teardrop piercing, 130
tears, traumatic, 262
tea tree oil, 239
third eye, 130–31
thread-locker products, 86
thrush, 240
Timorese tribe, 200
Tinglit, 10
tipping, 61
titanium jewelry, 93
tongue piercings, 11, 17,
    133–40, 149
tragus piercing, 106, 110
transdermal implants, 299
transfer pins, 72
travel, 32, 306–7
triangle piercing, 170, 178–81

tribal cultures, 10–11
Triclosan, 235
T-shirt trick, 229
Tutankhamun (King Tut), 9

U
Ukok, Princess of, 9
ultrasonic cleaning units, 45
upret piercing. See philtrum
    piercing
U-rings, 87

V
Vedas, 9
venoms, 136
Venus piercing. See Christina
    piercing
vermillion piercings, 147
vertical bridge, 130–31
vertical clitoral hood (VCH)
    piercing, 170, 171–75
vipers, 136
vitamins
  A, 229
  B complex, 229
  C, 229
  E, 57, 229, 286
  K, 57, 229
vulva piercings
  anatomy and, 169–70
  childbirth and, 309
  Christina, 187–89
  clitoris, 170, 189–91
  Duke, 175–76
  fourchette, 170, 185–87, 205
  horizontal clitoral hood
    (HCH), 170, 176–78
  hypersensitivity and, 170–71
  infibulation and, 316–17
  labia majora, 170, 182–84
  labia minora, 170, 184–85
  Princess Albertina, 191–92
  Princess Diana, 175–76
  risky, 26
  sex and, 315
  startle response to, 170–71
  triangle, 170, 178–81
  vertical clitoral hood (VCH),
    170, 171–75
  See also genital piercings

W
waivers, 63
Ward, Jim, 12, 13, 14, 15, 79,
    98, 330
weight
  loss/gain, 302–3
  as obstacle to piercing, 33
wood jewelry, 287
workplace, piercings in, 32,
    321–22
wound shaping, 291
wrecking ball fractures, 132

Y
yeast infections, 171, 240